PSYCHOLOGY RESEARCH PROGRESS

RECENT HISPANIC PSYCHOLOGICAL RESEARCH ON FEEDING BEHAVIOR AND HIV PATIENTS

PSYCHOLOGY RESEARCH PROGRESS

Additional books in this series can be found on Nova's website
under the Series tab.

Additional e-books in this series can be found on Nova's website
under the e-book tab.

PSYCHOLOGY RESEARCH PROGRESS

RECENT HISPANIC PSYCHOLOGICAL RESEARCH ON FEEDING BEHAVIOR AND HIV PATIENTS

CIRILO H. GARCIA CADENA
ANTONIO LOPEZ-ESPINOZA
AND
JULIO A. PIÑA LOPEZ
EDITORS

nova publishers
New York

For permission to use material from this book please contact us:
Telephone 631-231-7269; Fax 631-231-8175
Web Site: http://www.novapublishers.com

Library of Congress Cataloging-in-Publication Data

ISBN: 978-1-62948-919-3

Published by Nova Science Publishers, Inc. † New York

CONTENTS

PREFACE

This book incorporates works of empirical research, derived from different conceptual models based on psychological or psychosocial theory. It presents scientific studies on psychology, done principally by Spanish-speaking researchers from different countries, and tries to include the best academic efforts of research as an easy way of communication with non-Latin researchers.

Chapter 1 - Direct or indirect stimulation of serotonin receptors (5-HT$_{2C}$R), 5-HT$_{1B}$R and 5-HT$_6$R subtypes decrease food intake while stimulation of 5-HT$_{1A}$R increases it. Using non-selective drugs or increasing 5-HT at the synaptic cleft may bind to different subtypes producing opposing effects on intake, if this would be the case, agonist action at 5-HT$_{1A}$R may obscure the anorectic effect. The authors tested the hypothesis that indorenate (INDO) an agonist with low affinity for 5-HT$_{1B/2C}$Rs that decreases food intake, but also with high affinity for 5-HT$_{1A}$R, may benefit from the blockade of 5-HT$_{1A}$R to clearly express its anorectic action. Male Wistar rats were trained to eat their food and water daily in a period of 4 h.

On test days mesulergide (non-selective 5-HT$_{2C/2A}$ antagonist, 1.0 mg/kg), mianserin (non-selective 5-HT$_{2A/2B/2C}$ antagonist, 3.0 mg/kg), methiothepin (non-selective 5-HT$_{1E/1F/1A}$ antagonist, 0.3 mg/kg) or saline were given before INDO (17.0 mg/kg); a control group received two injections of saline.

INDO decreased food intake; mesulergide and mianserin prevented its anorectic effect, although only the antagonism of mesulergide reached statistical significance. Methiothepin enhanced the anorectic effect of INDO. Blockade of 5-HT$_{1A}$R allowed the observation of the full participation of the 5-HT$_{2C}$R on the anorectic action of INDO.

Chapter 2 - The present study investigates whether the exposure to acute or chronic foot-shocks and the possibility of escape of them differentially affect food and water intake in rats deprived of water or both food and water in females and males rats. The rats were deprived of water 23.5 hours a day (partial deprivation) or for three consecutive days of food and water (total deprivation) and after to baseline condition they were exposed to acute (60 for two days) or chronic (10 for 12 days) escapable or inescapable electric shocks. The subjects exposed to acute and chronic shocks reduced food and water intake when the deprivation was partial and water was available in the stress context, that is, in the chamber where shocks occurred. However, when the animals were total deprived, no stress-induced reduction of food and water intake was observed, suggesting that level of deprivation was a crucial variable. Additionally, a slight difference between escapable or inescapable shocks was suggested, but results are not clear.

Chapter 3 - Obesity is a pathology often associated with the genesis of diseases such as hypertension, diabetes, heart problems, etc. Research in this field has focused on understanding the different factors that promote the beginning and maintenance of obesity, one of them are the hedonic properties of food. Thus, the aim of this research was to evaluate the effect of administration of the selective CB1 receptor agonist ACEA in the nucleus *accumbens* shell (NAcS) on palatable food intake in pre-satiated male wistar rats. During a 4-day period of habituation, the animals were deprived of food for 22 hours, and then they had access to the standard food (solid) during 1 hour, and finally they had access to the experimental food (sweetened condensed milk, 10% sucrose) for 1 hour. In the experimental sessions, the animals were injected with vehicle and 2 different doses of ACEA (0.25, 0.5 or 0.75 μg, multidose crossover design, where dose was determined by a Latin square with an inter-test interval of 2 days, each rat was registered in 3 independent experimental sessions) before having access to experimental food (rats were in the same feeding paradigm as in the habituation period). According to the obtained results, ACEA administration had a dose-dependent stimulatory effect of palatable food ingestion. The authors' findings suggest that activation of CB1 receptors in the NAcS stimulate intake via increasing the hedonic properties of food.

Chapter 4 - The purpose of this review was to describe the origin and development of the study of food-intake control in rats by exteroceptive stimuli. The strategy followed was to group the different studies according to similarities in their procedures, which arose mainly from a hypothetical-deductive line aimed to support or refute several motivational theories. First, studies in which the procedure consisted of pairing stimuli with a state of food-deprivation and that determined the effect of presenting these stimuli on eating are described. Subsequently, studies in which stimuli related to food were presented on subjects with or without food deprivation are described. It is concluded that the fundamental operation to control food intake by stimuli presentation is to pair them with food. It is also concluded that regardless of the origin of the different studies reviewed, they share the same operations of presenting food-access periods interpolated with periods without access to food and that they vary the moment of presentation of the stimuli. It is proposed that these variables can be used to integrate the results of different studies in the area.

Chapter 5 - Obesity is a public health problem associated with chronic degenerative diseases. In order to study this pathology, several murine models have been development based on high-calorie diet, neuroendocrine and genetic changes or brain lesions. The objective is to offer proposals for treatment and prevention for this disease. The authors describe the role of monosodium glutamate in the development of murine obesity models. This model has been related to neuronal death of hypothalamus arcuate nucleus, structure that regulates hormonal signals as insulin and leptin which are involved in food intake.

Chapter 6 - The patterns of eating, drinking and running in rats were studied under free access to food, water and an activity wheel conditions. In order to obtain food, the subjects had to press a lever, to obtain water the rats had to lick a tube. For both behaviors, to drink and to eat, a continuous reinforcement schedule was operating during the whole study. The subjects lived in the experimental boxes with a 12 h light/dark cycle during 20 sessions. Subjects showed activity increases in the running wheels during the light cycle along sessions, the activity during the dark cycle was relatively stable. There were no differences in presses for food and licks between light cycle and dark cycle. Body weight did not show changes along sessions. The results represent an exploratory approach, as a base line to study the activity-based anorexia phenomenon.

Chapter 7 - The experimental evidence shows that modification of the physical space has effects on behavior; among the most evident are the alterations in body weight and food intake. With the purpose of determining the effect of space modifications on body weight and food intake, eight male rats from the same litter were used and two groups of four subjects each were formed. They remained in free food and water access conditions. During 40 days their body weight, food, and water intake was registered daily by group. The experiment was divided into two phases with duration of 20 days each. During the first phase group 1 was placed in a 16x28x18 size box and group 2 in a 20x38.5x23.5 size box. At the end of the first phase, group 1 was moved into the box that group 2 was in and group 2 was moved to the box group 1 was in. The obtained results did not show significant changes between the groups in spite of the space modifications and the concentration of subjects.

Chapter 8 - Purpose of this study was to evaluate effects on water and food intake when exposed to a variety of foods. 12 Wistar rats were used, six females and 6 males. Three groups were created: Norm-Caloric Group, Hypo-Caloric Group, and Hyper-Caloric Group, each were assigned two females and two males. Experiment was divided in 7 phases. Phases 1, 3, 5, and 7 lasted 10 days. In these phases the norm-caloric group was exposed to a norm-caloric diet, the hypo-caloric group to a hypo-caloric diet, and the hyper-caloric group to a hyper-caloric diet. Phases 2, 4, and 6 lasted three days, and all subjects were exposed to three diets simultaneously (Variety of foods). Results showed that subjects in norm-caloric and hypo-caloric groups, and also females of the hyper-caloric group, increased their food intake during the exposure periods to the variety of foods, regardless of the type of diet they previously received. However, hyper-caloric group maintained its intake. Evidence shows that when exposed to a variety of foods the rats did not regulate their food or calorie intake.

Chapter 9 - Tourism areas are increasingly characterized as environments of increased HIV risk. Alcohol venues located in tourism areas have been implicated in facilitating HIV transmission; however few studies have spatially characterized alcohol venues and their potential relationship with elevated HIV risk. The limited attention to how HIV transmission is facilitated by social and spatial aspects of alcohol venues warrants further attention. The authors systematically assessed the social, spatial and behavioral characteristics of alcohol venues in a Dominican tourism town. A venue-based survey was completed for 135 alcohol venues located within the targeted area. Additionally, the authors employed geographic information systems (GIS) to spatially describe the venues in relation to HIV risk factors.

Results suggest the Sosúa tourism area is characterized by: 1) a high concentration of alcohol venues; 2) widespread population mixing between risk groups; 3) spatial co-occurrence of alcohol venues, sexual commerce, and drug transactions, and 4) low availability of HIV prevention services.

Our results suggest alcohol venues should be targeted for HIV prevention efforts in Dominican tourism areas. Data underscore the importance of context in shaping individual risk behavior. HIV prevention interventions and policies should consider the broader social dynamics of alcohol venues and target such venues for structural interventions.

Chapter 10 - Preventive interventions for HIV/AIDS within a school context have increased in the last few years, although no recent data on the quality and impact of these actions are available. In this paper the authors aimed to describe and assess school HIV/AIDS prevention programs administered in Spain from 1995 to 2010, which have been evaluated. Preventive interventions for HIV/AIDS and sexual health programs targeting adolescents in schools lasting more than 1 hour. The authors evaluated the quality and impact of programs following quality criteria associated with successful interventions. Fourteen controlled studies were identified, of which 4 were high quality (28%), 3 intermediate-high quality (21%), 4 intermediate-low quality (28%) and 3 low quality (21%). No progressive evolution in the quality of interventions was observed. Evaluative deficiencies and lack of follow-up on the intervention effects in the medium to long term do not allow for learning about their impact upon adolescents. The authors discuss the strengths and weaknesses of prevention programs and propose measures for the future.

Chapter 11 - The main purpose of this study was to examine how women's constructions about sexual pleasure configure high-risk behaviors during sexual encounters. Results emerge from a qualitative study. Using the technique of discourse analysis stemming from a *post*-structuralist perspective the authors analyze women's discourses during sexual encounters. Finally, they point out the scope of this work for psychology, some conclusions to be drawn from this research and recommendations for future research and interventions for HIV /AIDS.

Chapter 12 - In this paper the authors summarize the central core of a psychological model for adherence behaviors (PMAB) in the context of HIV-positive persons. First, they justify the importance of a conceptual analysis approaching a formal model. Second, the authors describe recent developments based on the model and the implications for future research to improve both, their knowledge on mechanisms underlying adherence behaviors, as well as designing and implementing intervention programs for behavior change from a psychological point of view.

Chapter 13 - Based on a psychological model, a cross-sectional study was carried out with the participation of fifty-four HIV persons under antiretroviral medication in Michoacán, Mexico, who answered three self-administered questionnaires: psychological variables and adherence behaviors, perceived social support, and depression. For data analysis a set of structural equation modeling was performed. The final model showed a direct effect of perceived social support on motives, and this one on medication-adherence behaviors, explaining both variables 61% of total variance (χ^2/df [5] = 0.368; GFI = 0.986; AGFI = 0.959; CFI = 1.000; RMSEA = 0.000); also, an effect of adherence behaviors on viral load was observed, explaining 35% of the variance; viral load in turn explains 29% of the variance of CD4+ cell count. The current study found valuable evidence of how interaction between two psychological and social variables influences positively on the consisting and efficient practice of adherence behaviors, with direct and mediated effects on both biomarkers, viral load levels and CD4+ lymphocytes cell count. The authors discuss the relevance of these variables in healthcare institutions context which provide specialized attention for HIV persons under antiretroviral medication in Mexico.

Chapter 14 - A retrospective and cross-sectional study was performed in order to identify gender differences in psychological variables associated with adherence behaviors among 74 HIV+ patients from Sonora, Mexico, who answered two self-administered questionnaires: 1) Psychological variables underlying adherence behaviors, and 2) Stress-related situations. Statistically significant differences were observed among non-adherent and 100% adherent patients (χ^2 [1] = 26.162; $p < .001$), as well as among men (83.7%) and women (72%) practicing adherence behaviors all days of the week ($Z = -4.907$; $p < .001$); finally, a multivariate logistic regression analysis showed that motivation variables (corrected OR =

1.75; 95% CI: 1.27-2.39), as well as current behavioral competencies (corrected OR = 1.12; 95% CI: 1.00-1.24) were psychological variables associated with adherence behaviors. Results show that motivation and optimal current competent performance are psychological variables operating in different way in both VIH+ men and women; this issue must be taken into account in order to improve the effectiveness of interdisciplinary intervention programs regarding Mexican health care institutions

Chapter 15 - Antiretroviral treatments (ARTs) stop the replication of HIV, but it is a major requirement for people with HIV/AIDS (PWHA) to display adherence behaviors equal to or higher than 90%. Since the disease and its treatment are considered highly stressful, PWHA are required for implementing a variety of coping skills (CSs) that enable to cope with them efficiently.

This study explores the relationship between adherence to the ART and CSs in a group of 158 PWHA receiving attention at Hospital Muñiz, in the Autonomous City of Buenos Aires, Argentina.

Two assessment methods were applied: an *ad hoc* questionnaire to measure adherence, and the Moos Coping Scale (form B). The main correlations were found between stress management strategies with problem-solving behaviors ($p = .00$), cognitions oriented towards problem-solving ($p = .00$), cognitive avoidance-resignation ($p = .04$), emotions oriented towards problem-solving ($p = .00$), and social support ($p = .00$). Meanwhile, social support turned out to be positively related to problem-solving behaviors ($p = .00$), negatively to strategies of problem-avoidance ($p = .00$), avoidance/emotional release ($p = .00$), as well as with an avoidance index ($p = .00$). This study revealed the relationship between adherence to the ART and different coping strategies, which lead to the conclusion that acquaintance with these strategies, could help to predict, with a reasonable degree of certainty, the probability of adherence to the ART by patients with HIV.

Chapter 16 - The convenience sample consisted of 325 gay men whose ages range from 18 to 64 years ($X = 32.8$; $SD = 9.81$). Of the total number of participants, 17.8% ($n = 58$) had been diagnosed with HIV and 78.8% ($n = 265$) had not. People living with HIV (PLWHIV) were compared with non-living HIV people. This study included different measures of homophobia (minority stress events, perceived discrimination and perceived victimization, stigma perceived by homosexual people), HIV stigma, and different measures concerning quality of life. Results show that the homophobia measures of the two groups may be regarded as similar. For general measures concerning quality of life, statistically meaningful differences were found in satisfaction with life and in some dimensions of psychological and social well-being. As to psychological and social well-being, significant differences were found in autonomy levels ($t_{[306]} = -3.82$; $p < .005$; $d = .50$) and social integration ($t_{[312]} = -2.34$; $p < .05$; $d = .35$) in the social well-being scale. Concerning clinical symptomatology, differences were found only in dimensions referring to somatization and depression, indicating that PLWHIV are more prone to show their discomfort in bodily dysfunctions and mood disorder. Finally, participants with high scores on the HIV stigma scale report significant higher levels of victimization and discrimination, lower levels of social well-being and high levels of clinical symptomatology.

Introduction: One Hundred Years of Beginning of Research in Feeding Behavior

Antonio López-Espinoza
Guest Editor
Director del Centro de Investigaciones en Comportamiento Alimentario y Nutrición (CICAN) CUSur- U. de G.
Zapotlán El Grande, Jalisco, a 20 de Junio del 2012, Mexico

One hundred years had been passed since feeding behavior research started. In 1912 the scientific works of Ramon Turró "Origins of Knowledge: Hunger" (1912) and the one of Walter B. Cannon and A.L Washburn "An Explanation of Hunger" (1912) were remarkable. These contributions are obligate reference for all that are dedicated to feeding behavior research. It is true that in the beginning of feeding behavior study most of contributions use to focus in hunger as first element in the eating act, last hundred years had permit characterize a great number of phenomenon's associate with feeding. Between them we can appoint: feeding preferences, food selection, binge eating, binge drinking, foraging, hoarding, among others.

It is necessary considerate that theory and experimental analysis of feeding behavior had been conjugate contributions of different sciences. This element is probably one distinctive characteristic of feeding behavior research in these first hundred years of work.

This monographic had as principal objective, present scientific contributions in feeding behavior researchers. However, a second objective is to form part of academic festivity that in the Centro de Investigaciones en Comportamiento Alimentario y Nutrición CICAN (Behaivoral Feeding and Nutrition Research Center) of CUSur, University Guadalajara, Mexico cooperating with research groups of others universities realize in this 2012 to commemorate first century of feeding behavior research.

Our commemoration is confirmed by next contributions. In the first article David N. Velazquez-Martinez of UNAM and Ana Maria Balboa-Verduzco of Instituto Politecnico Nacional presents their job named "A 5-HT_{1A} antagonist may enhance the anorectic effect of a 5-HT_{2C} receptor agonist". Our second job is presented by Marina Liliana Gonzales-Torres, Antonio Lopez-Espinoza and Cristiano Valerio Dos Santos of Guadalajara University; in it they prove a "Possible interaction between the effects of stress and deprivation on eating behavior in rats". In the next contribution conjunction UNAM researchers and Autonomus University Of Nuevo Leon integrated by Felipe Cortes-Salazar, Juan Manuel Mancilla-Diaz, Veronica Elsa Lopez-Alonso, Brenda Gonzales-Hernandez and Rodrigo Erick Escartín-Perez present us "Relationship between cb1 receptors in the nucleus *accumbens* shell and the hedonic value of food". Varsovia Hernández of UNAM presents the article "The study of stimulus control of food intake in rats: A review". Monica Navarro-Meza of Guadalajara University and Omar Arroyo-Helguera of University Veracruzana describe us "Role of monosodium glutamate in the development of murine obesity models". Carlos Flores Aguirre, Luis Fernando Zárate Molina and Rebeca Mateos of University of Guadalajara and University of Valle de México Campus Zapopan present "Activity patterns, food intake, and water consumption in rats: an exploratory analysis". Alma Gabriela Martínez Moreno, Diana Merced Venancio-López, Antonio López-Espinoza and Carmen Livier García Flores of CICAN - University of Guadalajara present us "Evaluating body weight and food intake in two sizes home box in rats". Finally, Antonio López-Espinoza, Alma Gabriela-Martinez, Virginia Aguilera, Alma Galindo, Asucena Cárdenas-Villalvazo, Elia Valdés, Ana Patricia Zepeda and Cristina Espinoza present the article called "Effects of a variety of foods on feeding behavior in rats".

For the conclusion I want to recognize the job of authors, reviewers and editorial group of International Journal of Hispanic Psychology, thanks to them it was possible the publication of this monographic number dedicated to feeding behavior research. In the name of all researchers that participate in this monographic, we invite the students, teachers and researchers to involve actively in study and research of feeding behavior; we know for sure that in this activity you will find satisfaction and sweet moments associated with their own feeding.

In: Recent Hispanic Psychological Research … ISBN: 978-1-62948-919-3
Editors: C. H. Garcia Cadena, A. Lopez-Espinoza et al.

Chapter 1

A 5-HT_{1A} Antagonist May Enhance the Anorectic Effect of A 5-HT_{2C} Receptor Agonist

David N. Velázquez-Martínez*[*1] and Ana Maria Balboa-Verduzco[2]

[1]Department of Psychophysiology, School of Psychology,
Universidad Nacional Autónoma de México, México
[2]Coordination of Graduate Studies,
Interdisciplinary Center of Sciences of Health,
"Santo Tomás" Unit, Instituto Politécnico Nacional, México

Abstract

Direct or indirect stimulation of serotonin receptors (5-HT_{2C}R), 5-HT_{1B}R and 5-HT_6R subtypes decrease food intake while stimulation of 5-HT_{1A}R increases it. Using non-selective drugs or increasing 5-HT at the synaptic cleft may bind to different subtypes producing opposing effects on intake, if this would be the case, agonist action at 5-HT_{1A}R may obscure the anorectic effect. We tested the hypothesis that indorenate (INDO) an agonist with low affinity for 5-$HT_{1B/2C}$Rs that decreases food intake, but also with high affinity for 5-HT_{1A}R, may benefit from the blockade of 5-HT_{1A}R to clearly express its anorectic action. Male Wistar rats were trained to eat their food and water daily in a period of 4 h.

On test days mesulergide (non-selective 5-$HT_{2C/2A}$ antagonist, 1.0 mg/kg), mianserin (non-selective 5-$HT_{2A/2B/2C}$ antagonist, 3.0 mg/kg), methiothepin (non-selective 5-$HT_{1E/1F/1A}$ antagonist, 0.3 mg/kg) or saline were given before INDO (17.0 mg/kg); a control group received two injections of saline.

INDO decreased food intake; mesulergide and mianserin prevented its anorectic effect, although only the antagonism of mesulergide reached statistical significance. Methiothepin enhanced the anorectic effect of INDO. Blockade of 5-HT_{1A}R allowed the observation of the full participation of the 5-HT_{2C}R on the anorectic action of INDO.

* Send correspondence to: David N. Velázquez Martínez. Laboratorio de Farmacología Conductual. Departamento de Psicofisiología. Facultad de Psicología. Universidad Nacional Autónoma de México. México, D.F. 04510. México. Mail: velazque@unam.mx. Tel. +(52) 55-5622 0555 ext #41214.

Keywords: Food Intake, indorenate, methiothepin, mesulergide, mianserin, rats

INTRODUCTION

Serotonin (5-Hydroxytryptamine, 5-HT) plays an important role in the regulation of food intake (see reviews of: Clifton and Kennett, 2006; Garfield and Heisler, 2009; Halford, Harrold, Boyland, Lawton, and Blundell, 2007). SINCE there are up to 14 different subtypes of serotonin receptors (5-HTRs) (Pytliak, Vargova, Mechirova, and Felsoci, 2011), interest arises to identify the differential participation of each of them on the modulation of eating behavior. Specifically, using pharmacological and genetic tools, it has been suggested that direct or indirect stimulation of 5-HT_{2C}R, 5-HT_{IB}R and 5-HT_6R subtypes may decrease food intake (Macor, Burkhart, Heym, Ives, Lebel, Newman, Nielsen, Ryan, Schulz, Torgersen, and et al., 1990; Martin, Bos, Jenck, Moreau, Mutel, Sleight, Wichmann, Andrews, Berendsen, Broekkamp, Ruigt, Kohler, and Delft, 1998; Woolley, Bentley, Sleight, Marsden, and Fone, 2001). In contrast, the stimulation of the somatodendritic 5-HT_{1A}R (involved in a negative feedback regulation of 5-HT release, see: Hutson, Dourish, and Curzon, 1986, 1988) and administration of 8-OH-DPAT induced an increase in the consumption of palatable diets (Dourish, Cooper, Gilbert, Coughlan, and Iversen, 1988; Dourish, Hutson, and Curzon, 1985). As the decrease or increase of intake depend on different receptor subtypes, and agents that increase the availability of 5-HT at the synaptic cleft or drugs that are not selective for a particular subtype may bind to different subtypes producing opposing effects on food intake. If this would be the case, the anorectic effect may be obscured if the same agent displays agonist action at 5-HT_{1A}R; in such case, the anorectic effect may benefit from the blockade of such receptors.

Indorenate (5-methoxytryptamine B-methylcarboxylate HCl, INDO) has high affinity for 5-HT_{1A}R, but also low affinity for 5-$HT_{1B/2C}$Rs (Benítez-King, Antón-Tay, and Hong, 1991; Dompert, Glaser, and Traber, 1985; Hoyer, Engel, and Kalkman, 1985). Its antihypertensive (Hong, Rión, Aceves, Benítez-King, and Antón-Tay, 1987) and anxiolytic activity (Fernández-Guasti and López-Rubalcava, 1990) has been related to the stimulation of 5-HT_{1A}R. Also, INDO induce a decrease in food consumption after intraventricular (López-Cabrera, Velázquez-Martínez, Prado, García, and Ortíz, 1991) or systemic administration (Velázquez-Martínez, Valencia, López, and Villarreal, 1995), despite such decrease was not expected considering its high affinity for 5-HT_{1A}R; this inhibition of food intake may be expressed since INDO may behave as partial agonist at the 5-HT_{1A}R, as some studies of drug discrimination have suggested (Miranda, Hong, López-Cabrera, and Velázquez-Martínez, 1998; Velázquez-Martínez, López, Sánchez, Ramírez, and Hong, 1999). Furthermore, the effect was prevented by cinanserin, cyproheptadine or metergoline, purported 5-HT_2R antagonists but not by haloperidol, a dopaminergic antagonist (Velázquez-Martínez et al., 1995). The anorectic action of INDO may be opposed by its affinity to 5-HT_{1A}R, it may benefit by the co-administration of methiothepin, a nonselective 5-HT_1R antagonist; therefore, the aim of the present chapter was to test the hypothesis that the anorectic action of a nonselective agonist may benefit from the co-administration of a low dose of a 5-HT_{1A}R antagonist; it was also explored the pretreatment with mesulergide and mianserin (nonselective 5-HT_2R antagonists) in order to show that the methiothepin effect was specific.

METHOD

Subjects

Subjects were 30 male Wistar rats, 3 months old and weighing 200-300 g at the start of the experiment, obtained from the breeding colony of the Faculty of Psychology (Universidad Nacional Autónoma de México). The animals were housed singly under a cycle of 12 h light and 12 h darkness, with lights on at 8:00 am and a temperature of 23 (+/-1) ºC.

Procedure

On arrival at the laboratory the subjects had *ad libitum* access to food (Laboratory Rodent Diet, Constant Nutrition 5001, Purina, St. Louis. MO. USA) and water for 3 days; then, they were trained over 2 weeks to consume their food and water daily in a period of 4 h (from 10 am to 2 pm). Independent groups were used to evaluate the interaction of the antagonists with the INDO; then, on experimental days the subjects were weighed and randomly assigned to 5 groups of 6 rats.

All groups received two injections, 3 groups received one injection of the antagonist and one group received vehicle; 30 min later the 4 groups received INDO (17.8 mg/kg, a dose close to the ED50, see: Velázquez-Martínez et al., 1995). The fifth group (control) received two injections of saline (separated by 30 min). The test of food intake started after 30 min of the last injection. The doses of the antagonists evaluated were chosen from the literature and were mesulergide (1.0 mg/kg: Aulakh, Hill, Yoney, and Murphy, 1992), mianserin (3.0 mg/kg: Kennett and Curzon, 1988) and methiothepin (0.3 mg/kg: Gardier, Kaakkola, Erfurth, and Wurtman, 1992). Mesulergide and mianserin had been used to prevent dyskensias (Shireen and Haleem, 2011); mesulergide has been used also as an antimigrane drug (Bolcskei, Farkas, Kocsis, and Tarnawa, 2009) and mianserin to treat depression (Serretti, Chiesa, Calati, Perna, Bellodi, and De Ronchi, 2011), while methiothepine may complete its development as an antipsychotic/antimigrane drug (Slassi, 2002).

Test of Food Consumption

On the days of testing a grid and blotting paper were added to the floor of the cage for collecting the spillage. Thirty min after the last injection (INDO or vehicle) the subjects had access to a weighted amount of food and water, which for the test occasion lasted for 24 h. The remaining water and food (including the correction for spillage that was carefully collected from the bottling paper) were determined after 1, 2, 4 and 24 h of access.

Drugs

Drugs used in this study were mesulergide HCl, mianserin HCl, methiothepin mesylate (Sigma Aldrich, St. Louis, MO, USA), and indorenate HCl (Miles-CINVESTAV, México). All drugs were dissolved in sterile isotonic saline and administered subcutaneously (s.c.) in a volume of 1.0 ml/kg.

Data Analysis

Food and water consumption on the test days were expressed as intake per 100 g of body weight (BW) and compared to the intake shown by the control group. For comparison between INDO-Saline conditions repeated measures two-way ANOVA was used with drug condition as one factor and the hours of access as the second factor (with 4 levels: 1,2, 4 and 24 h). For comparison between drug conditions (5 conditions), one-way ANOVA was used. When significant results were obtained ($p<0.05$) *a posteriori* comparisons with the Bonferroni's test were performed to determine the direction of the difference ($p<0.05$).

RESULTS

Figure 1 shows the effects of the administration of 17.8 mg/kg of INDO on food and water intake. After the administration of saline and during the first hour of access the subjects ate about 5.7 g/100g BW and drank 3.9 ml/100g BW; after 24 h of continued access they ate 14.8 g and drank 16.3 ml. The administration of 17.8 mg/kg of INDO decreased food intake to 2.0 g for the first hour of access, to 6.0 g after 4 h of access, but only a slight decrement was observed after the end of the 24 h of access. The administration of INDO produced no alterations in water consumption; but a small increase in water intake was observed after 24 h of access (from 16.3 to 24.8 ml). Two-way ANOVA indicated significant differences for food in both the hours-of-access factor ($F[3,30]=170.6$, $p<0.001$) and in the drug-condition factor ($F[1,10]=25.70$, $p<0.001$) but not in their interaction ($F[3,30]=2.30$, $p>0.05$), the *a posteriori* Bonferroni tests indicated that INDO produced a significant decrease in food intake after 1 ($p<0.001$), 2 ($p<0.01$) and 4 ($p<0.001$) h of access. For water intake, two-way ANOVA indicated significant differences in the hours-of-access factor ($F[3,30]=391.4$, $p<0.001$) and the interaction ($F[3,30]=30.09$, $p<0.001$), but not for the drug-condition factor ($F[1,10]=3.95$, $p=0.075$), the Bonferroni tests indicated that the increase was significant ($p<0.001$) only for the intake of water cumulated for 24 h of access. In food and water intake, the differences in the hours-of-access factor were related to the increase in consumption as time of access elapsed and were not further explored.

Figure 2 shows the interaction of the antagonist's mesulergide, methiothepin and mianserin with INDO on food intake after 1 and 2 h of access. The pretreatment with mesulergide or mianserin prevented the decrease in food intake induced by the administration of INDO, As shown, during the first hour of access and after the pretreatment with methiothepin, INDO induced a further decrease in food intake (from 2.0 g/100g BW to 0.9 g/100g BW). For the consumption during the first hour of access, one-way ANOVA confirmed the significant differences between the drug-treated groups ($F\ [4,\ 29]=32.2$, $P<0.001$). The *a posteriori* Bonferroni tests confirmed that with mesulergide although the intake did not return to the control level it reached significance from effect of INDO alone ($p<0.05$), but with mianserin the antagonism did not reach statistical significance. The Bonferroni test also confirmed that the increase observed in the anorectic effect of INDO after methiothepin was significant ($p<0.05$).

Figure 2 also shows that after 2 h of access to food the initial antagonism after the pretreatment with mesulergide or mianserin faded away with time; however, it persisted the increase in the anorectic effect of INDO observed after the pretreatment with methiothepin.

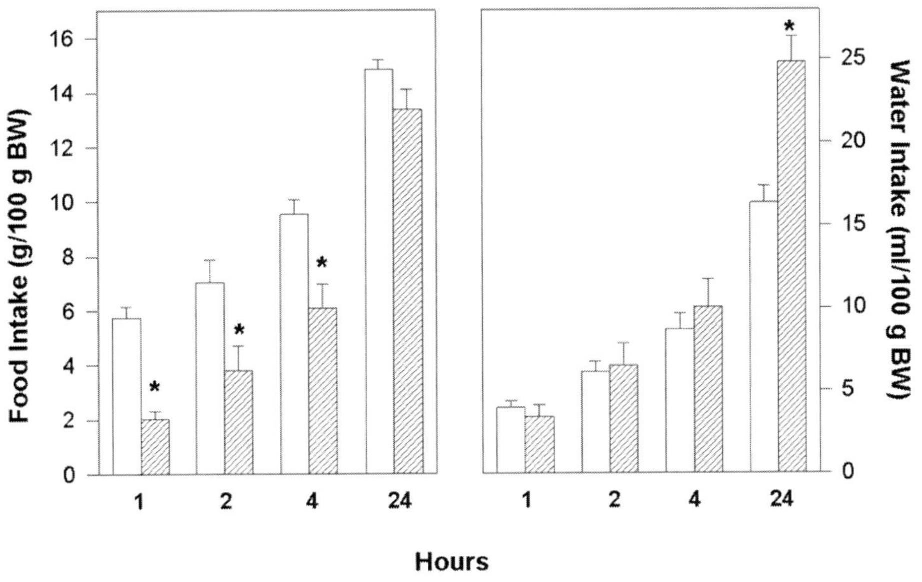

Figure 1. Cumulated food (left panel) or water (right panel) intake of rats treated with indorenate or vehicle. Open bars indicate consumption after saline administration, while shadowed bars indicate consumption after indorenate. Significant differences to the vehicle group at the corresponding time is indicated with *. Mean Mean ± S.E. of 6 subjects.

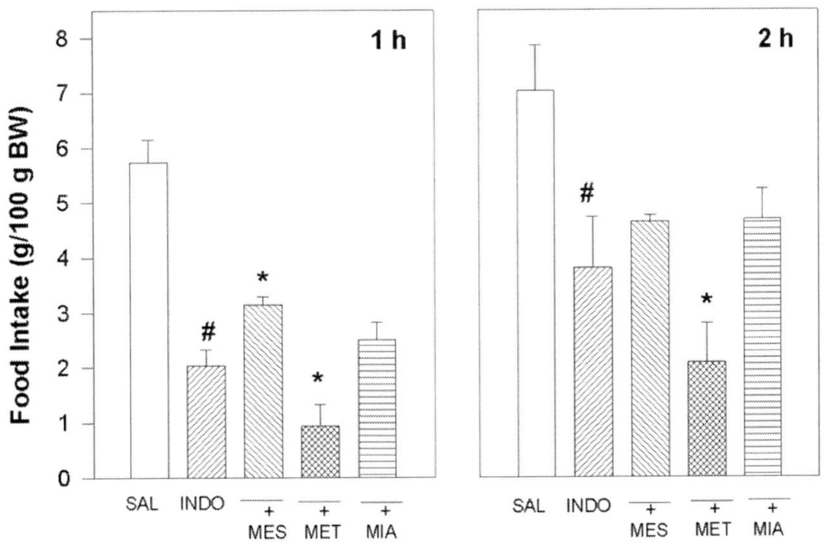

Figure 2. Affects of indorenate administration or vehicle and the pretreatment with methiothepin, mianserin and mesulergide on food intake of rats. Left panel shows food consumption during the first hour of access to food following the administration of indorenate or vehicle. Right panel shows consumption during the second h of access. Abscissa shows drug or vehicle conditions. Ordinates show consumption by 100 g of body weight. Significant difference to vehicle administration is indicated with #, while * indicates significant difference to indorenate-alone administration. Mean ± S.E. of 6 subjects.

One-way ANOVA indicated significant differences between the groups ($F[4,29]=7.48$, $p<0.001$); the *a posteriori* Bonferroni tests confirmed that the changes induced by mesulergide or mianserin did not reach statistical significance ($p>0.05$), but the increase in the anorectic effect of INDO after the pretreatment with methiothepin was significant ($p<0.05$); although the anorectic effect decreases with time, the enhancing effect exerted on the INDO remained.

After 4 h of access to food persisted the decrease in food intake induced by INDO that vanished by 24 h of access; the effects of the pretreatment with any of the antagonists vanished by 4 or 24 h of access (not shown). One-way ANOVA indicated significant differences between the groups by 4 h ($F[4,29]=8.90$, $p<0.001$) or 24 h ($F[4,29]=12.15$, $p<0.001$); however, the *a posteriori* Bonferroni tests indicated that experimental groups had differences only to the saline control group and none of them had differences to the INDO group.

Figure 3 shows the effect of INDO and its interactions with serotonin antagonists on water intake. As shown INDO had no effect on water intake: rats drank 3.9 ml/100g BW after saline and 3.4 ml/100g BW after the administration of INDO. However, INDO induced a decrease in water intake after the pretreatment with mesulergide (to 2.5 ml/100 g BW), mianserin (to 1.33 ml/100 g BW) or methiothepin (intake decrease to 0.85 ml/100 g BW). One-way ANOVA revealed significant differences between the groups ($F[4,29]=13.52$ $p<0.001$), the Bonferroni tests indicated that when INDO was administered alone, it did not produce a significant decrease in water intake ($p>0.05$); however, only when it was given after mianserin or methiothepin induced a significant ($p<0.05$) decrement in water intake.

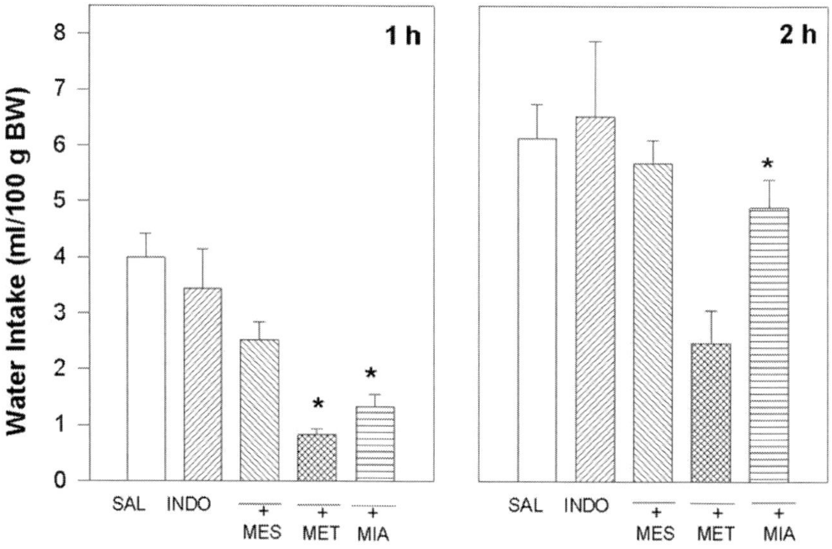

Figure 3. Effects of indorenate administration or vehicle and the pretreatment with methiothepin, mianserin and mesulergide on water intake of rats. Left panel shows water consumption during the first hour of access to food following the administration of indorenate or vehicle. Right panel shows consumption during the second h of access. Abscissa shows drug or vehicle conditions. Significant difference to indorenate-alone administration is indicated with *. Mean ± S.E. of 6 subjects.

Figure 3 also shows that after 2 h of access the effect of the pretreatment with mesulergide or mianserin vanished, while the effect of the pretreatment with methiothepin persisted. One-way ANOVA indicated significant differences between the groups ($F[4,29]=5.533$, $p<0.001$) and the *a posteriori* Bonferroni tests confirmed that the effect after the pretreatment with mesulergide and mianserin did not reach statistical significance while only the combined administration of INDO and methiothepin induced a significant ($p<0.01$) decrease in water intake. One-way ANOVA indicated no significant differences on water intake after 4 h of access ($F[4,29]=1.08$, $p>0.1$) (not shown). After 24 h of access to water (not shown), one-way ANOVA indicated significant differences between the groups ($F[4,29]=12.38$, $p<0.001$); however, the *a posteriori* Bonferroni tests indicated that experimental groups had differences only to the saline control group and none of them had differences to the INDO group.

DISCUSSION

The serotonergic receptors most directly implicated in the control of food intake are the postsynaptic 5-HT_{2C}R, 5-HT_{1B}R and 5-HT_6R, associated with an inhibition of food intake (Garfield and Heisler, 2009; Halford et al., 2007), while the stimulation of 5-HT_{1A}R is associated with the increases in the consumption of food intake (Dourish et al., 1985; Vickers and Dourish, 2004). Since the anorectic effect of an agonist at 5-HT_{2C}R, 5-HT_{1B}R or 5-HT_6R may decrease if the agent also binds at the 5-HT_{1A}R, we tested the hypothesis that the anorectic activity of a 5-HT_{2C}R agonist may benefit with the co-administration of a 5-HT_{1A}R antagonist. Previously, it was found that the systemic administration of INDO produced a dose-dependent decrease in food intake with an ED_{50} of 91.7 mmol/kg (roughly 17 mg/kg, close to the dose used in this study) (Velázquez-Martínez et al., 1995). When the anorectic action of INDO was compared to that of fenfluramine or amphetamine, it was found that the potency of INDO was of less magnitude than that of amphetamine or fenfluramine after systemic administration (Velázquez-Martínez et al., 1995) but similar to that of fenfluramine after central administration . This study confirmed that the administration of INDO produced a decrease in food intake that although faded away, was still visible after 4 hours of continued access to food. The decrease in food intake faded away by 24 hours of access. It is noteworthy that the decrease in food intake induced by INDO was unrelated to an alteration of locomotor activity and was limited to food intake while no significant decrements in water intake were observed as documented by present results and previous observations (López-Cabrera et al., 1991). Previously, it was postulated that serotonin mechanisms are involved in the anorectic action of INDO as its effect was prevented by the 5-HT antagonists cinanserin, cyproheptadine or metergoline but not by the dopaminergic antagonist haloperidol (Velázquez-Martínez et al., 1995) or by cholinergic or adrenergic antagonists (unpublished observations). As the anorectic action of INDO has been related to 5-$HT_{1B/2C}$Rs but it also has affinity for the 5-HT_{1A}R; INDO was used to test the hypothesis that its co-administration with a 5-HT_{1A}R antagonist would increase its anorectic action. The remarkable observation was that after the pretreatment with methiothepin, that has been described as a nonselective antagonist of some of the 5-HT_1Rs family (5-$HT_{1A/1E/1F/6}$), INDO induced a further decrease in food intake during the first and second hours of access. Previously, it was described that mianserin was able to prevent the decrease in 5-HIAA brain levels induced by fluoxetine or d-fenfluramine (Gardier et al., 1992), this action of fenfluramine had been related to the stimulation of the 5-HT_1Rs family. The enhancement seems to be specific to methiothepine, as the pretreatment with mesulergide prevented the decrease in food intake induced by the administration of INDO. Previously it was described that mesulergide is able to prevent the decrease in food intake induced by the administration of the 5-$HT_{2A/2C}$ agonist DOI (Aulakh et al., 1992) and the hyperthermic effect of DOM (Aulakh, Mazzola-Pomietto, Wozniak, Hill, and Murphy, 1994). It has been suggested that the binding of [^{3}H]-mesulergide in the presence of spiperone is likely to be an accurate reflection of 5-HT_{2C} binding (López-Gimenez, Tecott, Palacios, Mengod, and Vilaro, 2002). The pretreatment with the nonspecific 5-$HT_{2A/2B/2C}$ antagonist mianserin blocks the discriminative stimulus properties of 5-HT_2 agonists (Dekeyne, Girardon, and Millan, 1999; Dekeyne, Lob, and Millan, 2001) and the anorectic action of the 5-$HT_{2C/1B}$R agonists mCPP (Kennett and Curzon, 1988), TFMPP (Klodzinska and Chojnacka-Wojcik, 1990) or that of the 5-$HT_{2A/2C}$ agonist DOI (Aulakh et al., 1992); however, in our experiment although mianserin reduced the anorectic action of INDO such reduction did not reach statistical significance; a different pretreatment time or dose of mianserin may reveal its antagonist action upon INDO. The interest in the participation of 5-HT in the regulation of food intake emerged after the description of the anorectic activity of fenfluramine, an amphetamine derivate, devoid of stimulant activity (Le Douarec, Schmitt, and Laubie, 1966; Rothman and Baumann, 2002), but able to produce a blockade of 5-HT reuptake concomitant to a decrease in the brain levels of 5-HT and 5-hydroxyindoleacetic acid (5-HIAA) (Duhault and Verdavainne, 1967; Rothman and Baumann, 2002). Anorectic activity has also been described after the systemic or intra-hypothalamic administration of 5-HT (Blundell and Latham, 1979; Fletcher and Paterson, 1989) and for indirect agonists that inhibit the re-uptake of 5-HT such as fluoxetine, paroxetine, sertraline, fluvoxamine and sibutramine (Konkle, Sreter, Baker, and Bielajew, 2003; Liu, Connoley, Harrison, Heal, and Stock, 2002; Nielsen, Chapin, Johnson, and Torgersen, 1992; Nonogaki, Nozue, Takahashi, Yamashita, Hiraoka, Kumano, Kuboki, and Oka, 2007; Yen, Wong, and Bemis, 1987). Since all these agents are not selective of the 5-HT_{2C}R, 5-HT_{1B}R or 5-HT_6Rs, and the enhanced anorectic effect of INDO induced by methiothepin confirms the suggestion that the blockade of 5-HT_{1A}R allow us to observe the full participation of the receptors related to the inhibition of food intake, then the blockade of 5-HT_{1A}R may also benefit the anorectic activity of the releasing agents or those that inhibit the reuptake mechanism.

Acknowledgments

Supported by DGAPA IN303209 and CONACYT 29337. Technical assistance of J.I. Ramirez-Labastida is appreciated.

References

Aulakh, C. S., Hill, J. L., Yoney, H. T., and Murphy, D. L. (1992). Evidence for involvement of 5-HT1C and 5-HT2 receptors in the food intake suppressant effects of 1-(2,5-

dimethoxy-4-iodophenyl)-2-aminopropane (DOI). *Psychopharmacology (Berl), 109*(4), 444-448.

Aulakh, C. S., Mazzola-Pomietto, P., Wozniak, K. M., Hill, J. L., and Murphy, D. L. (1994). Evidence that 1-(2,5-dimethoxy-4-methylphenyl)-2-aminopropane-induced hypophagia and hyperthermia in rats is mediated by serotonin-2A receptors. *Journal of Pharmacology and Experimental Therapeutics, 270*(1), 127-132.

Benítez-King, G., Antón-Tay, F., and Hong, E. (1991). Characterization of indorenate effects on brain monoamine metabolism. *Drug Development Research, 23*, 325-331.

Blundell, J. E., and Latham, C. J. (1979). Serotonergic influences on food intake: effect of 5-hydroxytryptophan on parameters of feeding behaviour in deprived and free-feeding rats. *Pharmacology, Biochemistry and Behavior, 11*(4), 431-437.

Bolcskei, H., Farkas, B., Kocsis, P., and Tarnawa, I. (2009). Recent advancements in anti-migraine drug research: focus on attempts to decrease neuronal hyperexcitability. *Recent Pat CNS Drug Discov, 4*(1), 14-36.

Clifton, P. G., and Kennett, G. A. (2006). Monoamine receptors in the regulation of feeding behaviour and energy balance. *CNS Neurol Disord Drug Targets, 5*(3), 293-312.

Dekeyne, A., Girardon, S., and Millan, M. J. (1999). Discriminative stimulus properties of the novel serotonin (5-HT)2C receptor agonist, RO 60-0175: a pharmacological analysis. *Neuropharmacology, 38*(3), 415-423. doi: S0028390898002032 [pii]

Dekeyne, A., Lob, L., and Millan, M. J. (2001). Following long-term training with citalopram, both mirtazapine and mianserin block its discriminative stimulus properties in rats. *Psychopharmacology (Berl), 153*(3), 389-392.

Dompert, W. U., Glaser, T., and Traber, J. (1985). 3H-TVX Q 7821: identification of 5-HT1 binding sites as target for a novel putative anxiolytic. *Naunyn-Schmiedebergs Archives of Pharmacology, 328*(4), 467-470.

Dourish, C. T., Cooper, S. J., Gilbert, F., Coughlan, J., and Iversen, S. D. (1988). The 5-HT1A agonist 8-OH-DPAT increases consumption of palatable wet mash and liquid diets in the rat. *Psychopharmacology (Berl), 94*(1), 58-63.

Dourish, C. T., Hutson, P. H., and Curzon, G. (1985). Characteristics of feeding induced by the serotonin agonist 8-hydroxy-2-(di-n-propylamino) tetralin (8-OH-DPAT). *Brain Research Bulletin, 15*(4), 377-384. doi: 0361-9230(85)90005-X [pii]

Duhault, J., and Verdavainne, C. (1967). [Modification of the cerebral serotonin level in the rat by trifluoromethyl-2-phenyl ethyl aminopropane (Fenfluramine 768 S)]. *Archives Internationales de Pharmacodynamie et de Therapie, 170*(2), 276-286.

Fernández-Guasti, A., and López-Rubalcava, C. (1990). Evidence for the involvement of the 5-HT1A receptor in the anxiolytic action of indorenate and ipsapirone. *Psychopharmacology (Berl), 101*(3), 354-358.

Fletcher, P. J., and Paterson, I. A. (1989). A comparison of the effects of tryptamine and 5-hydroxytryptamine on feeding following injection into the paraventricular nucleus of the hypothalamus. *Pharmacology, Biochemistry and Behavior, 32*(4), 907-911.

Gardier, A. M., Kaakkola, S., Erfurth, A., and Wurtman, R. J. (1992). Effects of methiothepin on changes in brain serotonin release induced by repeated administration of high doses of anorectic serotoninergic drugs. *Brain Research, 588*(1), 67-74.

Garfield, A. S., and Heisler, L. K. (2009). Pharmacological targeting of the serotonergic system for the treatment of obesity. *Journal of Physiology, 587*(Pt 1), 49-60. doi: jphysiol.2008.164152 [pii], 10.1113/jphysiol.2008.164152 [doi]

Halford, J. C., Harrold, J. A., Boyland, E. J., Lawton, C. L., and Blundell, J. E. (2007). Serotonergic drugs : effects on appetite expression and use for the treatment of obesity. *Drugs, 67*(1), 27-55. doi: 6714 [pii]

Hong, E., Rión, R., Aceves, J., Benítez-King, G., and Antón-Tay, F. (1987). Further evidence for a central antihypertensive effect of indorenate. *Proceedings of the Western Pharmacology Society, 30*, 1-3.

Hoyer, D., Engel, G., and Kalkman, H. O. (1985). Molecular pharmacology of 5-HT1 and 5-HT2 recognition sites in rat and pig brain membranes: radioligand binding studies with [3H]5-HT, [3H]8-OH-DPAT, (-)[125I]iodocyanopindolol, [3H]mesulergine and [3H]ketanserin. *European Journal of Pharmacology, 118*(1-2), 13-23. doi: 0014-2999(85)90658-2 [pii]

Hutson, P. H., Dourish, C. T., and Curzon, G. (1986). Neurochemical and behavioural evidence for mediation of the hyperphagic action of 8-OH-DPAT by 5-HT cell body autoreceptors. *European Journal of Pharmacology, 129*(3), 347-352.

Hutson, P. H., Dourish, C. T., and Curzon, G. (1988). Evidence that the hyperphagic response to 8-OH-DPAT is mediated by 5-HT1A receptors. *European Journal of Pharmacology, 150*(3), 361-366.

Kennett, G. A., and Curzon, G. (1988). Evidence that hypophagia induced by mCPP and TFMPP requires 5-HT1C and 5-HT1B receptors; hypophagia induced by RU 24969 only requires 5-HT1B receptors. *Psychopharmacology (Berl), 96*(1), 93-100.

Klodzinska, A., and Chojnacka-Wojcik, E. (1990). Anorexia induced by M-trifluoromethylphenylpiperazine (TFMPP) in rats. *Polish Journal of Pharmacology and Pharmacy, 42*(1), 13-17.

Konkle, A. T., Sreter, K. B., Baker, S. L., and Bielajew, C. (2003). Chronic paroxetine infusion influences macronutrient selection in male Sprague-Dawley rats. *Pharmacology, Biochemistry and Behavior, 74*(4), 883-890.

Le Douarec, J. C., Schmitt, H., and Laubie, M. (1966). [Pharmacologic study of fenfluramine and its optical isomers]. *Archives Internationales de Pharmacodynamie et de Therapie, 161*(1), 206-232.

Liu, Y. L., Connoley, I. P., Harrison, J., Heal, D. J., and Stock, M. J. (2002). Comparison of the thermogenic and hypophagic effects of sibutramine's metabolite 2 and other monoamine reuptake inhibitors. *European Journal of Pharmacology, 452*(1), 49-56.

López-Cabrera, M., Velázquez-Martínez, D. N., Prado, R., García, G., and Ortíz, R. (1991). Effects of the intracerebroventricular administration of indorenate and fenfluramine on spontaneous behavior and food intake in rats. *Proceedings of the Western Pharmacology Society, 34*, 468.

López-Gimenez, J. F., Tecott, L. H., Palacios, J. M., Mengod, G., and Vilaro, M. T. (2002). Serotonin 5- HT (2C) receptor knockout mice: autoradiographic analysis of multiple serotonin receptors. *Journal of Neuroscience Research, 67*(1), 69-85. doi: 10.1002/jnr.10072 [pii]

Macor, J. E., Burkhart, C. A., Heym, J. H., Ives, J. L., Lebel, L. A., Newman, M. E., Nielsen, J. A., Ryan, K., Schulz, D. W. and Torgersen, L. K. (1990). 3-(1,2,5,6-Tetrahydropyrid-4-yl)pyrrolo[3,2-b]pyrid-5-one: a potent and selective serotonin (5-HT1B) agonist and rotationally restricted phenolic analogue of 5-methoxy-3-(1,2,5,6-tetrahydropyrid-4-yl)indole. *Journal of Medicinal Chemistry*, 33(8), 2087-2093.

Martin, J. R. Bos, M. Jenck, F. Moreau, J. Mutel, V. Sleight, A. J. Wichmann, J. Andrews, J. S. Berendsen, H. H. Broekkamp, C. L. Ruigt, G. S. Kohler, C. and Delft, A. M.(1998). 5-HT2C receptor agonists: pharmacological characteristics and therapeutic potential. *Journal of Pharmacology And Experimental Therapeutics*, 286(2), 913-924.

Miranda, F., Hong, E., López-Cabrera, M., and Velázquez-Martínez, D. N. (1998). Modulation of the discriminative stimulus properties of indorenate by 5-HT receptors. *Proceedings of the Western Pharmacology Society, 41*, 60.

Nielsen, J. A., Chapin, D. S., Johnson, J. L., Jr., and Torgersen, L. K. (1992). Sertraline, a serotonin-uptake inhibitor, reduces food intake and body weight in lean rats and genetically obese mice. *American Journal of Clinical Nutrition, 55*(1 Suppl), 185S-189S.

Nonogaki, K. Nozue, K. Takahashi, Y. Yamashita, N. Hiraoka, S. Kumano, H. Kuboki, T. and Oka, Y.(2007). Fluvoxamine, a selective serotonin reuptake inhibitor, and 5-HT2C receptor inactivation induce appetite-suppressing effects in mice via 5-HT1B receptors. *International Journal of Neuropsychopharmacology,* 10(5), 675-681. doi: 10.1017/s1461145706007206.

Pytliak, M., Vargova, V., Mechirova, V., and Felsoci, M. (2011). Serotonin receptors - from molecular biology to clinical applications. *Physiological Research, 60*(1), 15-25.

Rothman, R. B., and Baumann, M. H. (2002). Serotonin releasing agents. Neurochemical, therapeutic and adverse effects. *Pharmacology, Biochemistry and Behavior, 71*(4), 825-836. doi: S0091305701006694 [pii]

Serretti, A., Chiesa, A., Calati, R., Perna, G., Bellodi, L., and De Ronchi, D. (2011). Novel antidepressants and panic disorder: evidence beyond current guidelines. *Neuropsychobiology, 63*(1), 1-7. doi: 10.1159/000321831

Shireen, E., and Haleem, D. J. (2011). Reversal of haloperidol-induced motor deficits by mianserin and mesulergine in rats. *Pak J Pharm Sci, 24*(1), 7-12.

Slassi, A. (2002). Recent advances in 5-HT1B/1D receptor antagonists and agonists and their potential therapeutic applications. *Curr Top Med Chem, 2*(6), 559-574.

Velázquez-Martínez, D. N., López, C. M., Sánchez, H., Ramírez, J. I., and Hong, E. (1999). Discriminative stimulus properties of indorenate, a serotonin agonist. *Journal of Psychiatry and Neuroscience, 24*(2), 130.

Velázquez-Martínez, D. N., Valencia, F. M., López, C. M., and Villarreal, J. E. (1995). Effects of indorenate on food intake: a comparison with fenfluramine and amphetamine. *Psychopharmacology (Berl), 117*(1), 91-101.

Vickers, S. P., and Dourish, C. T. (2004). Serotonin receptor ligands and the treatment of obesity. *Current Opinion in Investigational Drugs, 5*(4), 377-388.

Woolley, M. L., Bentley, J. C., Sleight, A. J., Marsden, C. A., and Fone, K. C. (2001). A role for 5-ht6 receptors in retention of spatial learning in the Morris water maze. *Neuropharmacology, 41*(2), 210-219.

Yen, T. T., Wong, D. T., and Bemis, K. G. (1987). Reduction of food-consumption and body-weight of normal and obese mice by chronic treatment with fluoxetine - a serotonin reuptake inhibitor. *Drug Development Research, 10*(1), 37-45. doi: 10.1002/ddr.430100106.

In: Recent Hispanic Psychological Research ... ISBN: 978-1-62948-919-3
Editors: C. H. Garcia Cadena, A. Lopez-Espinoza et al.

Chapter 2

POSSIBLE INTERACTION BETWEEN THE EFFECTS OF STRESS AND DEPRIVATION ON EATING BEHAVIOR IN RATS

***Marina Liliana González-Torres*[*1], *Antonio López-Espinoza*[2] *and Cristiano Valerio dos Santos*[1]**
[1]Studies and Researches in Behavior Center, University of Guadalajara, Mexico
[2]Behavioral Feeding and Nutrition Research Center. CUSur, University of Guadalajara, México

ABSTRACT

The present study investigates whether the exposure to acute or chronic foot-shocks and the possibility of escape of them differentially affect food and water intake in rats deprived of water or both food and water in females and males rats. The rats were deprived of water 23.5 hours a day (partial deprivation) or for three consecutive days of food and water (total deprivation) and after to baseline condition they were exposed to acute (60 for two days) or chronic (10 for 12 days) escapable or inescapable electric shocks. The subjects exposed to acute and chronic shocks reduced food and water intake when the deprivation was partial and water was available in the stress context, that is, in the chamber where shocks occurred. However, when the animals were total deprived, no stress-induced reduction of food and water intake was observed, suggesting that level of deprivation was a crucial variable. Additionally, a slight difference between escapable or inescapable shocks was suggested, but results are not clear.

Keywords: Eating behavior, escapable foot-shocks, inescapable foot-shocks, deprivation, rats

* Address for correspondence: Marina Liliana González-Torres Centro de Estudios e Investigaciones en Comportamiento (CEIC) Universidad de Guadalajara. Calle Francisco de Quevedo # 180 Col. Arcos Vallarta 44130. E-mail: liliglz@hotmail.com.

INTRODUCTION

Organisms react to stress with physiological and behavioral changes in order to maintain homeostasis and increase chances of survival (Tsigos and Chrousos, 2002). Stress can be either acute or chronic depending on its duration and sometimes on its intensity. Chronic stress is defined by the repeated exposure to a stressor for a long period of time, while acute stress usually refers to one or two exposures to a possibly more intense stressor. Chronically stressed animals don't experience all the hormonal consequences that animals exposed to one single stress event do (Harris, Gu, Mitchell, Endale, Russo and Ryan, 2004), but repeated exposure to stress may represent a severe threat to health, leading to the development of physiological and behavioral dysfunctions, including changes in feeding behavior (Fachin, Silva, Boschang, Pettenuzzo, Bertinetti, Billodre, Peres, Busnello, and Dalmaz, 2008). Studies evaluating animal models of stress have suggested that food intake may either increase or decrease during stressful periods (Dallman, 2010; González-Torres, López-Espinoza and dos Santos, 2010; Ortolani, Oyama, Ferrari, Melo and Spadari-Bratfisch, 2011). This difference in the results may be in part due to the use of different stressors, different types of food or levels of deprivation.

One of the procedures most widely used to study of stress is the learned helplessness paradigm. This paradigm uses a triadic design with groups, which have a possibility to finish or avoidance the stressor (controllable), other groups yoked to prior but with no this possibility (uncontrollable), and finally, groups naïve (control). This paradigm states that the most stressful situation and one that produces the greatest effect is uncontrollable situation (Overmier, 2002, Seligman and Maier, 1967).

Recently, Gonzalez-Torres et al. (2010) reported that rats exposed to both, either escapable or inescapable electric foot-shocks, that is, the subject have the possibility of finished to stressor with some specific behavior or nothing of they do will finish to stressor, respectively, reduced their body weight gain and food and water intake. This reduction in water intake in stressed animals was inconsistent with the results observed in other studies (Dess, Chapman and Minor, 1988; Job and Barnes, 1995), which reported no effect on water consumption. This difference was likely due to differences in the schedules of access to food and water. González-Torres et al. (2010) restricted access to water and food for 14 hours a day and reported that the consumption was similar to a condition of free access. Dess, Chapman and Minor (1988) and Job and Barnes (1995), restricted access to water for 30 minutes, which may have led to a higher state of water deprivation and made it more necessary for the body to consume water than respond to stress by reducing intake.

If the effect of the stressor on eating behavior is due to shocks per se or its uncontrollability has not yet been clarified. Job and Barnes (1995) reported that the inescapable shock evoked the most effect, but Dess, Minor and Brewer (1989) and González-Torres, et al. (2010) not observed differences between escapable or inescapable shocks.

Additionally, it has been proposed that the simultaneous presentation of food or water with stimuli associated with the stressful situation can result in an inhibition of behavior required to obtain food (Jackson and Delprato, 1974). In the experiment by González-Torres et al. (2010), food and water were offered in a context different from the stressful situation. Then, it is conceivable that when the food or water is available in the stress context, that is, in the same place where stressful stimuli occurred, consumption will be reduced even more than when they are available in a different context. The context associated with the stress presents danger signals for the subject and the regulatory change hypothesis proposed by Dess (1991) predicts that subjects tend to employ a conservative strategy, reducing the external energy expense and using energy reserves of the body, that is reflected for a reduction in the food intake and body weight gain, thereby reducing risk exposure. However, if the deprivation is a crucial variable, no changes or an increase in the consumption should be observed, despite water being available in the stress context.

The aim of the present study was to evaluate the effects of acute or chronic stress (electric foot shocks) on food and water intake in female and male rats deprived of water or both food and water, when the water was available in the stress context. In addition, the possible differences between the effects of escapable or inescapable shocks were investigated.

METHOD

Subjects

Forty experimentally naïve male *Wistar* rats (twenty males and twenty females) eight weeks old at the beginning of the experiment, were used. The animals were housed in a temperature-controlled room (22±2 °C), with a 12 h light/dark cycle (lights on at 8:00 hrs).

Apparatus

The rats were placed in individual home-cages (13 cm high, 27 cm wide and 38 cm large). To record food intake and body weight, a precision electronic scale was used. Two 200-ml graduated bottles were used to measure water intake daily. Rodent laboratory chow Purina® and purified water were provided.

During the shocks sessions, the rats were placed in a Plexiglas chamber (26×21×26 cm) provided with a grid floor made of stainless-steel (4.8 mm) rods spaced 1.6 cm apart (MED-VFC-model RS-NIRU, Video Fear Conditioning for rats - Near Infrared Unit). The chambers were isolated from external noise and light. The floor was connected to an ENV-414S shock generator (aversive stimulator standalone / scrambler). One of the lateral panels of these chambers had an orifice through which the rat could insert its snout or any other body part. This orifice was provided with a photobeam whose interruption was registered as an escape response.

Also a computer with MED-PC for Windows was used, which scheduled shock delivery to each chamber and recorded latency and numbers of escape responses.

Procedure

Prior to the start of the experiment, records on body weight and consumption of freely available chow (Purina®) and water were taken for ten days.

Subjects were randomly assigned to one of five groups of 8 rats each (4 females and 4 males). The first group was exposed to two sessions of 60 escapable electric shocks each one. The second group was yoked the first group and exposed to the same amount of sessions and shocks, but they were inescapable. The third group received the same amount of shocks but these were dispersed over 12 sessions of 10 escapable shocks. The fourth group was yoked to the third groups and exposed to 10 inescapable shocks. Finally, the control group was kept in its home-cages throughout the experiment. In addition, each group was subdivided in partial or total deprivation subgroups (n=4). The subgroups of partial deprivation had free access to food and just 30 min daily access to water throughout the experiment. The subgroups of total deprivation were exposed to a phase with no access to food and water for three days prior to shock sessions.

The experimental design consisted of four phases. The first phase was a baseline condition in which all subjects remained in the home-cages with access to food restricted to 14 hours, from 20:00 hrs to 10:00 hrs of the next day and records of body weight and food and water consumption taken daily for 10 days between 10:00 and 11:00 hrs. In this phase, water was available only for 30 minutes prior to the onset of the dark period for partial deprivation subgroups, and for 14 hours like food for total deprivation. Total deprivation subgroups were allowed access to neither food nor water for the last three consecutive days of this phase. In the second phase, rats were kept under the same feeding conditions of baseline, but they were exposed to sessions of electric foot-shocks according to their experimental protocol. In the third phase, groups exposed to acute stress were returned to baseline conditions for 10 days, and two other sessions of acute foot-shocks after that. Groups exposed to chronic stress were maintained in the stress phase, but this phase was divided into two phases of 12 sessions each for comparison purposes. During this phase, the partial deprivation subgroups had access to water available inside the chamber where they received shocks for 30 minutes, immediately after the session ended. The total deprivation subgroups had access to water in the home-cage along with food for 14 hours.

Foot-Shock Stress Protocol

Dyads of rats were formed, one of which was assigned to one escapable group and the other to an inescapable group. The shock sessions lasted approximately 60 or 10 minutes for acute and chronic stress groups respectively and were conducted between 18:00 and 20:00 hrs. The shock had an intensity of 0.6 mA and a maximum duration of 10 seconds and they were scheduled according to a variable time 60 seconds. When the "escapable" subject emitted the required response, the electric shock was switched off both for itself and for the "inescapable" rat yoked to it.

Data Analysis

The average of food and water intake and body weight of the last five days of each phase was considered in the analysis, except for acute stress groups, whose stress phase lasted two days; in this case, both days were included. For chronic groups, the first and the last five days of all 24 days of stress were considered. Statistical analysis was performed using SPSS version 16 for Windows. Non-parametric tests were performed to assess normality and homogeneity of variance (One-Sample Kolmogorov-Smirnov Test and Levene Test, respectively). Separate analyses were conducted for partial and total deprivation groups. Generalized Estimating Equations (GEE) was used to analysis of food and water intake. The within-subject variable was the phases of experiment and the interactions between group and phases and pairwise padjust contrasts were explored with Bonferroni tests. The normal distribution was used since non-parametric tests confirmed it. The identity link function and unstructured correlation matrix were selected. Separate one-way ANOVAs were used to compare body weight gain in each phase between groups. The differences were considered significant when $p \leq 0.05$.

RESULTS

Food Intake

The mean food intake of each group was calculated separately for females and males, then data from male and female subjects were grouped in Figure 1 depending on shock controllability (n=4). Although females showed consumption of food, water and body weight slowly lower than males in all conditions (e.g. mean of food intake in baseline for females 11.27±0.68 and 13.42±1.3 for males) the clustering of the data did not change the trend observed individually, and it made easier the statistical analysis. The mean food intake for the partial deprivation group was lower than for total deprivation groups during baseline. Food intake decreased in the groups exposed to foot-shocks during stress for both partial deprivation groups (Figure 1A and 1B) and for the group with total deprivation exposed to acute stress (Figure 1C). The GEE analysis revealed significant differences between phases for the acute and chronic groups with partial deprivation (Wald chi-square = 108.93, $p < 0.001$; Wald chi-square = 111.37, $p < 0.001$, respectively) and for acute groups with total deprivation (Wald chi-square = 17.044, $p = 0.001$). An interaction group*phase for the acute and chronic groups with partial deprivation and for the groups exposed to acute shocks with total deprivation was observed (Wald chi-square = 127.97, $p < 0.001$; Wald chi square = 5949. 81, $p < 0.001$; Wald chi-square = 26.396, $p < 0.001$, respectively).

Additionally, post hoc Bonferroni tests indicated that average food intake in the first stress phase for the acute stress groups with partial deprivation was significantly lower than the previous phase (baseline), regardless of shock controllability (escapable $p = 0.000$; inescapable $p = 0.000$), but no difference was observed in groups with total deprivation. In the second exposure to foot-shocks, the inescapable groups with partial and total deprivation significantly reduced food intake ($p = 0.003$; $p=0.007$, respectively). For the groups exposed to chronic shock sessions, partial deprivation groups had lower food intakes, but only in the first five days regardless of shock controllability (escapable $p = 0.025$; inescapable $p = 0.011$) (Figure 1B).

Water Intake

Figure 2 presents the mean water intake in each group (escapable, inescapable, and control groups), for partial deprivation (2A and 2B) and total deprivation (2C and 2D) groups. Water intake was reduced in the groups with partial deprivation, but it was increased in the groups with total deprivation.

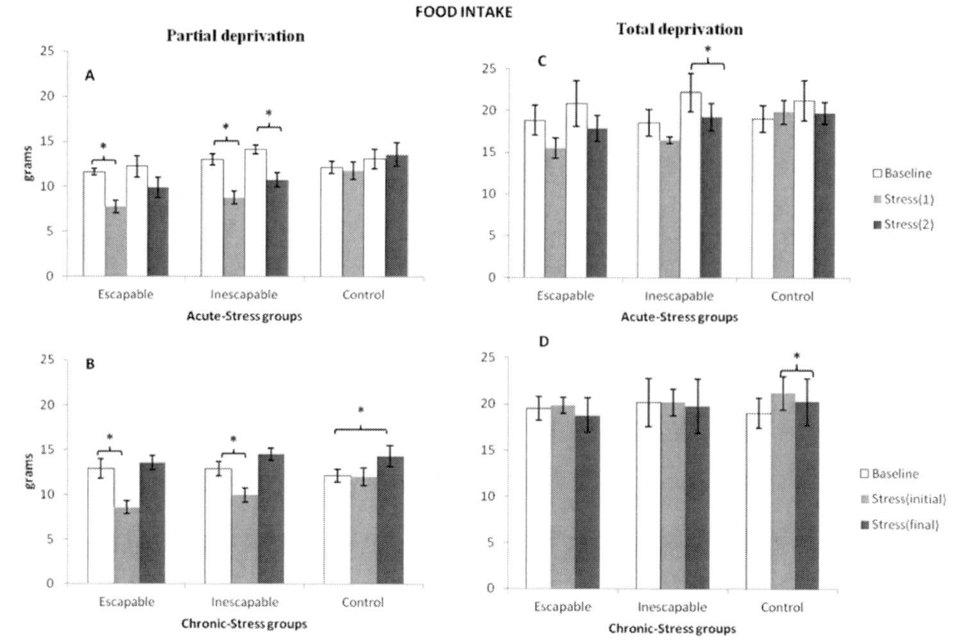

Figure 1. Average of food intake of females and males together with partial deprivation (left panel) and total deprivation (right panel) in each phase for acute (A and C, respectively) and chronic groups (B and D, respectively). (*) Significantly different from previous phase (GEE, $p < 0.05$).

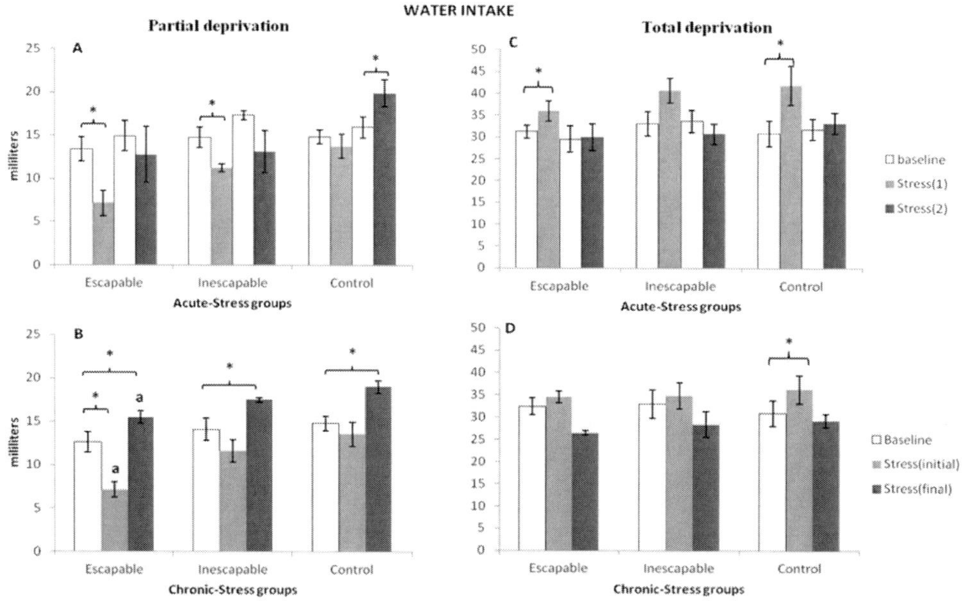

Figure 2. Average of water intake of females and males together with partial deprivation (left panel) and total deprivation (right panel) in each phase for acute (A and C, respectively) and chronic groups (B and D, respectively). (*) Significantly different from previous phase (GEE, $p < 0.05$). (a) Significantly different from control group (GEE, $p < 0.05$).

Significant difference between phases were observed in all groups exposed to shocks with partial deprivation (acute, Wald chi-square = 86.641, $p < 0.001$; chronic, Wald chi-square = 157.961, $p < 0.001$), and with total deprivation (acute, Wald chi-square = 81.454, $p < 0.001$; chronic, Wald chi-square = 63. 749, $p < 0.001$). Additionally, Bonferroni tests revealed that escapable, inescapable or control groups in acute stress (p= 0.003), in chronic stress (p= 0.001) with partial deprivation and acute stress with total deprivation (p= 0.022) were significantly different. An interaction group*phases was observed in groups exposed to acute shocks (partial deprivation, Wald chi-square = 63.595, $p < 0.0001$; total deprivation, Wald chi-square = 47.563, $p< 0.001$), but not for chronic stress groups with partial and total deprivation. In the first exposure to shocks, water intake significantly decreased in comparison with baseline for acute and chronic escapable groups with partial deprivation (p= 0.000; p= 0.003, respectively) and in the acute inescapable group with partial deprivation (p=0.002) according to the Boferroni test. For groups with total deprivation, water intake was higher than the previous phase in the first exposure to shocks for the acute and chronic escapable groups, as well as for the control group with total deprivation (escapable, p= 0.038; inescapable, p= 0.022; control, p= 0.000). In the second exposure to the acute shocks, control subjects with partial deprivation increased their water intake (p = 0.000). In the last five days of chronic shocks, all groups with total deprivation decreased their water intake and this reduction was significant in comparison to consumption in the first exposure to the stress (escapable, p= 0.000; inescapable, p= 0.000; control, p= 0.007). The chronic escapable group with partial deprivation was significantly different from the control group in both the first and second exposure to stress ($p < 0.05$).

Body Weight Gain

Body weight gain was calculated by dividing the average body weight of each phase into the average body weight of the previous phase and it was expressed in terms of percentage and represented in Figure 3. All subjects with partial deprivation reduced their body weight gain in the “Baseline” phase in comparison to the *ad libitum* condition (Figure 3A and 3B). All subjects with total deprivation gained around 12 - 14% of body weight in the first condition of baseline in comparison with previous condition (*ad libitum*) (Figure 3C and 3D). In the deprivation phases, all subjects reduced their body weight. An ANOVA was used to compare the body weight gain during stress and revealed a significant difference between the groups exposed to acute stress with partial deprivation in the first exposure ($F_{2,9}$= 5.345, p= 0.030) (Figure 3A). Post hoc Bonferroni test showed that acute escapable group with partial deprivation was significant different from control group at a marginal level (p=0.05). However, no difference between groups exposed to chronic shocks was found (Figure 3B). Body weight gain in the phases of acute and chronic shock sessions decreased in all groups with total deprivation in both exposures, included control group and no significant difference between groups was revealed (Figure 3C and 3D). In the last days of exposure to chronic stressor an ANOVA revealed significant differences between groups ($F_{2,9}$ = 5.757, p= 0.025), this difference occurred between inescapable and control group (Bonferroni, p = 0.03), since the body weight gain of inescapable group decreased respect to baseline more than control group (Figure 3D). The rats of control group with total deprivation recuperated the body weight gain at the same level that baseline, but in escapable and inescapable groups it didn't happen.

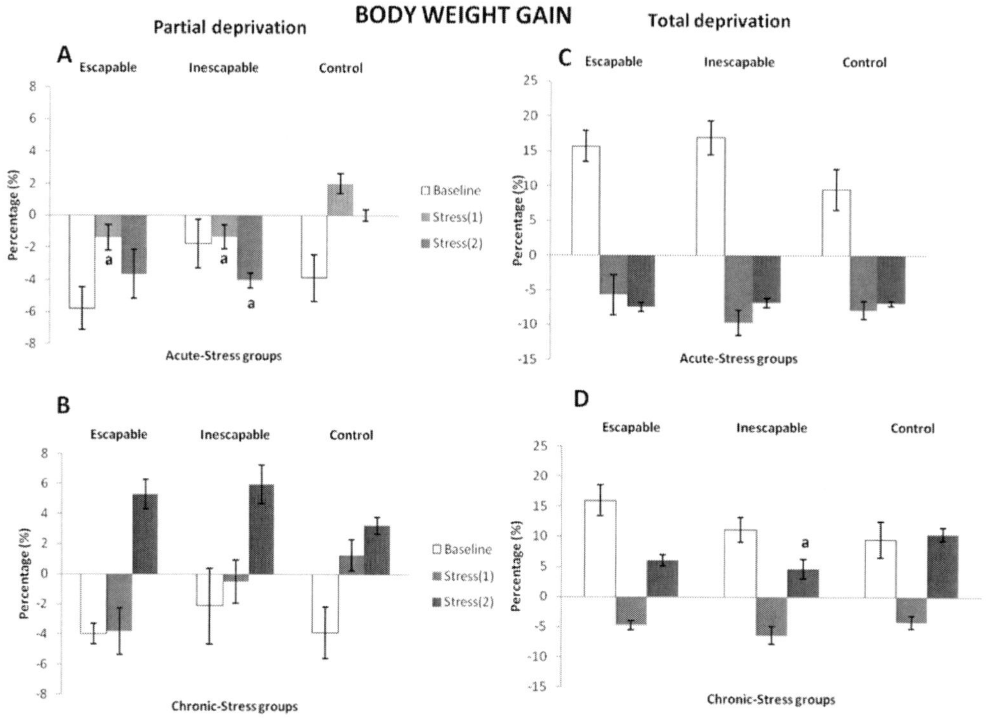

Figure 3. Average of body weight gain of subjects with partial deprivation (left panel) and total deprivation (right panel) in each phase for acute (A and C, respectively) and chronic groups (B and D, respectively). (a) Significantly different from control group (ANOVA, post hoc Bonferroni, $p < 0.05$).

Acquisition of Escape Response

All subjects acquired escape response during the first 60 shocks. In general, the latencies of the males (1 second) are smaller than the latencies for females (4 seconds) exposed to both, acute and chronic stressor. Lower latencies were also recorded during the second phase of stress in both, acute and chronic exposure to shocks. The mean percentage of escaped shocks for all subjects in the last 60 shocks was around of 85% and the mean latency of escape responses was around 2 seconds.

Discussion

Similar to previous studies, the reduction in food intake induced by electric shocks was found both in acute and chronic groups with partial deprivation (Dess, Chapman and Minor, 1988; Job and Barnes, 1995; González-Torres, López-Espinoza and dos Santos, 2010; Ortolani et al., 2011). However, no reduction in food intake was observed in the groups exposed to chronic shocks when the animals were deprived for three consecutive days before stress, but the increase observed in the control group did not occur either. The high level of deprivation appears to have reduced the effects of shocks on food intake.

The reduction in the water intake observed in the first exposure to foot-shocks in rats with partial deprivation is inconsistent with the results reported by Dess, Chaman and Minor (1988) and, Job and Barnes (1995). Although water was available for the same 30 minutes, it was presented in the shocks chambers (stress context), and maybe this is responsible for the reduction observed. In the second exposure to foot-shocks or the final sessions of chronic stress, however, the reduction was not observed, and some subjects even increased their water intake with respect to the baseline.

In order to evaluate this hypothesis, half of subjects were deprived of water for three consecutive days, resulting in a severe state of water deprivation before being exposed to shocks. With this manipulation, no stress-induced reduction was observed; instead, an increase was observed in all groups, suggesting that level of deprivation was a crucial variable. However, subjects in the chronic stress group with total deprivation reduced their intake only in the last days of the stress phase, which suggests two interesting hypotheses. First, chronic stress may have a stronger effect than acute stress, as Fachin et al. (2008) suggested. They argued that several factors involved in the response to stress may also be involved in feeding behavior, such as the activation of the autonomic nervous system (Berthoud and Morrison, 2008, Torres and Nowson, 2007) and the release of glucocorticoids (Adam and Epel, 2007; Tsigas and Chrousos, 2002; Ortolani et al., 2011), leptin (Baranowska, Baranowska-Bik, Bik, and Klein, 2006) and opioids (Bodnar and Klein, 2006). Second, the effects of deprivation were stronger than the effects of the shocks. Therefore, the first days of shocks no changes were observed. Then, as the state of deprivation diminished, the effect of stress could be visible by the end of the stress phase.

Body weight gain decreased in all groups exposed to shocks, as reported in other studies (González-Torres, López,-Espinoza, and dos Santos, 2010), but when the deprivation lasted three days, the animals recovered their body weight gradually and no effects of stress was evidenced.

These findings are well explained by the hypothesis of regulatory change (Dess, 1991). It claims that individuals under stress reduce their regular food intake to avoid the danger and thus consume their energy reserves, so they lose body weight. Nevertheless, when the organism has little energy left, this strategy can be dangerous.

Additionally, some differences between escapable or inescapable shocks were suggested by the results, but these not are clear. The reduction in food and water intake appeared stronger for the escapable groups with partial deprivation in the first exposure to stress. In the second exposure to acute stress, the inescapable group with partial deprivation showed a more pronounced reduction than its escapable counterpart did. Dess, Minor and Brewer (1989) failed to observe a difference between escapable and inescapable stress, in contrast with the observations of Job and Barnes (1995), whose experiments showed a stronger suppression of water intake adulterated with quinine only for subjects exposed to inescapable shocks. Dess et al.(1989) suggested that their failure to observe a difference in this respect was due to subjects' being older than those used generally in the learned helplessness paradigm, while subjects used by Job and Barnes (1995) were younger and possibly more vulnerable to stress. Subjects used in these experiments were younger than those used by Job and Barnes (1995), but no clear difference was observed. One possibility is that the escape response used in this study caused latencies to be short and the differences between escapable and inescapable shocks were minimized.

Finally, the animals exposed to total deprivation increased water consumption despite exposure to stress after the deprivation phase. However, the regularly reported increases in food intake after a period of deprivation with total deprivation periods similar to these (López-Espinoza and Martínez, 2001, 2004) did not occur in any subject exposed to the shocks. These results suggest that water intake was essential for the survival of the organism and the response to stress (intake reduction) did not matter.

REFERENCES

Adam, T. C. and Epel, S. E. (2007). Stress, eating and the reward system. *Physiology and Behavior, 91,* 449-458.

Baranowska, B., Baranowska-Bik, A., Bik, W., and Martynska, L. (2008). The role of leptin and orexins in the dysfunction of hypothalamo-pituitary-gonadal regulation and in the mechanism of hyperactivity inpatients with anorexia nervosa. *NeuroEndocrinology Letters, 29,* 37-40.

Berthoud, H. R. and Morrison, C. (2008). The brain, appetite, and obesity. *Annual Review of Psychology, 59, 55-92.*

Bodnar, R. J. and Klein, G. E. (2006). Endogenous opiates and behavior: 2005. *Peptides, 27,* 3391-3478.

Dallman, M.F. (2010). Stress-induced obesity and the emotional nervous system. *Trends in Endocrinology and Metabolism, 21,* 159-165.

Dess, N. K. (1991). Ingestion and emotional health. *Human Nature, 2,* 235-269.

Dess, N. K., Chapman, C. D., and Minor, T. R. (1988). Inescapable shock increases finickiness about drinking quinine-adulterated water in rats. *Learning and Motivation, 19,* 408-424.

Dess, N. K., Minor, T. R., and Brewer, J. (1989). Suppression of feeding and body weight by inescapable shock: Modulation by quinine adulteration, stress reinstatement, and controllability. *Physiology and Behavior, 45*, 975-983.

Fachin, A., Silva, R. K., Boschang, C. G., Pettenuzzo, L., Bertinetti, L., Billodre M. N., Peres, W., Busnello, F., and Dalmaz, C. (2008). Stress effects on rats chronically receiving a highly palatable diet are sex-specific. *Appetite, 51*(3), *592-598.*

González-Torres, M.L., López-Espinoza, A., and dos Santos, C.V. (2010) Efecto del tipo y controlabilidad del estrés sobre la conducta alimentaria en ratas. *Revista Mexicana de Análisis de la Conducta, 36,* 111-127.

Harris, R. B., Gu, H., Mitchell, T. D., Endale, L., Russo, M., and Ryan, D. H. (2004). Increased glucocorticoid response to a novel stress in rats that have been restrained. *Physiology and Behavior, 81,* 557-568.

Jackson, D. E. and Delprato, D. J. (1974). Aversive CSs supress lever pressing for food but not the eating of free food. *Learning and Motivation, 5*, 448-458.

Job, R. F. S. and Barnes, B. W. (1995). Stress and consumption: inescapable shock, neophobia, and quinine finickiness in rats. *Behavioral Neuroscience, 109*, 106-116.

López-Espinoza, A. and Martínez, H. (2001). Efectos de dos programas de privación alimentaria sobre el peso corporal de ratas Wistar. *Revista Mexicana de Análisis de la Conducta, 27*, 35-46.

López-Espinoza, A. and Martínez, H. (2004). Cambios en el patrón alimentario como efecto de la privación de agua o alimento en ratas en crecimiento. *International Journal of Psychology and Psychological Therapy, 4*, 93-104.

Ortolani, D., Oyama, L.M., Ferrari, E.M., Melo, L.L, and Spadari-Bratfisch, R.C. (2011). Effects of comfort food on food intake, anxiety-like behavior and the stress response in rats. *Physiology and Behavior 103,* 487-492.

Overmier, J. B. (2002). On learned helplessness. *Integrative Physiological and Behavioral Science, 37*, 4–8.

Seligman, M. E. P. and Maier, S. F. (1967). Failure to escape traumatic shock. *Journal of Experimental Psychology, 74,* 1-9.

Torres, S. J. and Nowson, C. A. (2007). Relationship between stress, eating behavior, and obesity. *Nutrition, 23,* 887-894.

Tsigos, C. and Chrousos, G. P. (2002). Hipotalamic-pituitary-adrenal axis, neuroendocrine factors and stress. *Journal of Psychosomatic Research, 53,* 865-871.

In: Recent Hispanic Psychological Research ... ISBN: 978-1-62948-919-3
Editors: C. H. Garcia Cadena, A. Lopez-Espinoza et al.

Chapter 3

RELATIONSHIP BETWEEN CB1 RECEPTORS IN THE NUCLEUS *ACCUMBENS* SHELL AND THE HEDONIC VALUE OF FOOD

***Felipe Cortés-Salazar*[1], *Juan Manuel Mancilla-Díaz*[1], *Verónica Elsa López-Alonso*[1], *Brenda González-Hernández*[2] and *Rodrigo Erick Escartín-Pérez*[1*]**

[1]Neurobiology of EatingLaboratory, Universidad Nacional Autónoma de México, FES Iztacala. Tlalnepantla, México, México

[2]Universidad Autónoma de Nuevo León, FCB, San Nicolás de los Garzas, Nuevo León, México

ABSTRACT

Obesity is a pathology often associated with the genesis of diseases such as hypertension, diabetes, heart problems, etc. Research in this field has focused on understanding the different factors that promote the beginning and maintenance of obesity, one of them are the hedonic properties of food. Thus, the aim of this research was to evaluate the effect of administration of the selective CB1 receptor agonist ACEA in the nucleus *accumbens* shell (NAcS) on palatable food intake in pre-satiated male wistar rats. During a 4-day period of habituation, the animals were deprived of food for 22 hours, and then they had access to the standard food (solid) during 1 hour, and finally they had access to the experimental food (sweetened condensed milk, 10% sucrose) for 1 hour. In the experimental sessions, the animals were injected with vehicle and 2 different doses of ACEA (0.25, 0.5 or 0.75 μg, multidose crossover design, where dose was determined by a Latin square with an inter-test interval of 2 days, each rat was registered in 3 independent experimental sessions) before having access to experimental food (rats were in the same feeding paradigm as in the habituation period). According to the obtained results, ACEA administration had a dose-dependent stimulatory effect of

*Address correspondence to: R. Erick Escartín-Pérez, Neurobiology of Eating Laboratory, UNAM FES Iztacala. 1 Av. de los Barrios, Los Reyes Iztacala, Tlalnepantla, México, 54090, México.E-mail address: escartin@ campus.iztacala.unam.mx.

palatable food ingestion. Our findings suggest that activation of CB1 receptors in the NAcS stimulate intake via increasing the hedonic properties of food.

Keywords: Palatability, Cannabinoids, *Accumbens*

Introduction

The endocannabinoid system plays an important role in energy homeostasis and food intake regulation (Di Marzo et al., 2001; Fride, 2005; Williams et al., 1998), and it is generally accepted that the hyperphagic effects of cannabinoid agonists are mediated by CB1 receptors (CB1R) (Williams and Kirkham, 1999). The CB1R are an integral component of energy balance at peripheral (Cota et al., 2003; Nakata and Yada, 2008) and central level (Gardner, 2005; Quarta et al., 2010). In the central nervous system (CNS), CB1R are widely expressed in areas related to the control of natural processes of appetite regulation, including the anterior cortex, several hypothalamic nuclei and the nucleus *accumbens* (Berry and Mechoulam, 2002; Herkenham et al., 1991; Pickel, Chan, Kash, Rodriguez and MacKie, 2004). Accordingly, it has been suggested that cannabinoids and endocannabinoids affect the feeding behavior modulating energy homeostasis and the reward system (Gardner, 2005; Quarta et al., 2010). Furthermore, recent evidence has demonstrated that CB1R in the CNS play a key role in the pathophysiological development of obesity, specifically when a high-energy diet is provided (usually a palatable diet), and according to these findings, clinical improvement produced by the antiobesity treatment with SR 141716 (Rimonabant, CB1R antagonist) may be initially explained by inhibition of food intake (a centrally mediated effect) and subsequently by increasing energy expenditure (a peripheral mediated effect) via sympathetic neurons (Quarta et al., 2010).

Obesity is often associated with the preference for palatable food, and the palatability itself may produce in some subjects over-consumption and weight gain. Particularly, the sensory characteristics of food (taste, smell, texture and appearance) may define its palatability (Kenny, 2011a). Most of the information related to the taste is integrated in the primary and secondary gustatory cortex, regions that are anatomically related to the nucleus *accumbens*, where consumption of both palatable food and drugs of abuse are regulated (Kenny, 2011b). Interestingly, anterior cortex expresses the CB1R's mRNA, specifically in regions that correspond to layers II, III and V, where perikarya of projection neurons are located, suggesting a presynaptic inhibition of glutamate release in the nucleus *accumbens* (Mailleux and Vanderhaeguen, 1992).

It has been proposed that dietary conditions (exposure to highly palatable diets with intermittent food restriction) may affect the expression pattern of CB1R in the medial region of the nucleus *accumbens* shell (NAcS), down-regulating the CB1R expression (Bello et al., 2011) as a probable consequence of higher endocannabinoid activity, since it has been shown that fasting increased levels of AEA (anandamide) and 2-AG (2-arachidonoylglycerol) in the limbic forebrain and, to a lesser extent, of 2-AG in the hypothalamus of rats (André and Gonthier, 2010). These findings support the hypothesis that cannabinoids and endocannabinoids in the NAcS may stimulate feeding by increasing the hedonically positive sensory properties of food.

In the present study, during a 4-day period rats were habituated to a food restriction program with limited access to a standard diet (pre-satiation phase) followed by exposure to a highly palatable food; this protocol causes an overeating pattern (re-exposure to food after 22 h of deprivation) that promotes satiety in a short period of time, and then the palatable food is offered and animals consume it by its palatability properties since they are in a pre-satiated state. Furthermore, the adaptation to the feeding paradigm was evaluated measuring (during 4 consecutive days) the food anticipatory activity, since it is well know that if animals are exposed to food for a limited period of time the meal is preceded by an increase in physical activity (Moran and Tamashiro, 2007).

It has been previously shown that activation of CB1R in the hypothalamus prevented the natural satiety sequence by modulating homeostatic mechanisms (Escartín-Pérez et al., 2009); however cannabinoids and endocannabinoids in the NAcS might also stimulate feeding by an independent (but not exclusive) mechanism, increasing the hedonically positive sensory properties of food. According to this rationale, the purpose of the present study was to evaluate the role of CB1R in the NAcS on the regulation of the hedonic value of food, by injecting to pre-satiated rats different doses of ACEA (CB1R agonist) before the exposure to a highly palatable food.

METHOD

Subjects

A total of 8 adult male Wistar rats (UNAM, FESI Mexico) weighting 220-240 g (9-10 weeks of age) at the beginning of testing were used. Rats were individually housed and kept in a temperature-controlled room at 21±1°C on a 12x12 h reversed light-dark cycle (lights on at 24.00 h) and had ad libitum access to food (standard rat chow) and water unless otherwise stated. All experimental procedures complied with the Official Mexican Norm (NOM-062-ZOO-1999), entitled Technical Specifications for the Production, Care, and Use of Laboratory Animals.

Diets

Standard laboratory chow: Harlan 2018S, fixed formula diet of 18% protein, 3.4% polyunsaturated fat, 1.3% monounsaturated fat, 0.9% saturated fat. The highly palatable food used was sweetened evaporated milk (Carnation®, 6% total fat, 3.75% saturated fat, 9.5% carbohydrates, 6% protein, blended with 10% sucrose).

Drugs

N-(2-Chloroethyl)-5Z,8Z,11Z,14Z-eicosatetraenamide (ACEA) was used (Tocris Bioscience). Since ACEA was supplied pre-dissolved in anhydrous ethanol, this solution was re-suspended in DMSO and ethanol was evaporated under a gentle stream of nitrogen, then the ethanol-free solution of ACEA was diluted in 0.9% saline solution. The final solution had

5% of DMSO and was injected in a volume of 0.5 μl at 0.2 μl/min. Fresh solution of drug was prepared on each test day.

Surgery

All animals were anaesthetized with ketamine and xylazine (112.5 mg/kg and 22.5 mg/kg I.P.) and were stereotaxically implanted with unilateral guide cannulaes for injection into the nucleus *accumbens* shell (coordinates AP + 1.52 mm and ML –0.7 mm relative to bregma, DV –6.0 mm relative to dura mater) according to Paxinos and Watson's Atlas (1998). Finally, animals were administered with benzathine penicillin (300,000 UI/kg, I.M.) in order to prevent infections and they had a surgical recovery period of 3 days with food (standard rat chow) and water ad libitum.

Feeding Paradigm

Rats were habituated (4 consecutive days) to a restricted feeding paradigm, with a period of 2 h of food access per day (standard diet 1 h, palatable diet 1 h) during the light phase of the light/dark cycle (always at the same time of the day). This procedure was performed in order to ensure that subjects were pre-satiated at the time of access to the palatable food, consuming it by its palatability properties. The adaptation to the feeding paradigm was evaluated measuring (during 4 days) the food anticipatory activity.

Behavioral Tests

During the habituation period (before experimental sessions, 4 consecutive days), activity was measured (s) 1 h before the time of food access considering different 3 mutually exclusive behavioral categories: activity (locomotion, non-ambulatory activity, and grooming), immobility, and sniffing. Standard food intake was measured (g) during a 60-min period (immediately after the activity registry); after standard food access, rats were provided with the experimental food, and its consumption was measured (ml) during a period of 1 hour. Both standard and experimental food intake as well as body weigth were measured during the complete habituation period (4 consecutive days). Baseline consumption of the experimental food was calculated by averaging the amount consumed each day during the habituation period. During the experimental sessions (post-habituation days), animals were injected intra-NAcS between the access to standard food and the exposure to the experimental food, and after 60 minutes, consumption of experimental food was assessed and compared to the baseline consumption; results are expressed in terms of percentage of change of baseline (baseline consumption of each animal was considered 100%). Rats remained all the time in their cages and measurements of the experimental food intake were always at the same time of the day (during the light phase of the light/dark cycle) and always after 1 hour of access to the standard diet (pre-satiated state).

Procedure

Following the habituation period, animals were randomly sorted into different conditions according to a multidose crossover design, where dose was determined by a Latin square with an inter-test interval of 2 days. Animals received intra-NAcS injections of vehicle (ACEA 0.0 µg) and 2 different doses of ACEA (0.25, 0.5 or 0.75 µg): each rat was injected in 3 independent sessions (one injection per session) with 2 days between injections. After experimental sessions, rats were sacrificed by a pentobarbital overdose, their brains were removed and subsequent histological verification of the injection site was performed. Data obtained from rats in which the cannulae were not placed correctly in the NAcS were excluded from the present report (Figure 1).

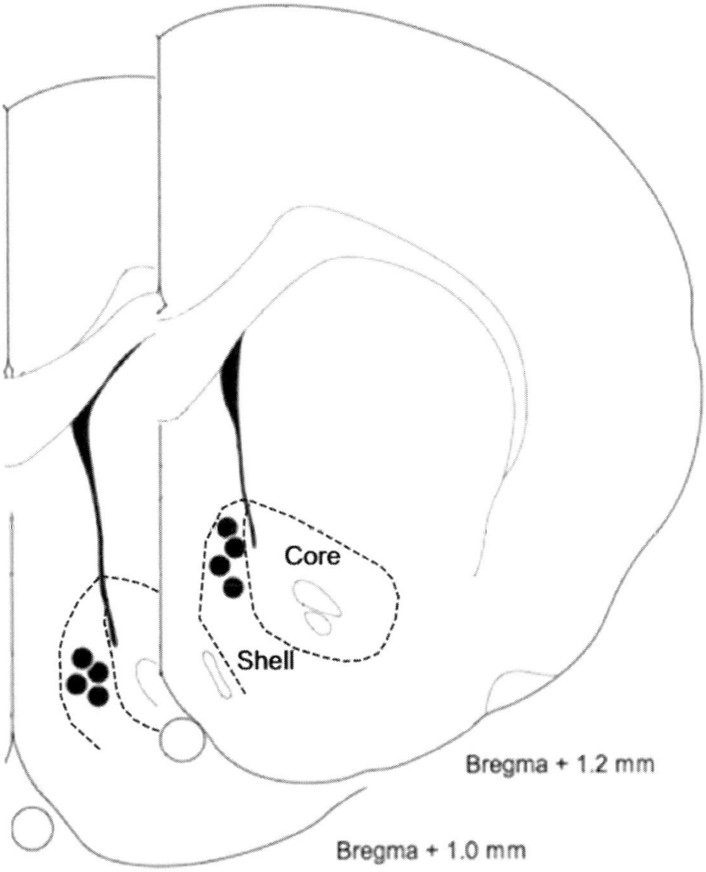

Figure 1. Schematic representation (black circles) of sites of injection in the nucleus *accumbens* shell. Anterior coordinates have been taken from the Atlas of Paxinos and Watson (1998).

Statistical Analysis

Data obtained in the habituation period was expressed in terms of means ± standard error of the mean (SEM) and was analyzed using repeated measures ANOVA (dose x time). The response to different doses of ACEA was expressed as percentage of change ± SEM, considering the average of palatable diet intake during the habituation period as the 100% (baseline consumption) and one-way ANOVA was used to evaluate the significance of differences; when appropriate, the Tukey's test was entered. The criterion for statistical significance was $p < .05$. Data were analyzed using GraphPad Prism Version 5.0.

RESULTS

Adaptation to the Feeding Paradigm

During the habituation period (4 consecutive days before experimental sessions), subjects increased their exploratory activity before they had access to the standard diet (food anticipatory activity), specifically sniffing increased significantly [$F_{(3,5)} = 6.54$; $p < .01$] and this behavioral measure remained steady through the days 3 and 4 (Figure 2 A). Immobility durations followed the opposite pattern, decreasing significantly [$F_{(3,5)} = 7.14$; $p < .01$] in the final 2 days of the habituation period (Figure 2 B). The behavioral category defined as activity (locomotion, non-ambulatory and grooming) did not changed significantly over time (data not showed).

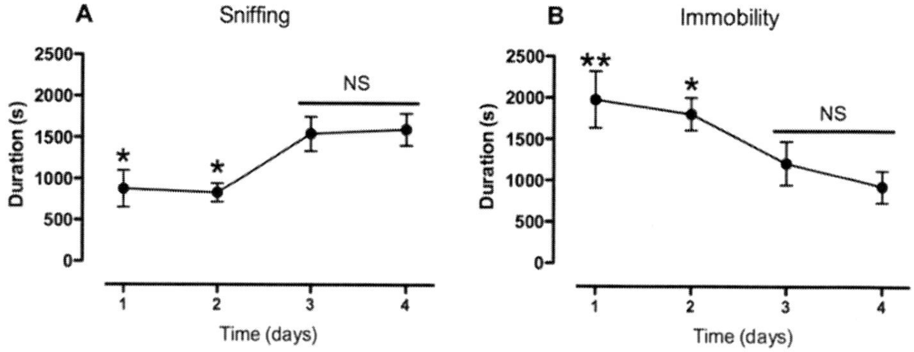

Figure 2. Food anticipatory activity measured in terms of means ± SEM of time (s) of immobility (A) and sniffing (B) during 1 hour before the access to the standard diet (4 days of habituation period). *$p < .05$; **$p < .01$; NS= Non significant.

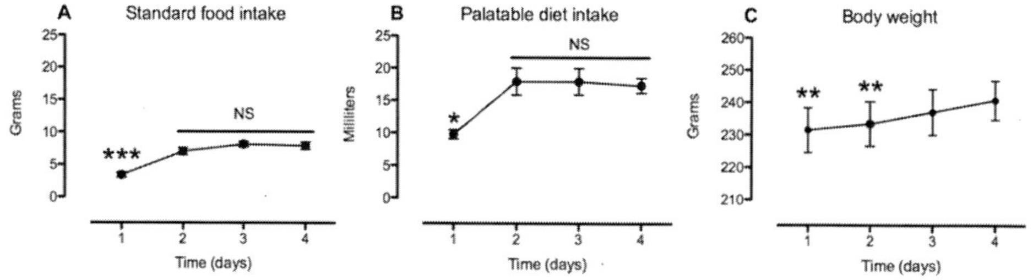

Figure 3. Adaptation to the feeding paradigm measured in terms of means ± SEM of the standard (A) and palatable (B) diets intake (g and ml respectively), and the body weight (g) during the habituation period (4 days). *$p < .05$; **$p < .01$; ***$p < .001$; NS= Non significant.

Standard food intake increased significantly [$F_{(3,7)} = 21.61$; $p < .001$] in the second day and remained steady to the end of the habituation period (Figure 3 A). Palatable food intake also increased in the second day [$F_{(3,7)} = 6.24$; $p < .001$] and remained high during the rest of the habituation (with no significant differences between days 2-4) (Figure 3 B); this period of steady intake of palatable food was averaged and was used as baseline consumption. Body weight was monitored to verify that the animals continued developing properly during the food-restricted paradigm (Figure 3 C).

Effects of Activation of CB1 Receptors in the NAcS on Palatable Food Intake

Figure 4 provides the mean percentage difference from baseline consumption of the palatable food intake of animals treated intra-NAcS with different doses of ACEA. The statistical analysis revealed that injections of ACEA in the nucleus accumbens leads to a dose-dependent increase the palatable food consumption [$F_{(3,24)} = 14.38$; $p < .001$].

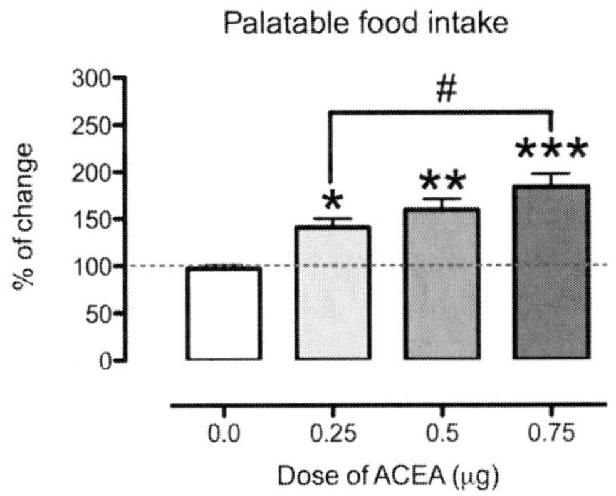

Figure 4. Effects of intra-NAcS injections of ACEA on palatable food intake expressed in terms of means ± SEM of the percentage of change on the average baseline consumption (expressed as the 100% in the vertical dotted line). *$p < .05$, **$p < .01$ and ***$p < .001$ vs dose of 0.0 μg of ACEA; #$p < .05$ dose of 0.25 vs 0.75 μg of ACEA; n= 6-8 per group.

DISCUSSION

The present study systematically evaluated the effects of intra-*accumbens* activation of CB1R on the hedonic value of food by injecting the CB1R agonist ACEA in the NAcS of pre-satiated rats exposed to a high palatable food in order to provide an insight into the mechanism underlying the cannabinoid-induced hyperphagia. Based on the well know phenomenon referred as food anticipatory activity (Moran and Tamashiro, 2007), we were able to design and test a protocol where specific changes in palatability-dependent consumption of food were evaluated; furthermore, rats in this study were appropriately adapted to the food-restricted paradigm since their patterns of food consumption (standard and palatable) were steady in a period of 3 days, and even when rats were food restricted, they continued gaining weight and the food anticipatory activity was observed. The fact that the animals were satiated before the access to the palatable diet ensured that they eat mainly because of the hedonic properties of food. While involvement of endogenous cannabinoid signaling in the nucleus *accumbens* has been previously reported (André and Gonthier, 2010; Bello et al., 2011), the finding that CB1 receptor activation in this nucleus induced hyperphagia is not fully understood. Previously published studies demonstrated an increase in food consumption as a result of intra-*accumbens* administration of anandamide or 2-AG (Kirkham, Williams, Fezza, and Di Marzo, 2002; Soria-Gómez et al., 2007); however, this results were observed with standard diets and using feeding protocols in which motivation to eat (homeostatic drive) can not be dissociated from the processing of positive sensory properties of food (hedonic properties). Consequently, the main finding of the present study was the cannabinoid-induced increase of palatable food intake in animals that were pre-satiated as a result of CB1R activation in the NAcS, effect that suggests that the cannabinoid-induced hyperphagia involves a strong hedonic component (Di Patrizio and Simansky, 2008). Additional work is needed to determine whether activation of CB1R stimulate food intake also by increasing the rewarding properties of food and not only by increasing its hedonically positive sensory properties. According to a recent review (Maccarrone et al., 2010), overactivity of the endocannabinoid system promotes an obese phenotype, and even before the onset of obesity endocannabinoid levels are increased, suggesting that this hyperactive neurotransmitter system could be a cause rather than a consequence of overweight. Indeed, complete deletion of CB1R (CB1R-KO mice) led to reduced body weight and resistance to develop obesity (Ravinet-Trillou, Delgorge, Menet, Arnone, and Soubrié, 2004), and also conditional deletion of CB1R in the forebrain (this animal model lacks CB1 protein in glutamatergic forebrain-projecting neurons and is referred as CaMK-CB1-KO) displayed a lean phenotype and resistance to diet-induced obesity (Quarta et al., 2010). Despite the fact that the clinical use of CB1R antagonist Rimonabant has been recently halted for the increased incidence of psychiatric side effects (Akbas, Gasteyger, Sjödin, Astrup and Larsen, 2009), the understanding of molecular, pharmacological and behavioral mechanisms related to the regulatory action of cannabinoids on feeding behavior might have an important impact on clinical practice. In conclusion, the present results provide experimental evidence that cannabinoids and endocannabinoids in the NAcS may stimulate feeding by increasing the hedonically positive sensory properties of food via CB1 receptors.

Acknowledgments

Funding for this study was provided by UNAM DGAPA grants IN224811-3, IN306711 and FESI PAPCA 53.

References

Akbas, F., Gasteyger, C., Sjödin, A., Astrup, A., and Larsen, T. M. (2009). A critical review of the cannabinoid receptor as a drug target for obesity management. *Obesity Reviews, 10*, 58–67.

André, A., and Gonthier, M. P. (2010). The endocannabinoid system: Its roles in energy balance and potential as a target for obesity treatment. *The International Journal of Biochemistry and Cell Biology, 42*(11), 1788–1801.

Bello, N. T., Coughlin, J. W., Redgrave, G. W., Ladenheim, E. E., Moran, T. H., and Guarda, A. S. (2011). Dietary conditions and highly palatable food access alter rat cannabinoid receptor expression and binding density. *Physiology and Behavior*, in press.

Berry, E. M., and Mechoulam, R. (2002). Tetrahydrocannabinol and endocannabinoids in feeding and appetite. *Pharmacology and Therapeutics, 95*, 185–190.

Cota, D., Marsicano, G., Tschöp, M., Grübler, Y., Flachskamm, C., Schubert, M., Auer, D., Yassouridis, A., Thöne-Reineke, C., Ortmann, S., Tomassoni, F., Cervino, C., Nisoli, E., Linthorst, A. C., Pasquali, R., Lutz, B., Stalla, G. K. andPagotto, U. (2003). The endogenouscannabinoid system affects energy balance via central orexigenic drive and peripherallipogenesis. *Journal of Clinical Investigation, 112*(3), 423–431.

Di Marzo, V., Goparaju, S. K., Wang, L., Liu, J., Batkai, S., Járai, Z., Fezza, F., Miura, G. I., Palmiter, R. D., Sugiura, T. and Kunos G. (2001). Leptin-regulated endocannabinoids are involved in maintaining food intake. *Nature, 410*(6830), 822–825.

Di Patrizio, N. V., andSimansky, K. J. (2008). Activating parabrachial cannabinoid CB1 receptors selectively stimulates feeding of palatable foods in rats. *Journal of Neuroscience, 28*(39), 9702–9709.

Escartín-Pérez, R. E., Cendejas-Trejo, N. M., Cruz-Martínez, A. M., González-Hernández, B., Mancilla-Díaz, J. M., and Florán-Garduño, B. (2009). Role of cannabinoid CB1 receptors on macronutrient selection and satiety in rats. *Physiology and Behavior, 96*, 646–650.

Fride, E. (2005). Endocannabinoids in the central nervous system: from neuronal networks to behavior. *Current Drug Targets - CNS and Neurological Disorders, 4*(6), 633–642.

Gardner, E. L. (2005). Endocannabinoid signaling system and brain reward: Emphasis on dopamine. *Pharmacology, Biochemistry and Behavior, 81*(2), 263–284.

Herkenham, M., Lynn, A. B., Johnson, M., Melvin, L., de Costa, B., and Rice, K. (1991). Characterization and localization of cannabinoid receptors in rat brain: A quantitative in vitro autoradiographic study. *The Journal of Neuroscience, 11*(2): 563–563.

Kenny, P. J. (2011a). Common cellular and molecular mechanisms in obesıty and drug addiction. *Nature Reviews Neuroscience, 12*(11), 638–651.

Kenny, P. J. (2011b). Reward mechanisms in obesity: new insights and future directions. *Neuron, 69*, 664–679.

Kirkham, T. C., Williams, C. M., Fezza, F., and Di Marzo, V. (2002). Endocannabinoid levels in rat limbic forebrain and hypothalamus in relation to fasting, feeding and satiation: stimulation of eating by 2-arachidonoyl glycerol. *British Journal of Pharmacology, 136*(4), 550–557.

Maccarrone, M., Gasperi, V., Catani, M. V., Diep, T. A., Dainese, E., Hansen, H. S., and Avigliano, L. (2010). The Endocannabinoid System and Its Relevance for Nutrition. *Annual Reviews of Nutrition, 30*, 423–440.

Mailleux, P., and Vanderhaechen, J. J. (1992). Distribution of neuronal cannabinoid receptor in the adult rat brain: a comparative receptor binding radioautography and in situ Hybridization histochemistry. *Neuroscience, 48*(3), 655–668.

Moran, T. H., and Tamashiro, K. L. K. (2007). Curt Richter: Spontaneous activity and food intake. *Appetite, 49*(2), 368–375.

Nakata, M., and Yada, T. (2008). Cannabinoids inhibit insulin secretion and cytosolic Ca 2+ oscillation in islet β-cells via CB1 receptors. *Regulatory Peptides, 145*, 49–53.

Paxinos, G. and Watson, Ch. (1998). *The brain in stereotaxic coordinates*. New York: Academic Press.

Pickel, V. M., Chan, J., Kash, T. L., Rodriguez, J. J., and MacKie, K. (2004). Compartment-specific localization of cannabinoid 1 (CB1) and mu-opioid receptors in rat nucleus *accumbens*. *Neuroscience 127*, 101–112.

Quarta, C., Bellocchio, L., Manzini, G., Mazza, R., Cervino, C., and Luzie, J. et al. (2010). CB1 Signaling in Forebrain and Sympathetic Neurons Is a Key Determinant of Endocannabinoid Actions on Energy Balance. *Cell Metabolism, 11*, 273–285.

Ravinet-Trillou, C., Delgorge, C., Menet, C., Arnone, M., and Soubrié, P. (2004). CB1 cannabinoid receptor knockout in mice leads to leanness, resistance to diet-induced obesity and enhanced leptin sensitivity. *International Journal of Obesity, 28*, 640–648.

Soria-Gómez, E., Matias, I., Rueda-Orozco, P. E., Cisneros, M., Petrosino, S., Navarro, L., Di Marzo, V.,and Prospéro-García, O. (2007). Pharmacological enhancement of the endocannabinoid system in the nucleus accumbens shell stimulates food intake and increases c-Fos expression in the hypothalamus. *British Journal of Pharmacology, 151*, 1109–1116.

Williams, C. M., and Kirkham, T. C. (1999). Anandamide induces overeating: mediation by central cannabinoid (CB1) receptors. *Psychopharmacology (Berl), 143*(3), 315–317.

Williams, C. M., Rogers, P. J., and Kirkham, T. C. (1998). Hyperphagia in pre-fed rats following oral delta9-THC. *Physiology and Behavior, 65*(2), 343–346.

In: Recent Hispanic Psychological Research ... ISBN: 978-1-62948-919-3
Editors: C. H. Garcia Cadena, A. Lopez-Espinoza et al.

Chapter 4

THE STUDY OF STIMULUS CONTROL OF FOOD INTAKE IN RATS: A REVIEW

*Varsovia Hernández**
Universidad Nacional Autónoma de México, Mexico

ABSTRACT

The purpose of this review was to describe the origin and development of the study of food-intake control in rats by exteroceptive stimuli. The strategy followed was to group the different studies according to similarities in their procedures, which arose mainly from a hypothetical-deductive line aimed to support or refute several motivational theories. First, studies in which the procedure consisted of pairing stimuli with a state of food-deprivation and that determined the effect of presenting these stimuli on eating are described. Subsequently, studies in which stimuli related to food were presented on subjects with or without food deprivation are described. It is concluded that the fundamental operation to control food intake by stimuli presentation is to pair them with food. It is also concluded that regardless of the origin of the different studies reviewed, they share the same operations of presenting food-access periods interpolated with periods without access to food and that they vary the moment of presentation of the stimuli. It is proposed that these variables can be used to integrate the results of different studies in the area.

Keywords: Stimulus control, exteroceptive stimuli, food-intake control, rats

INTRODUCTION

The variables that determine the beginning and the end of a food-intake period have been subject to debate for different researchers. Most of the formulations regarding food-intake control can be grouped under the depletion- repletion paradigm (Weingarten, 1985).

* Address for correspondence: Varsovia Hernández. School of Psychology, Universidad Nacional Autónoma de México. Laboratory of Operant Conditioning, Edificio C 2° Piso. Ave. Universidad 3004, Cd. Universitaria. México, D.F. C.P. 04510. Email: varsovia07@gmail.com.

According to this paradigm, when the storage of energy in the subject is under certain threshold, food-intake behavior begins and once the level of energy exceeds the upper threshold food-intake behavior ends. A corollary of the theories that follow that approach is that one way to ensure the occurrence of the beginning of a food-intake episode in an organism is through food deprivation. However, several studies found that the beginning of a food-intake episode and the amount of food eaten, besides being able to be controlled by food deprivation, can be controlled by antecedent stimuli presentation to a food access period. Despite that control of eating by stimulus presentation is an already established fact; there isn't a comprehensive review that clarifies the origin of this line of research.

The purpose of the present review is to describe the origin and development of the study of the control of the amount of food eaten and of the beginning of a food-intake episode by exteroceptive stimuli. The strategy followed in this review was to focus on the procedures used in different studies that evaluated control of food ingestion by stimuli presented before food accesses; these procedures in turn are consistent with the development of the study of this area. First, studies are discussed that attempt to condition food intake to the presentation of stimulus paired with periods without access to food. Second, studies that evaluated the effect of presenting stimulus paired with food on food intake in food-deprived subjects are described, and finally, I describe studies addressing the effect of presenting stimulus paired with food in subjects without food deprivation. Due to much of the stimulus control research on food intake has been done with rats, the review is restricted to research with this kind of subjects although it should be noted that applications of the findings of these studies are extended to other animals, including humans (cf., Herman and Polivy, 2008).

Effect of Presentation of Stimuli Paired with Periods without Food Access on Food Intake

The question regarding stimulus control on food intake has been present in psychology since the time of learning theorists (e.g., Hull, 1943; Anderson, 1941a), albeit indirectly. The first theoretical proposals and empirical studies on this topic focused on the possibility of conditioning hunger[1] and its behavioral effects (e.g. food intake) and are part of a more general topic of study on conditioned motivations.

Among the first antecedents in this area of study we can mention Hull (1943) with his principles regarding secondary motivations. As part of his system of behavior Hull postulated two kinds of drives: primary and secondary. The primary drives are related to inherent states of bodily needs (e. g. hunger, thirst, and sex); these drives cause activity and in turn are stimuli that elicit responses which may lead to reduce the state of necessity. The secondary drives refer to those that arise when a neutral stimulus repeatedly accompanied the evocation of a primary drive and a sharp decline in this. In this case, the previously neutral stimulus becomes a condition of drive in itself. For example, if a rat were exposed to a maze while food deprived, the condition of drive originated by the deprivation would condition to the stimuli of the maze (Bolles, 1967). Though Hull postulated the existence and the way a drive

[1] The use of the terms hunger, satiety and motivation in psychology has been debated by several authors, in this review to the extent possible, I tried such terms in the same sense as were used by the authors of the papers mentioned in the different sections.

is conditioned to environmental stimuli, apparently he didn't conduct studies to determine empirically his proposal. However, Hull (1951, cited in Cofer and Appley, 1964) cited the work of Anderson (1941a) to support his asseverations.

Anderson (1941a) proposed that there are internal and external components of motivation. An example of the internal components is the stomach contraction while external components refer to a situation or set of stimulus present at any given time. According to Anderson, if an internal stimulus such as stomach contractions (which produces a motivation) is removed when food is eaten and this happens repeatedly in a constant external situation, a motivation may be produced in the presence of the external situation even without internal stimulation. Because of this, it is said that the originally internalized motivation is now externalized. This theory is known as externalization of drive. Anderson conducted several studies to test some hypotheses derived from his theory (Anderson, 1941a, b, c). For example, in one study Anderson (1951c) placed food-deprived rats in a maze in which he gave them food when they reached the goal box. Subsequently he divided the rats in 4 different groups and he exposed them to a second maze. Two groups were exposed to the maze in conditions of food deprivation; one received food in the goal box and the other group didn't receive food. Two other groups run the maze without food deprivation, also one of them received food in the goal box and the other didn't receive food there. Anderson found that all the groups learned to navigate the maze, although the satiated groups had a higher number of mistakes compared to groups with food deprivation. According to Anderson, these results gave support to the externalization of drive theory.

Even though Anderson conducted several studies with results that support his theory, his experiments were subject to different critiques (Brown and Farber, 1968). Bolles (1967) mentioned some reasons to question Anderson´s results. First, the differences in the results between different experimental groups were not large so it is not known if they were statistically significant. Second, the subjects had different reinforcement histories so it is not clear if this history had any effect on the execution of the task. Finally, Bolles mentioned that in an attempt to replicate the results of Anderson, Siegel (1943) found negative results. Added to the criticism made by Bolles is the vagueness in the use of the concept of drive since in the externalization of drive theory it is treated as a variable that can depend of external an internal stimulation and also, occasionally plays the role of independent variable regulating the behavior of the subjects in the maze.

Is important to mention that the studies conducted by Anderson (1941a, b, c) do not explicitly address the topic of eating behavior, however these are the first studies in which the behavioral effects related to food-deprivation (among these food intake) tried to be controlled.

Parallel to the studies of Anderson are other series of experiments that also emerged in order to determine whether it was possible to condition motivational states like hunger to the presentation of stimuli paired with those states. Conditioning hunger states was important because "No purer realization of the latter concept [acquired motivation] seems possible than to show that, through appropriate conditioning techniques, hunger and thirst can be produced in an organism at will" (D´Amato, 1974, p. 84). These studies are known as conditioned drive studies and are the first that tried directly to control food intake through the presentation of stimuli. Within these studies, the experimental paradigm of conditioned hunger was the most widely used. In this paradigm two groups of subjects were food deprived, one for a short time and one for a long time and an external stimulus (frequently an experimental chamber) was paired with each level of deprivation. Later, the amount of food the groups consumed was measured in the presence of the stimulus under an intermediate level of deprivation. It was taken as evidence of conditioned hunger that the rats consumed more food in the presence of the stimulus previously paired with the strong drive than the other group of rats in the present of the stimulus paired with the weak drive.

A study that reported evidence for the conditioning of drives was that of Calvin, Bicknell and Sperling (1953a). These authors placed one group of rats in a particular box under 22 hours of food deprivation. Another group was placed in the box under one hour of food-deprivation. Later, for both groups food consumption was measured in the box under 11.5 hours of food-deprivation. It was found that the group placed previously in the box with the strong deprivation ate more food than the other group. However, several studies that sought to replicate this finding had negative results (see Cravens and Renner, 1970 as a review of this literature).

Some researchers suggested several reasons why in most studies about conditioned drive-states food intake could not be conditioned to exteroceptive stimuli paired with states of deprivation (e.g., Cravens and Renner, 1970). Among these they mention the slow establishment of the condition of hunger (Brown and Farber, 1968; Cravens and Renner, 1969; 1970) and the type of stimulus used (Mineka, 1975). Regarding the first criticism, it was mentioned that since the establishment of the condition of hunger is gradual and slow it would be difficult to condition it to the presentation of stimuli. However, D´Amato (1974) in a review of the literature of secondary motivations mentioned that even in studies that tried to condition the intake with insulin injections (which control that the subjects ingest food quickly after the injection), no data was found to support the idea that conditioned hunger could be established.

Concerning the type of stimulus used, the criticism was that it has been reported that conditioning is affected by the type of stimulus used (see Domjan, 2005). For example, in a conditioned aversion procedure establishing an aversion to a gustatory stimulus is faster than to an auditory or visual stimulus (García and Koelling, 1966). Since the studies of conditioned hunger used predominantly as stimulus characteristics of the experimental chambers, which may be assumed that are not ecologically relevant (Domjan, 2005), the lack of positive findings can be explained due to the type of stimuli used. However, Mineka (1975) conducted a study in which she used as stimuli different flavors paired with periods of deprivation and no conclusive results were obtained.

Because most of the results of studies evaluating food-intake control by presenting paired stimuli with periods of deprivation were negative, several authors concluded that either the phenomenon does not exist or its existence has yet to be established. (Bolles, 1967; Brown and Farber, 1968; Cofer and Appley, 1964; D´Amato, 1974). At present the questions regarding the existence of conditioned motivational states seem to have reemerged since Michael's (1982; 2007) ideas of unconditioned and conditioned motivational operations (see Tapper, 2005 in reference to this point); however by the time the existence of conditioned hunger seems to be purely theoretical.

It is important to note in the different studies described in this section, the vagueness of the term hunger. In the experimental analysis of behavior that concept is understood as an intervening variable that is used as a way to keep economy of expression in the relations between the variable that describes (see Díaz and Hernández, 2009).

In studies on conditioned motivation and conditioned hunger at times seems to be synonymous with the operation of deprivation and sometimes seems to be a hypothetical construct or source of behavior that can be conditioned in itself, which further hinders the interpretation of such investigations (see MacCorquodale and Meehl, 1948 for arguments regarding the use of intervening variables and hypothetical constructs in psychology).

EFFECT OF PRESENTATION OF STIMULI PAIRED WITH FOOD ON INTAKE IN FOOD-DEPRIVED SUBJECTS

Alternatively to studies on conditioned hunger, several studies that evaluated the effect of stimulus presentation paired with food on food intake were conducted. These studies came from different perspectives; for example, to determine the effects of presenting a conditioned reinforcer prior to access to food on food intake or to determine the energizing effect of conditioned incentive stimulus paired with food. Research emerging on these lines has proven to be fruitful giving rise to several experiments on stimulus control on food intake (cf. Weingarten, 1985), which are described below.

One of the first studies that evaluated the possibility to control food intake by stimuli paired with food was that of Calvin, Bicknell, and Sperling (1953b). These authors were interested in determining whether a conditioned reinforcer has the same effect on behavior than a primary reinforcer. Specifically, if the presentation of a conditioned reinforcer prior to a food-access period would reduce food intake in the same way that presenting food would do it. Three groups of rats were formed, the first was exposed to an experimental chamber and was given food there, the second was not exposed to the experimental chamber and the third group was exposed to the experimental chamber but no food was given in it. Subsequently, they measured the intake of all groups in the experimental chamber. Contrary to what the authors expected, the group that consumed a greater amount of food was the one that received food in the experimental chamber in the first phase. The authors concluded that the presentation of food-related stimulus had an energizing effect on food intake.

From the study of Calvin, et al. (1953b), Valle (1968) conducted another study to determine whether exposure to food-related stimulus has cumulative effects on food-intake. The procedure consisted of presenting food to rats for one hour in a white chamber and then transfer them to a black chamber. After exposing the subjects for 14 days to this procedure the researcher placed all subjects in the white chamber for 0, 15 or 60 minutes before put them into the black chamber with food available. He found that increasing the duration of exposure to the stimulus increased food intake, so he concluded that the effect of exposure to food-related stimulus is accumulated. In this study Valle also found that the handling of the rats by the experimenter can serve as a stimulus that controls food intake.

Apart from the studies of Calvin, Bicknell, and Sperling (1953b) and Valle (1968), there were other studies that evaluated the effect of presenting stimuli paired with food on food intake but they focused on determine if food related stimulus acquired properties of conditioned incentive (Lovibond, 1980) and if its presentation affected food-intake (Zamble, 1973).

Zamble's study (1973) was based on the results of other studies that found that presenting stimuli paired with food increases general activity in rats to wonder if this conditioned excitement affects food intake. In a first experiment Zamble formed two groups; both of them had 30 minutes of access to food every 24 hours on average. For one group there was a light presented 15 minutes before the access to food and for the other group the light was presented randomly. Zamble found that the group with stimulus presentations before the access to food ingested a greater amount of food compared to the group with the random stimulus. The second experiment was similar to the first but for the control group the stimulus was presented after the meal. Again, Zamble found that the group with the stimulus presented prior to food access consumed between 10 and 15% more food compared with the control group. The author concluded that the stimulus acquired excitatory properties on eating and increased food consumption compared to presentations of stimulus not paired with food.

It is noteworthy that in the study of Zamble there was no reference to the study of Calvin, Bicknell, and Sperling (1953b) or Valle's (1968), and even the author asserts that his study was the first to report increases in intake controlled by stimulus presentation paired with food. This shows that at this point the area seemed to be composed of isolated demonstrations of stimulus control of food-intake.

Another study that came to test the assumptions of different motivational theories (Bindra, 1968 and Konorsky, 1967) was that of Lovibond (1980). In this study he determined if stimuli with a long duration (five minutes) paired with food have effects on general activity, lever-pressing and the amount of food consumed in rats. In Experiment 1 he used as stimuli four different types of experimental chambers with different visual, olfactory and tactile properties. The subjects were placed in two chambers while food deprived and in other two while not food deprived. In each condition of deprivation Lovibond gave food to the rats between 30 and 300 seconds after placing the rats in one chamber but not in the other. In different phases he measured activity, lever-pressing and food consumption during the five minutes of presentation of the different stimulus. The rats were more active and pressed more the lever when they were in chambers related to food and while food deprived. The amount of food eaten was on average 11.5% more in food related chambers than in chambers nor related to food.

In the second experiment, Lovibond used a variant of Zamble's (1973) procedure. In the training phase, on different days, the subjects were presented with a five-minutes tone before access to food or with a flashing light that ocurred randomly during the day. Food access was every 24 hours on average. In the test phase on different days each stimulus was presented before the food or just the food without stimuli. The amount of food consumed after the presentation of food-related stimulus was 11% greater than the intake with the food without related stimulus and 13% above the level consumed without stimulus presentation. Lovibond considered that with long intervals between the stimuli and food delivery the stimuli elicit food-related behaviors, while stimuli with short intervals inhibit behaviors related to search for food and elicit consummatory responses; this is similar to that proposed by Konorsky (1967).

Other researchers suggested that even the time of day when a rat is fed can act as a stimulus that controls food intake (Valle, 1981; Weingarten, 1985). This idea came from some studies that found that when restricting the period of access to food and presenting the food at a specific time, the intake of the subjects increased progressively (e.g., Baker, 1955). Valle (1981) conducted a study to determine whether food intake is conditioned to temporary stimuli. One group of rats could eat for two hours every 22 hours. Other group of rats could eat for the same amount of time but at irregular intervals with an average of 22 hours. Valle found that rats with irregular intervals between foods ate less and had a lesser growing rate in comparison to rats with regular periods of access to food. Valle concluded that the temporal stimuli acquired motivational properties.

Valle's findings highlight the importance of taking into account the effect of temporary variables when conducting experiments on feeding behavior and, in general, experiments in which food is delivered to the subjects as a reinforcer of some behavior. It is possible that in an attempt to maintain constant the experimental conditions, such as time of day to perform the experimental sessions, the experimenter also introduce variables that may explain some of his results.

The studies reviewed in this section show without doubt that the presentation of stimulus paired with food before the period of access to it control increases in food intake compared to stimulus presentation in a retrograde or random manner with respect to food. The stimuli used were of various modalities, such as lights, sounds, experimental chambers and even the passage of time, which shows the ubiquity of stimulus control on food intake. With regard to the explanations given to this finding, they have been mixed but mainly focused on the role of stimuli as conditioned incentives. Regardless of the explanation given by the authors to their findings, the fact that antecedent stimuli presentations to a food-access period increases the amount of food intake had the implication of questioning which operations, besides food deprivation control this behavior.

Effect of Presentation of Stimuli Paired with Food on Intake in Subjects without Food Deprivation

Having demonstrated that stimuli paired with food controls food intake in subjects with food deprivation, the question of whether this control is maintained after removal of the state of deprivation appeared to be a logical consequence. The studies described below allude to the effect of presenting stimuli paired with food on non-deprived conditions. The importance of the studies that used this procedure is that clearly showed that food intake can be controlled not only by food deprivation (or the decline in the level of a substance in the body) but also by exteroceptive stimuli paired with food.

One of the first studies that reported control of food intake in non-deprived rats by stimulus presentation was that of Grant and Milgram (1973). In this study they first presented food on a distinctive environment to food-deprived rats. Subsequently, food deprivation was eliminated and the rats were placed in the same environment with the food that was presented before. Grant and Milgram found that exposing the rats to the distinctive environment controlled food intake even if they were not food deprived.

A subsequent study was conducted by Weingarten (1983). This author determined whether stimulus paired with food controls the occurrence of a period of access to food. In the first phase Weingarten presented a stimulus consisting of a tone and a light for 4.5 minutes before delivering food to the rats. In the middle of each interval between meals a second stimulus (an intermittently tone) was presented.

In the second phase, the access to food was unrestricted. Once a day, both stimuli were presented followed by a meal delivery. Weingarten found that in the second phase the average latency to start an eating episode after the stimulus presentation was the same as in the first phase and less than to presentations to the other stimulus. He also found that subjects spent more time at the trough during the presentation of the stimulus antecedent to the delivery of food compared to the time when the other stimulus was presented. The author concluded that in the presence of stimuli that signal food access the subjects can initiate an episode of intake and that a complete theory of the onset of eating should incorporate the concept of learned controls as a determinant of food intake.

In subsequent studies, Weingarten used the procedure described above but focusing on the control of behavior classified as appetitive and consummatory (Craig, 1918; Weingarten, 1990; Weingarten and Martin, 1989). The first classification refers to pre-intake behaviors which are measured by the time subjects introduce the head into the feeder before food delivery and the latency to consume it. The second classification refers to behaviors that end a behavioral sequence and are measured through the amount of food eaten. According to this author, conditioned food studies are ideal for studying appetitive and consummatory behaviors as "it reveals the entire repertoire of responses associated with the feeding bout" (Weingarten, 1990, p. 20).

Weingarten and Martin (1989) conducted a study that used the distinction between appetitive and consummatory behaviors. In the first experiment they used a conditioned aversion procedure and found that presenting a stimulus associated with aversive food reduced subject's intake but appetitive behaviors not differed compared with a control group. In the second experiment they found that using physiological procedures it is possible to control separately appetitive and consummatory behaviors. In the third experiment they found that food entering the stomach before presenting a stimulus paired with food decreased appetitive and consummatory behavior. The authors suggested that appetitive behavior is controlled by stimuli associated with food and these direct the subject to the first contact with food. Once the subject comes into contact with food, consumption depends on their properties.

From his studies and other evidence about stimulus control over eating Weingarten (1985) proposed a two-factor theory of hunger. According to this theory there are two controls of food intake, one related to physiological events that indicate a low energy level in some nutrient (depletion-induced hunger) and another that involves the relationships between stimulus and food (incentive-induced hunger). Both controls differ in their onset properties, depletion-induced hunger is slow to develop, while incentive-induced hunger tends to be rapid. Likewise, depletion-induced hunger is general in the type of food eaten, while incentive-induced hunger is specific to the food that was paired with the stimulus. Weingarten said that there may be interaction between the two types of controls, even though, he mentioned that more research was needed in this area.

More recent studies have shown that according to what was postulated by Weingarten (1985), the effect of the presentation of stimulus paired with food on intake in subjects without deprivation is specific to the type of food that is paired with the stimulus (Galarce, Crombag and Holland, 2007, Experiment 2; Petrovich, Ross, Gallagher and Holland, 2007). For example, Petrovich, Ross, Gallagher and Holland (2007) conducted a study that determined if the experimental chamber can act as a stimulus that controls food-intake in subjects without food-deprivation and if the effect of stimulus presentation on intake is specific to the type of food that is paired with the stimulus. In the first phase of training they formed two groups of subjects, both deprived of food. One group was exposed to an experimental chamber with food inside while the other group was exposed to the same chamber but without delivery of food. After exposure to the experimental chamber both groups were taken to the home cages where they were given a different type of food. In the test phase food deprivation was removed for both groups and they were introduced to the experimental chamber which contained food. The food could be of the same type used in the training phase or the type used in the home cages. It was found that the group who had food present in the experimental chamber in the first phase consumed a greater amount of it compared to the other group, but only when food was of the same type that was delivered in the training phase in the experimental chamber. The authors concluded that the contextual stimulus served as conditioned stimulus that promotes eating and that this stimulation is specific to the food that was presented as unconditioned stimulus.

The procedure of Weingarten (1983) has also been used by researchers looking for the forebrain circuit that controls food intake through stimuli paired with food in non-deprived subjects (Holland and Petrovich, 2005; Petrovich, 2011; Petrovich and Gallagher, 2007). According to what was proposed by these authors, the lateral hypothalamus is the place to integrate internal physiological signals and external signals which control food-intake (Petrovich, 2011). Several studies determined the effect of lesioning certain regions of the basolateral amygdala (Holland, Petrovich and Gallagher, 2002), or other areas that connect the lateral hypothalamus with the basolateral amygdala (Petrovich, Ross and Holland, 2007), on food-intake in rats when presented with stimuli paired with food. Some researchers have concluded that the lateral hypothalamus communication with the basolateral amygdala is necessary for the occurrence of stimulus-controlled eating without food deprivation (Petrovich, 2011; Petrovich, Setlow, Holland and Gallagher, 2002).

In summary, the studies described in this section showed that control of stimulus paired with food on eating is maintained even when food-deprivation is remove and that this control is specific to the type of food that was paired with the stimulus. In addition, added the description of antecedent food-intake behaviors as entrances to the feeder and time on it. With respect to these behaviors, it was shown that using different procedures it is possible to control differentially appetitive and consummatory behaviors. Finally, one point to note is that now a prevailing trend in this area of study seems to be to find out the neural basis of this phenomenon.

Discussion

A brief review of the origin and development of the study of stimulus control of eating was made throughout this paper. The strategy followed was to describe the origin of this area based on the procedures used. I described some studies in which it was determined the effect of presenting stimuli previously paired with periods of food deprivation, of presenting stimuli paired with food on food-deprived subjects and finally, to present stimuli paired with food on subjects without food deprivation. Even though the review focused on the procedures used in different experiments, the way in which they were conducted corresponds to the different questions that the researchers sought to answer in each. As to the first set of studies and procedures, the underlying question was if it was possible to condition eating to stimuli paired with a motivational sate (hunger). In the studies in which the stimulus was paired with food, the question was if eating could be controlled by conditioned stimuli and also about the excitatory effect of stimuli paired with food.

In general, the vast majority of studies emerged from a hypothetical-deductive line designed to support or refute different theories of learning and motivation in force at the time. However, despite the differences in the origins of each study is possible to see that they all shared essentially the same operations: interpolated periods of access to food with periods without access. The main difference between the groups of studies described in the different sections in this review lay in the location where the stimulus was presented, either in periods of access or no access to food. In previous reviews of the literature on eating behavior has been mentioned that it is possible to integrate the findings of different studies based on the variables intervals between access and access to food (Bruner, 2010; Díaz-Reséndiz, Franco-Paredes, Martínez-Moreno, López-Espinoza and Aguilera-Cervantes, 2009). This tactic seems to be equally useful to integrate the various studies reviewed in this paper regardless of their origin in some particular theory. Following this approach, in further studies will be interesting to explore the manner in which food-intake can be controlled by the duration of periods of access and no access to food in combination with the presentation of stimuli paired with food (e.g., Hernández and Bruner, 2011). This is reminiscent of the proposed by Weingarten (1985) to study how stimulus presentation interacts with food-deprivation.

While this review was focused on the stimulus control on food- intake in rats, there are several studies that demonstrate that humans are sensitive to the same principles (Birch, McPhee and Johnson, 1988; Cornel, Rodin and Weingarten, 1989). In humans there is a wide line of research in this area, starting with the studies of Schachter (1968; 1971) about the influence of various types of stimuli on intake in obese and normal weight people, which has been of great influence in the area (e.g. Herman and Polivy, 2008; Polivy, Herman and Coelho, 2008). Due to the fact that humans are exposed daily to different food-related stimuli a deeper understanding of how stimulus control their intake is essential and can be beneficial, especially to people with eating disorders.

References

Anderson, E. E. (1941a). Externalization of drive: I. Theoretical considerations. *Psychological Review*, 48, 204-224.

Anderson, E. E. (1941b). The externalization of drive: II. The effect of satiation and removal of reward at different stages in the learning process of the rat. *The Journal of Genetic Psychology*, 59, 359-376.

Anderson, E. E. (1941c). The externalization of drive: III. Maze learning by non-rewarded and by satiated rats. *The Journal of Genetic Psychology*, 59, 397-426.

Baker, R. (1955). The effects of repeated deprivation experience on feeding behavior. *Journal of Comparative and Physiological Psychology*, 48, 37-42.

Bindra, D. (1968). Neuropsychological interpretation of the effects of drive and incentive-motivation on general activity and instrumental behavior. *Psychological Review*, 75, 1-22.

Birch, L. McPhee, L. and Johnson, S. (1988). Conditioned meal initiation in young children. *Appetite*, 13, 105-113.

Bolles, R. (1967). *Theory of motivation*. New York: Harper and Row.

Brown, J. and Farber, I. (1968). Secondary motivational systems. *Annual Review of Psychology*, 19, 99-134.

Bruner, C. A. (2010). Conducta de comer: variables comunes a través del condicionamiento y la motivación. *Revista Mexicana de Análisis de la Conducta*, 36(2), 1-11.

Calvin, J. S., Bicknell, E. A., and Sperling, D. S. (1953a). Establishment of a conditioned drive based on the hunger drive. *Journal of Comparative and Physiological Psychology*, 46, 173-175.

Calvin, J. S., Bicknell, E. A., and Sperling, D. S. (1953b). Effect of a secondary reinforcer on consummatory behavior. *Journal of Comparative and Physiological Psychology*, 46, 176-179.

Cofer, C. N. and Appley, M. H. (1964). *Motivation: Theory and research*. New York: Wiley.

Cornell, C. Rodin, J. and Weingarten, H. (1989). Stimulus-Induced eating when satiated. *Physiology and Behavior*, 45, 695-704.

Craig, W. (1918). Appetites and aversions as constituents of instincts. *Biological Bulletin*, 34, 91-107.

Cravens, R., and Renner, K. E.(1970). Conditioned appetitive drive states: Empirical evidence and theoretical status. *Psychological Bulletin*,73, 212- 220.

Cravens, R. and Renner, K.E. (1969). Conditioned hunger. *Journal of Experimental Psychology*, 2, 312-316.

D'Amato, M. (1974). Derived Motives. *Annual Review of Psychology*, 25, 83-106.

Díaz, F. and Hernández, V. (2009). Análisis de la conducta y teoría de la motivación: el caso de la conducta alimentaria. In A. López Espinoza and K. Franco Paredes (Eds.), *Comportamiento alimentario: una perspectiva multidisciplinar* (pp.123-137). Guadalajara, Jal.: Editorial Universitaria.

Díaz-Reséndiz, F., Franco-Paredes, K., Martínez-Moreno, A., López-Espinoza, A. and Aguilera-Cervantes, V., (2009). La ingesta de alimento en ratas: Una revision histórico-conceptual. *Universitas Psychologica*, 8, 519-532.

Domjan, M. (2005). Pavlovian conditioning: A functional perspective. *Annual Review of Psychology*, 56, 179-206.

Galarce, E. M., Crombag, H. S. and Holland, P. C. (2007). Reinforcer-specificity of appetitive and consummatory behavior of rats after Pavlovian conditioning with food reinforcers. *Physiology and Behavior*, 91, 95-105.

García, J. and Koelling, R. A. (1966). Relation of cue consequence in avoidance learning. *Psychonomic Science*, 4, 123-124.

Grant, D. and Milgram, N. (1973). Plasticity of normal feeding: Situational and individual factors. *Canadian Journal of Psychology*, 27, 305-316.

Hernández, V. and Bruner, C. A. (2011). El consumo de comida en ratas controlado por un estímulo neutral. Manuscript submitted for publication.

Herman, C. and Polivy, J. (2008). External cues in the control of food intake in humans: The sensory-normative distinction. *Physiology and Behavior*, 94, 722-728.

Holland, P. C. and Petrovich, G. D. (2005). A neural systems analysis of the potentiation of feeding by conditioned stimuli. *Physiology and Behavior*, 86, 747 -761.

Holland, P. C., Petrovich, G. D., and Gallagher, M. (2002). The effects of amygdala lesions on conditioned stimulus-potentiated eating in rats. *Physiology and Behavior*, 76, 117-129.

Hull, C. (1943). *Principles of behavior. An introduction to behavior Theory*. New York: Appleton Century Company.

Konorski, J. (1967). Integrative activity of the brain. An interdisciplinary approach. Chicago, Ill.: The University of Chicago Press.

Lovibond, P. F. (1980). Effects of long- and variable-duration signals for food on activity, instrumental responding and eating. *Learning and Motivation*, 11, 164-184.

MacCorquodale, K. and Meehl, P. (1948). On a distinction between hypothetical constructs and intervening variables. *Psychological Review*, 55, 95-107

Mineka, S. (1975). Some new perspectives on conditioned hunger. Journal of Experimental psychology: *Animal Behavior Processes*, 104, 134-148.

Michael, J. (1982). Distinguishing between discriminative and motivational functions of stimuli. *Journal of the Experimental Analysis of Behavior*, 37, 149–155.

Michael, J. (2007). Motivating Operations. In J. O. Cooper, T. E. Heron, and W. L. Heward (Eds.), *Applied behavior analysis* (pp. 374-391). Upper Saddle River, NJ: Prentice Hall/Merrill.

Petrovich, G. D., and Gallagher, M. (2007). Control of food consumption by learned cues: A forebrain-hypothalamic network. *Physiology and Behavior*, 91, 397-403.

Petrovich, G. D. (2011). Forebrain circuits and control of feeding by learned cues. *Neurobiology of Learning and Memory*, 95, 152-158.

Petrovich, G. D., Ross, C. A., Gallagher, M., and Holland, P. (2007). Learned contextual cue potentiates eating in rats. *Physiology and Behavior*, 90, 362-367.

Petrovich, D., Setlow, B., Holland, P. and Gallagher, M. (2002). Amygdalo-Hypothalamic circuit allows learned cues to override satiety and promote eating. *The Journal of Neuroscience*, 22(19), 8748-8753.

Polivy, J., Herman, C. P. and Coelho, J. S. (2008). Caloric restriction in the presence of attractive food cues: external cues, eating, and weight. *Physiology and Behavior*, 94, 729-733.

Siegel, P. (1943). Drive shift, a conceptual and experimental analysis. *Journal of Comparative Psychology*, 35, 139-148.

Schachter, S. (1968). Obesity and Eating. *Science*, 161, 751-756.

Schachter, S. (1971). Some extraordinary facts about obese humans and rats. *American Psychologist*, 26, 129-144.

Tapper, K. (2005). Motivating operations in appetite research. *Appetite*, 45, 95-107.

Valle, F. (1968). Effect of exposure to feeding-related stimuli on food consumption in rats. *Journal of Comparative and Physiological Psychology*, 66, 773-776.

Weingarten, H. P. (1985). Stimulus control of eating. Implications for a two-factor theory of hunger. *Appetite*, 6, 387-401.

Weingarten, H. P. (1983). Conditioned cues elicit feeding in sated rats: A role for learning in meal initiation. *Science*, 220, 431-433.

Weingarten, H. P. and Martin G. M. (1989). Mechanisms of conditioned meal initiation. *Physiology and Behavior*, 45, 735-740.

Weingarten, H. P. (1990). Learning, Homeostasis and the control of feeding behavior. In E. Capaldi (Ed.), *Taste, experience and feeding* (pp. 14-27). Washington, D.C: American Psychological Association.

Zamble, E. (1973). Augmentation of eating following a signal for feeding in rats. *Learning and Motivation*, 4, 138-147.

In: Recent Hispanic Psychological Research ... ISBN: 978-1-62948-919-3
Editors: C. H. Garcia Cadena, A. Lopez-Espinoza et al.

Chapter 5

ROLE OF MONOSODIUM GLUTAMATE IN THE DEVELOPMENT OF MURINE OBESITY MODELS

Mónica Navarro-Meza[*1] *and Omar Arroyo-Helguera*[2]
[1]Laboratory of Molecular Biology and Immunology, South University Center. Universidad de Guadalajara. Avenida Colón S/N. Ciudad Guzmán, Jalisco, México
[2]Institute of Public Health, Universidad Veracruzana, Avenida Luís Castelazo Ayala S/N, Col. Industrial Animas, Xalapa, Veracruz, México

ABSTRACT

Obesity is a public health problem associated with chronic degenerative diseases. In order to study this pathology, several murine models have been development based on high-calorie diet, neuroendocrine and genetic changes or brain lesions. The objective is to offer proposals for treatment and prevention for this disease. We describe the role of monosodium glutamate in the development of murine obesity models. This model has been related to neuronal death of hypothalamus arcuate nucleus, structure that regulates hormonal signals as insulin and leptin which are involved in food intake.

Keywords: Obesity model, monosodium glutamate

INTRODUCTION

The prevalence of obesity is increasing, in 2010, 43 million children under five years old presented overweight and obesity (De-Onis, Blossner, and Borghi, 2010), so that, is necessary to understand this for control and treatment. Epidemiological data indicate that formerly

* Address for correspondence: PhD. Mónica Navarro Meza. Laboratory of Molecular Biology and Immunology. South University Center. Universidad de Guadalajara. Avenida Colón S/N. Ciudad Guzmán, Jalisco, México. 49000. Tel: +52 341 41 575 22 22 ext 46134. Fax: +52 341 41 575 22 22. e-mail: monica.navarro@cusur.udg.mx.

obesity dominated in cities with a high socio-economic level, however, now also occurs in cities with low and medium socio-economic and environment levels, particularly in urban areas, World Health Organization (Ogden, Yanovski, Carroll, and Flegal, 2007; WHO, 2011; Finucane, et al., 2011). On the other hand, has be reported that overweight and obesity causes are due and imbalance between the consumer and the caloric expenditure, so it is suggested that physical exercise in combination with dietary restriction could be decline this alteration. Every year, over 2, 8 millions of adults died due to overweight or obesity: 44% because of diabetes, 23% of ischemic heart disease and between 7% and 41% of some cancers are associated with overweight and obesity (WHO, 2011; Yanovski, S., Z., and Yanovski, J., A., 2011). Epidemiological data indicate that the previously dominant obesity in high socioeconomic status, but now also comes in low and middle levels, particularly in urban areas (WHO, 2011). In order to understand the obesity pathophysiologies have been development experimental murine models based on high-calorie diet, neuroendocrine and genetic changes or brain lesions (Diemen, Trindade, and Trindade, 2006). A model of obesity that is often used in the laboratory is one that involves the administration of monosodium glutamate (MSG) during the neonatal period (Bunyan, Murrell, and Shah, 1976; Dolnikoff, Martin-Hidalgo, Machado, Lima, and Herrera, 2001). In the present review will address a description of the model on the administration of MSG in the development of obesity, describes the effects of MSG model in relate of the arcuate nucleus and ventromedial nucleus in adult organism complications, as well as advantages and disadvantages in this model.

Glutamate Is Synthesized through of Metabolic Pathways from Glucose

In nature, Glu is a non-essential amino acid that it is synthesized through several metabolic pathways from glucose, and then is stored in vesicles (Watkins, and Jane, 2006; Nedergaard, Takano, and Hansen, 2002). The Glu is released in the synaptic space as a result of membrane depolarization by Ca^{2+} mechanisms, after is subsequently recaptured in the synaptic cleft by a Na^{+} gradient dependent on neurotransmitter transporters located in the membrane, either neurons or glial cells (Hertz, Dringen, Schousboe, and Robinson, 1999; Hertz, Yu, Kala, and Schousboe, 2000; Fonseca, Monteiro, Alves, Carrondo, and Santos, 2005; Albrecht, Sonnewald, Waagepetersen, and Schousboe, 2011). In glial cells, the Glu is converted to glutamine by glutamine synthetase enzyme activity and released through Ca^{2+} pumps and Na^{+}/Ca^{2+} exchangers, and then is recaptured by neurons where it becomes again Glu by mitochondrial glutaminasa (Hertz, et al., 1999; Albrecht, et al., 2011). The Glu is considered the primary central nervous system (CNS) neurotrasmisor; its excitatory effects depend on its interaction with two types of postsynaptic receptors: the metabotropic (R-Glu_m) and ionotropic (R-Glu_i) (Nedergaard, et al., 2002; Kew, and Kemp, 2005). The R-Glu_m is activated by G proteins and promote the synthesis of second messengers. In the nervous system (NS) have been described eight subtypes of R-Glu_m 1-8 and are classified into three classes based on the homology of the amino acid sequence, agonists or antagonists affinity and by signal transduction pathways that regulate (Michaelis, 1998; Kew, and Kemp, 2005). R-Glu_i are integral membrane proteins that consist of 4 or 5 subunits constituted by about 900 amino acids and 3 known as transmembrane domains: M1, M3 and M4, and M2 which does not cross completely the membrane (Rosenmund, Stern-Bach, and Stevens, 1998). During embryonic development, the Glu modulates processes such as the synaptogenesis, growth and neuronal proliferation, in the adult participates in synaptic plasticity, posttetanic long-term potentiation (LTP), and in learning and memory (Nedergaard, et al., 2002). On the other hand, R-Glu over activation causes neuronal death through the process known as excitotoxicity in the CNS (Ankarcrona, et al., 1995; Olney, 2002; Lau, and Tymianski, 2010, which is considered a pathological cellular event characterized by intracellular Ca^{2+} accumulation, with the consequent activation of cellular damage processes (Choi, 1992; Choi, 1988; Olney, 2002). The Glu in the cells (cytosol) is at millimolar concentrations and has been reported to have important effects on taste perception, as intermediary metabolism and neurotransmission stimulant (Nedergaard, et al., 2002). In taste, Glu has an addictive effect and recent studies suggest the existence of Glu sensors, as wells as signal transduction pathways in the intestinal mucosa and in cavity molecules mouth (Kitamura, Tsurugizawa, and Torii, 2011). In addition, several studies have shown that the major fuels for the small intestinal mucosa are amino acids, as wells as essential biosynthetic precursors by intestinal lactaldehyde, nitric oxide, polyamines, and nucleotide as purine, pyrimidine and amino acids, necessary for the maintenance of the intestinal mucosa integrity and mass (Uematsu, Tsurugizawa, Kondoh, and Torii, 2009; Uematsu, Tsurugizawa, Uneyama, and Torii, 2010; Kitamura, et al., 2011). The Glu treatment induced neuronal death of hypothalamus arcuate nucleus in brain this structure regulates hormonal signals as insulin and leptin which are involved in food intake, causing a deficient control between measurement and energy spending (Dube, Xu, Kalra, Sninsky and Kalra, 1999; Schwartz, Woods, Porte, Seeley, and Baskin, 2000).

Glutamate in Peripheral Tissues

Food intake induces the activation of physiological responses that provide neural signals, endocrine, regulating digestion, absorption and assimilation of ingested nutrients (Uematsu, et al., 2010). The Glu is an amino acid in natural protein foods including meat, fish and milk (Giacometti, 1979; Young, and Ajami, 2000). The Glu is found in the blood and other fluids at micromolar level is also present in organs like the intestines, lungs, muscles and liver and has been reported that these organs express the Glu transport systems (Bertrand, Gross, Puech, Loubatieres-Mariani, and Bockaert, 1992; Young, and Ajami 2000; Gill, and Pulido, 2001). Experimental reports indicate that Glu receptors are expressed in testes, ovaries, kidneys, bone, spleen, pancreas cells, intestine, esophagus and liver cells (Gill, and Pulido, 2001). The Glu accumulates in secretory granules of α-pancreatic cells because of the vesicular Glu transporters. Additionally, Glu can activate the autocrine signaling pathways in these cells. Pancreatic β-cells have been observed in the R-AMPA, which are comparable to neuronal cells (Bertrand, et al., 1992). The Glu is present in the cells (cytosol) at millimolar and it has been reported that its role in taste perception, intermediary metabolism and neurotransmission stimulating is important (Kitamura, et al., 2011). The Glu has an addictive effect, and recent studies suggest the presence of Glu sensors and transduction molecules in intestinal mucosa and in the oral cavity (Niijima, 2000). The vagus nerve afferents respond to Glu in the stomach and regulate autonomic reflexes (Niijima, 1991).

MONOSODIUM GLUTAMATE (MSG)

The MSG is the sodium salt of Glu (Glu, water and sodium), the Glu was first isolated from plants and was found to be an essential component to enhance the flavor, nowadays, MSG is produced by a natural fermentation process, Institute of Food Technology (IFT). There is research to indicate that the taste of MSG is a good and there is a specific receptor Glu taste on the tongue. The GMS increased food consumption, so it is proposed that is an important ingredient in the alterations of eating behavior (Ninomiya, 2001). The body has the ability to metabolize MSG added in the same manner in metabolizing Glu found naturally in some foods (Beyreuther et al., 2007). Neonatal of MSG induces obesity (Olney, 1969; Bunyan, et al., 1976), it has been shown that administration of 4 mg/g (2 to 8 days postnatal) in rodents (4-10 doses) induces obesity in adulthood, it has been linked to damage to the hypothalamic nuclei (ventromedial and arcuate), which alters the intake, absorption and energy expenditure (Macho, Fickova, Jezova, and Zorad, 2000; Kanarek, Meyers, Meade, and Mayer, 1979; Beyreuther, et al., 2007 The administration of GMS as a single dose causes inhibition of dopamine in the hypothalamus (Lorden, and Caudle, 1996). In contrast, it has been reported in adult rats when administered various doses (4-10) of MSG, there is an increase in leptin levels, this results in loss of inhibitory effect exerted by leptin on the adrenal gland, and induces the release of glucocorticoids (Lorden, and Caudle, 1986; Tokuyama, and Himms-Hagen, 1989; Lorden, and Caudle, 1996; Perello, Gaillard, Chisari, and Spinedi, 2003). The participation of the adrenal gland in the induction of obesity is part of the changes in the hypothalamic-pituitary-adrenal axis that mediates neuroendocrine response in situations of imbalance, which is associated with increased synthesis of the hormone corticotropin releasing (CRH) in the nucleus of the hypothalamus pareventricular (Martins, et al., 2004; Meister, et al., 1989). The activation of neurons that synthesize and release CRH is modulated by neurotransmitters and neuropeptides, including NPY (neuropeptide Y) from the arcuate nucleus of hypothalamus (Lorden, and Caudle, 1986; Abe, Saito, and Shimazu, 1990). The release of glucocorticoids results in a negative feedback mechanism on neuronal activity in the synthesis of CRH, when binding to CRH-R1 receptors produces adenocorticotropina hormone secretion (ACTH) which leads to the release of glucocorticoids by the adrenal glands (Lorden, and Caudle, 1996; Guimaraes, et al., 2002). Glucocorticoids lead to increase hepatic gluconeogenesis, so that the response to hormones such as glucagon and catecholamines, have also been associated with increased lipolysis in adipocytes and therefore fat distribution (Martins, et al., 2004). It has also been reported that the increase in food intake induced metabolic disorders associated with oxidative stress is related with the increased levels of glucose, insulin, triglycerides and leptin (Heiman, et al., 1997; Dawson, Pelleymounter, Millard, Liu, and Eppler, 1997; De-Mello, et al. 2001; De-Souza, Nunes, Gobatto, and De-Mello, 2003; Della-Fera, Qian, and Baile, 2001)

INJURIES IN THE VENTROMEDIAL NUCLEUS AND THE HYPOTHALAMIC ARCUATE

In the CNS there are found nuclei that are needed to regulate the food intake through regulating signs in the digestive system (Dube, et al., 1999; Elefteriou, Takeda, Liu,

Armstrong, and Karsenty, 2003; Balbo, Grassiolli, and Ribeiro, 2007). The hypothalamus develops signals of satiety which contains multiple neural systems that contribute to the regulation of homeostasis energy balance (Miskowiak, and Partyka, 1993; Kalra, et al., 1999; Schwartz, Woods, Porte, Seeley, and Baskin, 2000).

Arcuate Nucleus

It is one of the hypothalamic nuclei that are associated with the integrative function of energy balance, this nucleus contains neurons that control the appetite (Schwartz et al., 2000; Dawson, et al., 1997). It has been reported that this nucleus has a weak blood-brain barrier and has direct communication with peripheral signals (Dawson, Pelleymounter, Millard, Liu, and Eppler, 1997). Among the chemicals that regulate the food that is eaten are the NPY, melanocyte stimulating hormone, γ-amino acid butyric acid (GABA) and Glu. NPY is produced mainly in the arcuate nucleus. It regulates appetite through two receptor subtypes, the Y1 and Y5, widely distributed in the hypothalamus (Schwartz, Baskin, Kaiyala, and Woods, 1999; Schwartz, et al., 2000). Another of the substances produced in this core is galanin and it has been reported that their receptors are distributed in the hypothalamus (Leibowitz., and Hoebel, 1998). Arcuate nucleus neurons contain receptors for glucocorticoids that regulate the increase in food intake and body weight (Schwartz, et al., 2000; Dawson, et al., 1997). In addition, there are leptin receptors in the arcuate nucleus that are related to the activation and inactivation of GABAergic neurons and NPY. CRH increased by leptin is associated with increased appetite (Cowley, Smart, and Rubinstein, 2001; De Araujo., et al., 2006). The arcuate nucleus is a brain structure that regulates food intake through hormonal signals, including adiposity signal (Lorden and Caudle, 1996). The arcuate nucleus integrates peripheral signals, this information is transmitted to the hypothalamus that in turn regulates the autonomic nervous system (ANS) (Redding, Schally, Arimura and Wakabayashi, 1971; Abe, et al., 1990). In this nucleus are two types of neuronal populations that regulate satiety signal, the population of neurons are sensitive to the feeling of hunger and population of neurons sensitive to the feeling of satiety (Olney, 1969; Dawson, et al., 1997; Schwartz, et al., 2000). The arcuate nucleus neurons receive their signals from the sense organs (smell, sight, taste) and the hormone ghrelin is produced by stomach cells, where it triggers gastric contractions. It has also been reported that this hormone is released in the brain as a neurotransmitter (Schwartz, et al., 2000). Bowel distension induces cholecystokinin increases the plasma insulin levels. The signal from the arcuate nucleus sends its message to the paraventricular nucleus of the hypothalamus so that signals of fullness can be sent. The signal that reaches the sensitive cells of the arcuate nucleus of hunger inhibits the activity of cells in the paraventricular nucleus and the cells sensitive to satiety. The inhibitory neurotransmitters such as GABA and NPY are inhibitory signals of satiety in the paraventricular nucleus and lead to overfeeding. The lateral hypothalamus controls the production of insulin and alters the responses to taste. As a consequence, the experimental model is associated with injury to this area and animals have alterations in eating behavior (Kalra, et al., 1999; Schwartz, et al., 2000 Batterham, Cowley, and Small, 2002; De Araujo., et al 2006; Diemen, et al., 2006). It has been reported that the administration of GMS reduces of neuronal cells (Choi, 1988; Cheung, Pascoe, Giardina, John, and Beart, 1998; Elefteriou, et al., 2003), it also occurs glucose tolerance, hyperinsulinemia, hypertriglyceridemia and hypertension, and the development of diabetes (De-Souza, Nunes, Gobatto, and De-Mello, 2003; Balbo, Grassiolli, and Ribeiro, 2007). It has been suggested that MSG-induced obesity could be a useful model for studying the accumulation of risk factors for the development of vascular disease (De-Mello, et al., 2006; Diemen, et al., 2006).

Ventromedial Nucleus

This nucleus has been named as the satiety center, it is considered as a signal site appetite control. It Receives projections from the arcuate nucleus and sent efferents to the paraventricular nucleus. It also presents projections inside and outside the hypothalamus which regulates the activity of the sympathetic and parasympathetic systems. Regarding the sympathetic pathway promotes the alteration in energy absorption and loss of body weight, stimulated by corticotropin (CRH) and inhibited by NPY (Redding, Schally, Arimura, and Wakabayashi, 1971; Dube, et al., 1999; Kalra, et al., 1999, Kitamura, et al., 2011). In contrast to the parasympathetic occurs via reverse balance determines the energy deposition by insulin secretion and induces lipogenesis in the liver and adipose tissue. Ventromedial nucleus stimulation induces satiety signals, meanwhile the vagus nerve sends information in the stomach wall to the brain (Redding, et al., 1971; Meister, et al., 1989). Thus, the stomach detects the intake of fats and other nutrients. It has been reported that distension of the duodenum also produces a feeling of satiety, in addition, the duodenum excreted cholecystokinin, a hormone that regulates hunger acting duodenal level. Other factors that influence hunger are glucose, insulin and glucagon (Redding, et al., 1971; De-Souza, Nunes, Gobatto, and De-Mello, et al., 2003; Diemen, et al., 2006). When glucose levels are high, the liver cells make fat cells into glycogen and fat. It has been reported that in obesity leptin resistance occurs is less sensitive to leptin levels (Ceddia, Koistinen, Zierath, and Sweeney, 2002). The GMS has affected the intake through the vagus nerve which influences the functions and homeostasis of the body. The relationship between the MSG-induced damage and metabolic changes that produce mild hypophagia is poorly known (Dawson, Pelleymounter, Millard, Liu, and Eppler, 1997). This model has shown that rats have decreased weight compared to control animals, yet they have an increased fat due to hypertrophy of adipocytes (Lorden, and Caudle, 1986; Moreno, et al., 2006). The damage in the arcuate nucleus is associated with a decrease in food intake stunted compared to the injury of the ventromedial nucleus of the hypothalamus (VMN) is associated with hyperphagia, but did not reduce growth. The MSG in rats shows significantly increased fat and serum triglycerides, insulin and total liver fat. Obesity is associated with diseases such as dyslipidemia and steatosis hepatitis. It has been reported high activation of the sympathetic system could be associated with the development of obesity-related hypertension (Lorden, and Caudle, 1986; Pelleymounter, Baker, McCaleb, and 1999; Moreno, et al., 2006). The lesion in the arcuate nucleus affects the production of growth hormone (GH) (Maiter, Underwood, Martin, and Koenig, 1991). In rodents, has shown that fat gain induced by the GMS, the increase in leptin levels is similar in both sexes, as well as in adipose tissue of rats treated with MSG has been observed angiotensin II receptor (Pinterova, et al., 2001). A mitochondrial level has been observed in a high calcium retention capacity. The excess of Ca^{2+} associated with neuronal death is explained by two fundamental mechanisms: the transition pore opening in mitochondria causing its swelling and the release of proteins such as cytochrome C. (Albert, Helmer-Matyjek, and Nairn, 1984; Choi, 1988; Choi, 1992). Once you open the pore in the mitochondria, is released more Ca^{2+} and an alteration in the synthesis of ATP is produced (Choi, 1992). In the obese rats it has been reported an increase in the secretion of catecholamines from adrenal glands. The beginning of obesity by GMS depends on the sympathetic adrenal axis activity that leads to decreased of catecholamines secretion (Bunyan, Murrell, and Shah, 1976; Astrup, 1995; Batterham, Cowley, and Small, 2002). Studies have reported a Glu-rich diet stimulates the sensory regions of the stomach and intestines causing alterations in bowel function (Kitamura, Tsurugizawa, and Torii, 2011).

Advantages

There are several obesity models; however, an excellent model must represent many or all pathophysiological features of this disease (Diemen, et al., 2006; Matyskova, et al., 2008). In this regard, GMS obesity murine model, in contrast with other models, produce several complications such as hypophagia, leptin and insulin resistance, hyperleptinemia, neural and metabolic alterations that cause obesity and type II diabetes as a consequence of neuronal death in the arcuate nucleus (Nagata, et al., 2006). The relationship between glutamate-induced damage of the arcuate nucleus and the metabolic changes that produce obesity is poorly understood. Another advantages is that it has not been explored its usefulness yet for studying the neural, neuroendocrine, metabolic and immunological mechanisms that lead to the development of obesity. Glutamate obese murine model had dramatically increased leptin levels resulting from attenuated leptin signaling in arcuate nucleus and being a good model of arcuate nucleus located leptin resistance (Dawson, 1997).

Disadvantages

Obesity is a consequence of polygenetic interaction with the environment, while, glutamate model is an artificial model that causes obesity due a metabolic imbalance, rather than to increased intake of food (WHO, 2003). Should be an excellent model whether fat gains were a result of a high-calorie diet, this could be a principal disadvantage. On the other hand, this model induces neuronal death in the arcuate nucleus an irreversible manner, in the opinion this should difficult to test the specificity of therapeutic compounds and its effect at this level. In conclusion the causes and effects of obesity induced for administration of MSG in experimental models may offer a better understanding of the physiopathogeny of obesity, and options for prevention and treatment.

REFERENCES

Abe, M., Saito, M., and Shimazu, T. (1990). Neuropeptide Y in the specific hypothalamic nuclei of rats treated neonatally with monosodium glutamate. *Brain Research Bulletin, 24,* 289–291.

Albert, K., A., Helmer-Matyjek, E., and Nairn, A., C. (1984). Calcium/phospholipid-depending protein kinase (protein kinase C) phosphorylates and activates tyrosine hydroxylase. *Proceedings of the National Academy of Sciences of the United States of America, 81,* 7713–7717.

Albrecht, J., Sonnewald, U., Waagepetersen,H.,S., and Schousboe, A. (2011). Glutamine in the central nervous system: function and dysfunction. Neuron Glia Biology, 21,1-14.

Altman, J. (2002) Weight in the balance. *Neuroendocrinology,76,* 131-6.

Ankarcrona, M., Dypbukt, J., M., Bonfoco, E., Zhivotovsky, B., Orrenius, S., Lipton, S. A., and Nicotera, P. (1995). Glutamate-induced neuronal death: a succession of necrosis or apoptosis depending on mitochondrial function. *Neuron*, 15, 961-973.

Astrup, A. (1995). The sympathetic nervous system as a target for intervention in obesity. *International Journal of Obesity,19,* S24–S28.

Batterham, R.L., Cowley, M., A., and Small, C. J. (2002). Gut hormone physiologically inhibits food intake. *Nature,418,* 650-4.

Bertrand, G., Gross, R. Puech, R., Loubatieres-Mariani M.M. and Bockaert, J. (1992) Evidence for a glutamate receptor of the AMPA subtype wich mediates insulin release from rat perfused pancreas. *British Journal of Pharmacology, 106*, 354-359.

Beyreuther, K., Biesalski, H. K., Fernstrom, J. D., Grimm, P., Hammes, W. P., Heinemann, U., Kempski, O. Stehle, P., Steinhart, H. and Walker, R. (2007). Consensus meeting. Monosodium glutamate. an update. *European Journal of Clinical Nutrition*, 3, 304–313.

Bunyan, J., Murrell, E., A., and Shah, P., P. (1976). The induction of obesity in rodents by means of monosodium glutamate. *The British journal of Nutrition, 1,* 25-39.

Ceddia, R.,B., Koistinen, H.,A., Zierath, J.,R., and Sweeney, G. (2002). Analysis of paradoxical observations on the association between leptin and insulin resistance. *The FASEB journal: official publication of the Federation of American Societies for Experimental Biology*, 6,1163-76.

Cheung, N., S., Pascoe, C., J., Giardina, S., F., John, C., A., and Beart, P.,M. (1998). Micromolar L glutamate induces extensive apoptosis in an apoptotic-necrotic continum of insult dependent excitotoxic injury in cultured cortical neurones. *Neuropharmacology, 37,*1419-29.

Choi, D., W. (1988). Glutamate neurotoxicity and diseases of the nervous system. *Neuron 1*, 623-634.

Choi, D. W. (1992). Excitotoxic cell death. *Journal of Neurobiology, 23,*1261-1276.

Cowley, M.,A., Smart, J.,L., and Rubinstein, M. (2001). Leptin activates anorexigenic POMC neurons through a neural network in the arcuate nucleus. *Nature,411,* 480-4.

Dawson, R., Pelleymounter, M., Millard, W., Liu, S., and Eppler, B. (1997). Attenuation of leptin-mediated effects by monosodium glutamate-induced arcuate nucleus damage. *The American Journal of Physiology, 273,* E202-E206.

Dawson, R., Pelleymounter, M.,A., Millard, W.,J., Liu, S., and Eppier, B. (1997). Attenuation of leptin-mediated effects by monosodium glutamate-induced arcuate nucleus damage. American journal of physiology. *Endocrinology and Metabolism, 273,* E202-E206.

De-Araujo I.,E., Gutierrez, R., Oliveira-Maia, A.,J., Pereira, A., Nicolelis, M.,A., and Simon S.,A. (2006). Neural ensemble coding of satiety states. *Neuron, 4,* 483-494.

De-Onis, M., Blossner, M., and Borghi, E. (2010). Global prevalence and trends of overweight and obesity among preschool children. *The American Journal of Clinical Nutrition, 5,* 1257-1264.

Della-Fera, M.,A., Qian, H., and Baile, C., A. (2001). Adipocyte apoptosis in the regulation of body fat mass by leptin. *Diabetes, Obesity and Metabolism, 5,* 299-310.

de-Mello, M.,A., De-Souza, C.,T., Braga, L.,R., Dos-Santos, J.,W., Ribeiro, I.,A., and Gobatto, C.,A. (2001). Glucose tolerance and insulin action in monosodium glutamate (MSG) obese exercisetrained rats. *Physiological Chemistry and Physics and Medical NMR, 1,* 63-71.

de-Souza, C.,T., Nunes, W.,M., Gobatto, C.,A., and De-Mello, M.,A. (2003). Insulin secretion in monosodium glutamate (MSG) obese rats submitted to aerobic exercise training. *Physiological Chemistry and Physics and Medical NMR, 1,* 43-53.

Diemen, V., V., Trindade, E., N., and Trindade, M., R. (2006). Experimental model to induce obesity in rats. *Acta Cirurgica Brasileir,. 21,* 425-429.

Dolnikoff, M., Martin-Hidalgo, A., Machado, U.,F., Lima, F.,B., and Herrera, E. (2001). Decreased lipolysis and enhanced glycerol and glucose utilization by adipose tissue prior to development of obesity in monosodium glutamate (MSG) treated-rats. *International Journal of Obesity and Related Metabolic Disorders, 3,* 426-33.

Dube, M.,G., Xu, B., Kalra, P.S., Sninsky, C.A., and Kalra, S.P. (1999). Disruption in neuropeptide Y and leptin signaling in obese ventromedial hypothalamic-lesioned rats. *Brain Research, 1,* 38-46.

Elefteriou, F., Takeda, S., Liu, X., Armstrong, D., and Karsenty, G. (2003). Monosodium glutamate-sensitive hypothalamic neurons contribute to the control of bone mass. *Endocrinology, 144,* 3842-3847.

Finucane, M., M., Stevens, G.,A., Cowan, M.,J., Danaei, G., Lin, J.,K., Paciorek, C.,J., Singh GM, Gutierrez HR, Lu Y, Bahalim AN, Farzadfar F, Riley, L.M., Ezzati, M. (2011). Global Burden of Metabolic Risk Factors of Chronic Diseases Collaborating Group (Body Mass Index). National, regional, and global trends in body-mass index since 1980: systematic analysis of health examination surveys and epidemiological studies with 960 country-years and 9.1 million participants. *Lancet Publishing Group*, 9765, 557-567.

Fonseca, L.,L., Monteiro, M.,A., Alves, P.,M., Carrondo, M.,J., and Santos, H. (2005). Cultures of rat astrocytes challenged with a steady supply of glutamate: new model to study flux distribution in the glutamate-glutamine cycle. *Glia, 51,* 286-296.

Giacometti, T. (1979). Free and bound glutamate in natural products. In Filer, L.J. Jr, Garattini, M. R, Kare, M.R., Reynolds, W.A. and, Wurtman, R.J. (Eds), *Glutamic Acid: Advances in Biochemistry and Physiology (pp. 25–34).* New York: Raven Press.

Gill, S., S., and Pulido, O., M. (2001). Glutamate receptors in peripheral tissues: corrent knowledge, future research and implications for toxicology. *Toxicolol. Pathol., 29,* 208-223.

Guimaraes, R.,B., Telles, M.,M., Coelho, V.,B., Mori, R.,C., Nascimento C.,M., and Ribeiro E.,B. (2002). Adrenalectomy abolishes the food-induced hypothalamic serotonin release in both normal and monosodium glutamate-obese rats. *Brain Research Bulletin, 4,* 363-9.

Hertz, L., Dringen, R., Schousboe, A., and Robinson, S.,R. (1999). Astrocytes: glutamate producers for neurons. *Journal of Neuroscience Research*, 57, 417-428.

Hertz, L., Yu, A.,C., Kala, G., and Schousboe, A. (2000). Neuronal-astrocytic and cytosolicmitochondrial metabolite trafficking during brain activation, hyperammonemia and energy deprivation. *Neurochemistry International, 37,*83-102.

Institute of Food Technology (IFT). (1987). Monosodium glutamate. *Food Technology, 41,* 134–135.

Kalra, S.,P., Dube, M.,G., Pu, S., Xu, B., Horvath, T.,L., and Kalra, P.,S. (1999). Interacting appetite-regulating pathways in the hypothalamic regulation of body weight. *Endocrine Reviews. 20,* 68-100.

Kanarek, R.,B., Meyers, J., Meade, R.,G., and Mayer, J.(1979). Juvenile-onset obesity and deficits in caloric regulation in MSG-treated rats. *Pharmacology, Biochemistry, and Behavior, 5,* 717-21.

Kew, J. N., and Kemp, J.,A. (2005). Ionotropic and metabotropic glutamate receptor structure and pharmacology. *Psychopharmacology, 179,* 4-29.

Kitamura, A., Tsurugizawa, T., and Torii, K. (2011) Biological significance of glutamate signaling during digestion of food through the gut-brain axis. *Digestion, 1,* 37-43.

Leibowitz., S., F., and Hoebel, B.,G. (1998). Behavioral neuroscience of obesity. In Bray, G. A., Bouchard, C., and James, W.P.T (Eds.), *Handbook of obesity: neuroscience of obesity* (pp. 313-358). New York: Marcel Dekker.

Lau, A. and Tymianski, M. (2010). Glutamate receptors, neurotoxicity and neurodegeneration. Pflügers Archiv. *European Journal of Physiology, 2,* 525-42.

Lorden, J.,F., and Caudle, A. (1986). Behavioral and endocrinological effects of single injections of monosodium glutamate in the mouse. *Neurobehavioral Toxicology and Teratology, 5,* 509-19.

Lorden, J.F., and Caudle, A. (1996). Behavioral and endocrinological effects of single injections of monosodium glutamate in the mouse. Neurobehav Toxicol Teratol. 1986 York DA. Lessons from animal models of obesity. *Endocrinology and Metabolism Clinics of North America, 4,* 781-800.

Macho, L., Fickova, M., Jezova, D., and Zorad, S. (2000). Late effect of postnatal administration of monosodium glutamate on insulin action in adult rats. *Physiological Research, 49,* S79-S85.

Maiter, D., Underwood, L., E., Martin, J., B., and Koenig J.I. (1991). Neonatal treatment with monosodium glutamate: effects of prolonged growth hormone (GH)-releasing hormone deficiency on pulsatile GH secretion and growth in female rats. *Endocrinology, 2,* 1100–1106.

Martins, A. C., Souza, K. L., Shio, M.,T. Mathias, P.C., Lelkes, P.I., and Garcia, R. M. (2004). Adrenal medullary function and expression of catecholamine-synthesizing enzymes in mice with hypothalamic obesity. *Life Sciences, 26,* 3211-22.

Matyskova, R., Maletinska, L., Maixnerova, J., Pirnik, Z., Kiss, A., and Zelezna, B., (2008). Comparison of the obesity phenotypes related to monosodium glutamate effect on arcuate nucleus and/or the high fat diet feeding in C57BL/6 and NMR1 mice. *Physiological Research, 57,* 727-734.

Meister, B., Ceccatelli, S., Hokfelt, T., Anden, N.,E., Anden, M., and Theodorsson, E. (1989) Neurotransmitters, neuropeptides and binding sites in the rat mediobasal hypothalamus: effects of monosodium glutamate (MSG) lesions. *Experimental Brain Research, 76,* 343-368.

Michaelis, E.,K., (1998) Molecular biology of glutamate receptors in the central nervous system and their role in excitotoxicity, oxidative stress and aging. *Progress in Neurobiology, 54,* 369-415.

Miskowiak, B., and Partyka, M. (1993). Effects of neonatal treatment with MSG (monosodium glutamate) on hypothalamopituitary- thyroid axis in adult male rats. *Histology and Histopathology, 4,* 731-4.

Moreno, G., Perello, M., Camihort, G., Luna, G., Console, G., Gaillard, R.C. and Spinedi, E. (2006) Impact of transient correction of increased adrenocortical activity in hypothalamo damaged, hyperadipose female rats. *International Journal of Obesity*, 1, 73-82.

Nagata, M., Susuki, W., Likusa, S., Tabuchi, M., Maruyama, H., Takeda, S., Aburada, M. and Miyamoto, K. (2006). Type 2 diabetes mellitus in obese mouse model induced by monosodium glutamate. *Experimental Animals*. 55,109-115.

Nedergaard, M., Takano, T., and Hansen, A. (2002). Beyond the role of glutamate as neurotransmitter. *Nature Reviews. Neuroscience,9,*748-55.

Niijima, A. (1991). Effects of taste stimulation on the efferent activity of the pancreatic vagus nerve in the rat. *Brain Res Bull.,*26, 161–164.

Niijima, A. (2000). Reflex effects of oral, gastrointestinal and hepatoportal glutamate sensors on vagal nerve activity. *J Nutr 130,* 971S– 973S.

Ninomiya, K. (2001). An overview of recent research on MSG. Sensory applications and safety. *Food Australia, 53,* 546–549.

Ogden, C. L., Yanovski, S., Z. Carroll, M., D. and Flegal, K., M. (2007). The epidemiology of obesity," *Gastroenterology, 6,* 2087–2102.

Olney, J. W. (2002). New insights and new issues in developmental neurotoxicology. *Neurotoxicology. 6,* 659-68.

Olney, J.W. (1969). Brain lesions, obesity, and other disturbances in mice treated with monosodium glutamate. *Science, 164,* 719-721.

Organización mundial de la Salud. Obesidad y sobrepeso. Retrieved from: http://www.who.int/mediacentre/factsheets/fs311/es/index.html

Perello, M., Gaillard, R.C., Chisari, A., and Spinedi, E. (2003) Adrenal enucleation in MSG-damaged hyperleptinemic male rats transiently restores adrenal sensitivity to leptin. *Neuroendocrinology,3,*176-84.

Pinterova, L., Zelezna, B., Fickova, M., Macho, L., Krizanova, O., Jezová, D. and Zórad, S. (2001). Elevated AT1 receptor protein but lower angiotensin II-binding in adipose tissue of rats with monosodium glutamate-induced obesity. *Hormone and Metabolic Research,* 33, 708-712.

Redding, T.W., Schally, A.V., Arimura, A., and Wakabayashi, I. (1971). Effect of monosodium glutamate on some endocrine functions. *Neuroendocrinology, 8,* 245-255.

Rosenmund, C., Stern-Bach, Y., and Stevens, C.,F. (1998). The tetrameric structure of a glutamate receptor channel. *Science, 280,*1596-9.

Schwartz, M.W., Baskin, D.G., Kaiyala, K.J., and Woods, S.C. (1999) Model for the regulation of energy balance and adiposity by the central nervous system. *The American Journal of Clinical Nutrition, 69,* 584-96.

Schwartz, M.,W., Woods, S.,C., Porte, D., Seeley, R.,J., and Baskin, D.,G.(2000). Central nervous system control of food intake. *Nature, 404,* 661-71.

Tokuyama, K., and Himms-Hagen, J. (1989). Adrenalectomy prevents obesity in glutamate-treated mice. *American Journal of Physiology, 257,* E139-44.

Watkins, J. C. and Jane, D.E. (2006). The glutamate story. *British Journal of Pharmacology, 147,* S100-S108.

World Health Organization (WHO) (2003). Diet, nutrition and prevention of chronic diseases," WHO Technical Report Series 916, WHO, Geneva, Switzerland.

World Health Organization (WHO), The WHO Child Growth Standards, http://www.who.int/childgrowth/in/.

Yanovski, S., Z. and Yanovski, J. A. (2011). Obesity prevalence in the United States--up, down, or sideways? *New England Journal of Medicine, 11,* 987-989.

Young, V.,R., and Ajami, A., M. (2000). Glutamate: an amino acid of particular distinction. *Journal Nutrition, 130,* 892S–900S.

In: Recent Hispanic Psychological Research ... ISBN: 978-1-62948-919-3
Editors: C. H. Garcia Cadena, A. Lopez-Espinoza et al. © 2014 Nova Science Publishers, Inc.

Chapter 6

ACTIVITY PATTERNS, FOOD INTAKE, AND WATER CONSUMPTION IN RATS: AN EXPLORATORY ANALYSIS*

Carlos Flores Aguirre[1,#], Luis Fernando Zárate Molina[1] and Rebeca Mateos Morfín[2]

[1]Universidad de Guadalajara, México
Center of Studies and Research on Behavior
[2]Universidad del Valle de México, Campus Zapopan
Coordination of graduate Studies and Executives Undergraduates

ABSTRACT

The patterns of eating, drinking and running in rats were studied under free access to food, water and an activity wheel conditions. In order to obtain food, the subjects had to press a lever, to obtain water the rats had to lick a tube. For both behaviors, to drink and to eat, a continuous reinforcement schedule was operating during the whole study. The subjects lived in the experimental boxes with a 12 h light/dark cycle during 20 sessions. Subjects showed activity increases in the running wheels during the light cycle along sessions, the activity during the dark cycle was relatively stable. There were no differences in presses for food and licks between light cycle and dark cycle. Body weight did not show changes along sessions. The results represent an exploratory approach, as a base line to study the activity-based anorexia phenomenon.

Keywords: Activity-based anorexia, food intake, water consumption, activity wheel, rats

---

* This research was funded by Grant 104902 from the Consejo Nacional de Ciencia y Tecnología (CONACYT).

Address for correspondence: Center of Studies and Research on Behavior. Francisco de Quevedo No. 180, Col Arcos Vallarta, Guadalajara, Jalisco, México, 44130. fac13489@cucba.udg.mx, Luys_f@hotmail.com, rebecamateos@gmail.com.

INTRODUCTION

In activity-based anorexia (ABA) studies, researchers have concentrated on observing the phenomenon considering two fundamental conditions: the access to food during one period of one hour a day and the access to an activity wheel the 23 remaining hours (Cano, Gutiérrez and Pellón, 2006; Dwyer and Boakes, 1997; Epling and Pierce, 1988; Lett, Grant, Smith and Koh, 2001; Pérez, Magalhäes and Pellón, 2010).

Under these conditions subjects show a loss of body weight, low food intake and increased activity in the running wheel. However, this manipulation has some difficulties since it does not allow the researcher to quantify the subjects' food intake during a complete light-dark cycle (due to the one hour a day food availability). Furthermore, it does not allow the subjects to choose between eating or running since both activities occur at a different time. Some works have contributed to the understanding of ABA even though their main objective/focus was not on the study of this phenomenon. At present, it has not been reported a study in which the rat has free access to food, water and the activity wheel all at the same time. There are some works that, although not having the study of ABA as the main purpose, have contributed indirectly to the understanding of this phenomenon. For example, Richter (1927) reported that rats with free access to food and water showed eating and drinking episodes during the day, but both activities were higher during the dark cycle. Also, Richter (1927) found that the daily pattern of feeding was sensitive to diverse environmental variables, for example the availability to develop some activities such as climbing towers, running in running wheels and nesting in their boxes, are factors that affect the duration and the frequency of eating episodes.

In a recent study, Díaz and Bruner (2007) studied the possible interactions between eating and drinking in rats. They placed their subjects in conditioning chambers in which the rats had free access to food and water during 24 hours. The results of their study were consistent with the results reported by Richter (1927), the rats showed alternate episodes of food and drink along the day, showing higher food intake and water consumption during the dark cycle. These two studies (Richter, 1927; Díaz and Bruner, 2007), allow to know the feeding pattern of the rat along a complete light-dark cycle, however, they do not provide information about the activity (for example the activity in the running wheels) developed by the subjects in a similar period.

In ABA studies, besides knowing the quantity of food intake by the rat and water consumption, it is also of interest to know the activity that the organisms deploy in the running wheels.

In those studies the access to food and the availability of wheels occur in different periods. In ABA studies it has been reported that the body weight is inversely proportional to the activity that the subjects develop in the running wheels (Routtenberg and Kuznesof, 1967). This result can be explained as follows: firstly it is known that a rat has several episodes of food per day (Díaz and Bruner, 2007; Richter, 1927), and in the procedure used to study the ABA their food intake is restricted to one hour a day; secondly, the activity in the wheel also contributes to the decrease in body weight (Boakes, 2007). Therefore, the phenomenon of ABA could be due to a failure to adapt to the restricted feeding schedule.

Moreover, the role that the running-wheel activity plays on the ABA is not completely clear, because it ignores how much of the animal's activity occurs in the activity-wheels under free feeding conditions, which makes difficult to know how food restriction and the animal's activity interact along the light-dark cycle in the development of the ABA phenomenon. The present study was designed to obtain a baseline of the natural eating, drinking and running patterns in order to advance in the study of some of the variables implied in the development of the activity-based anorexia phenomenon.

METHOD

Subjects

Four experimentally naive female Wistar rats were used. All animals were monitored and fed daily, and at 180 days of age began the experiment. Subjects were individually housed in their home cages with free access to purified water and food (Purina rat chow). A 12 h light/dark cycle was programmed (lights on from 8:00 to 20:00). All animal care procedures were in accordance with the NOM-062-ZOO-1999.

Apparatus

Four experimental boxes equipped with running wheels (MED ENV-042A) were used. Each box was located in soundproof shells with a fan that served as white noise and facilitated the circulation from the air to the interior of the box. Each box had in the side wall an opening (7 cm x 10 cm) that allowed the access to an activity wheel (9 cm wide and 34 cm of diameter) that could rotate freely, 12 g tension were required to rotate the wheel and to activate the counter.

Inside each chamber there was an operative panel in which a lever was placed (MED-ENV-112CM) sensitive to a force of 0.15 N to close the micro switch. The lever was located at 6.5 cm regarding the floor and to 2 cm regarding the left wall of the box. The pellet receptacle was located 2.5 cm regarding the floor. The pellet dispenser provided 45 mg of food (MED-ENV-203M-45). During the light cycle (from 8:00 to 20:00) a lamp of 28 V placed 22 cm of the floor in the opposed wall to the operative panel illuminated the box. Access to water was provided by a lickometer pipe (ENV-251L) that registered the number of licks and daily water consumption. The control of events and data were recorder by an interface MED Associates Inc. (Model SG-610D) coupled to a computer equipped with MED-PC IV for Windows software.

Procedure

The subjects were moved from their home cages to the experimental boxes without having any type of training neither to press the lever to receive food nor to lick the lickometer tube to obtain water. At 10:30 a.m. the subjects were weighed, and the water bottles and pellet dispensers were filled. At 11:00 a.m. the program was restarted and the session finished at 10:30 a.m. of the following day. A continuous reinforcement schedule was effective during 20 sessions and the subjects had free access to the running-wheel.

RESULTS

Figure 1 shows the running activity measured in number of wheel turns for each subject in each daily session. The functions with white circles represents the subjects activity along the light cycle, complementarily the functions with black circles corresponds the subjects activity during the dark cycle. As a whole, the four subjects showed more activity during the light cycle than the dark cycle. During the light cycle, the number of wheel turns was gradually increasing along sessions in all the rats. However, during the dark cycle the number of wheel turns was relatively constant along sessions. A paired t test showed a higher activity in the wheel turns during the light cycle (M = 824.4, SE = 128.8) than the dark cycle (M = 403.3, SE = 48.9), t (3) = 5.09, $p < 0.05$.

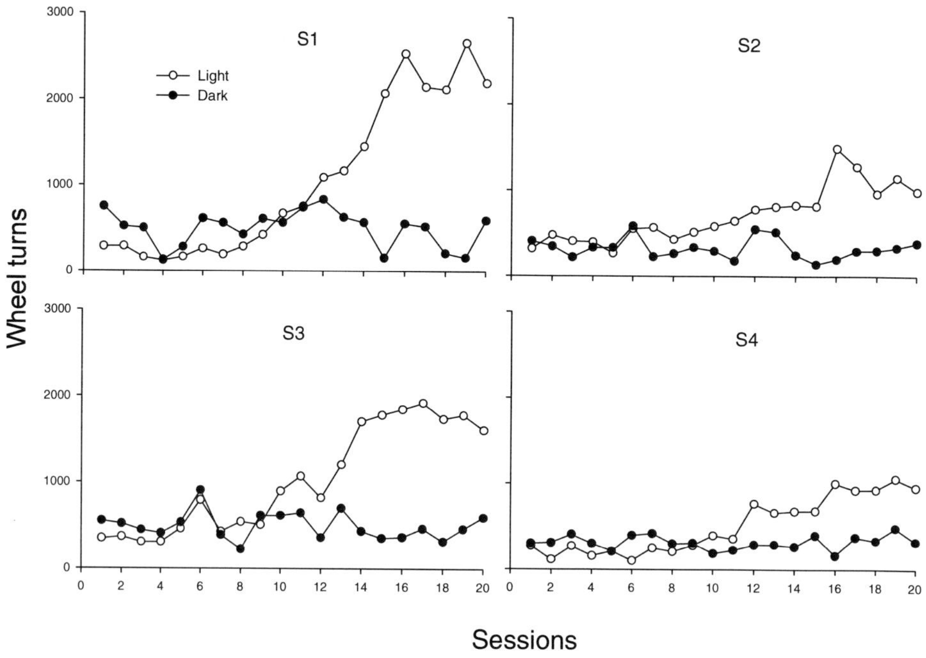

Figure 1. Wheel turns per session for each rat; white circles corresponds light cycle while black circles corresponds dark cycle.

The Figure 2 shows the number of bar-presses for food by subjects in each session. As Figure 1, white circles corresponds presses during light cycle, whereas black circles corresponds presses during dark cycle. All the subjects maintained a relatively stable pattern of bar-pressing along sessions. A paired t test did not showed differences between presses for food during the light (M = 368.7, SE = 12.6) and dark cycles (M = 359.4, SE = 24.4), t (3) = 0.306, $p > 0.05$.

Figure 3 shows the number of licks by subjects in each daily session. All the subjects showed irregular licking patterns along sessions. A paired t test did not showed differences between number of licks during the light (M = 4371.2, SE = 423.8) and dark cycles (M = 4535.9, SE = 270.2), t (3) = - 0.564, $p > 0.05$.

Figure 4 shows the body weight by subject in each daily session. In a general way, all the rats maintained its body weights relatively stable along the sessions. Mean body weight were 213.1, 212.5, 216.7, 215.4 for S1, S2, S3 and S4, respectively.

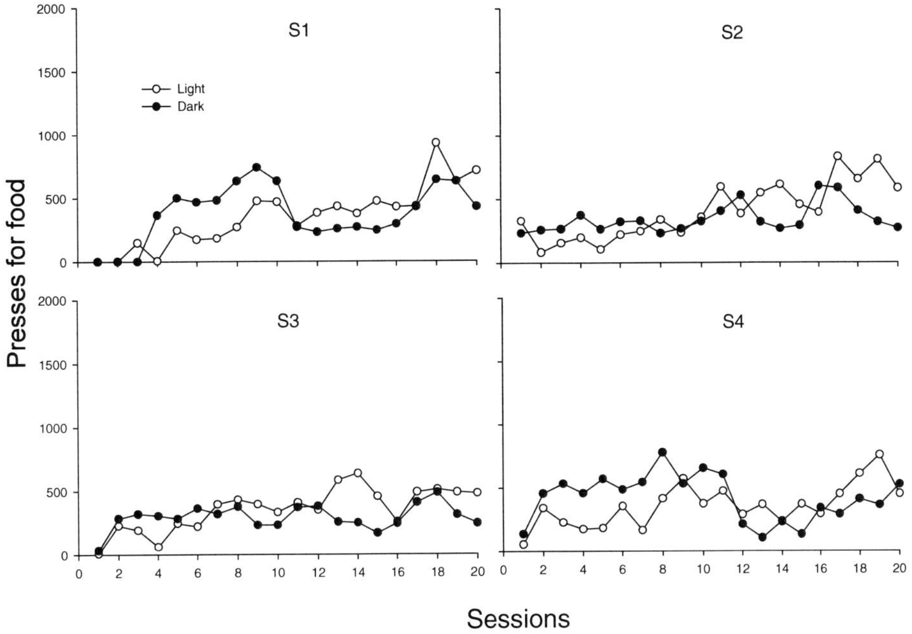

Figure 2. Bar presses for food per session for each rat; white circles corresponds light cycle while black circles corresponds dark cycle.

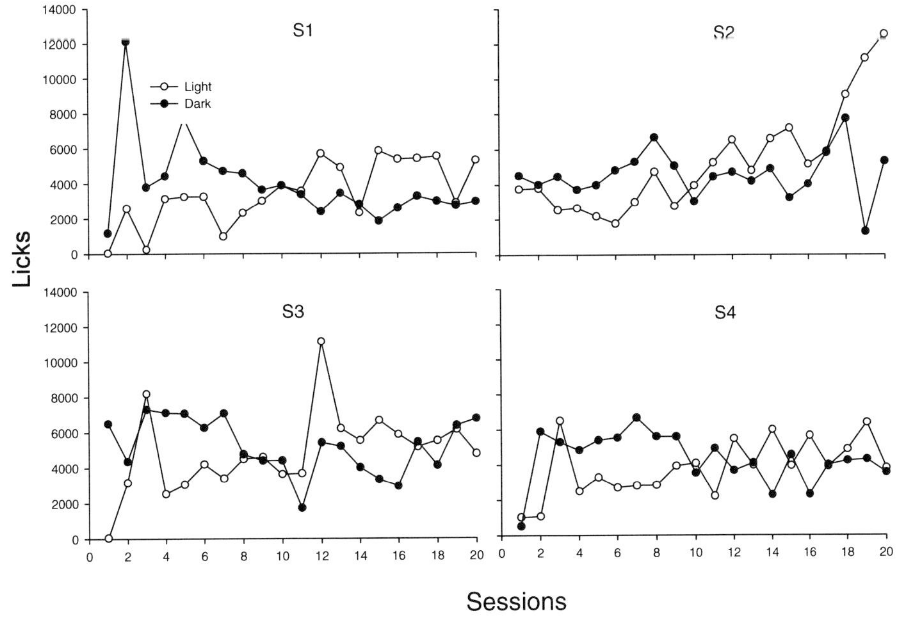

Figure 3. Licks per session for each rat; white circles corresponds light cycle while black circles corresponds dark cycle.

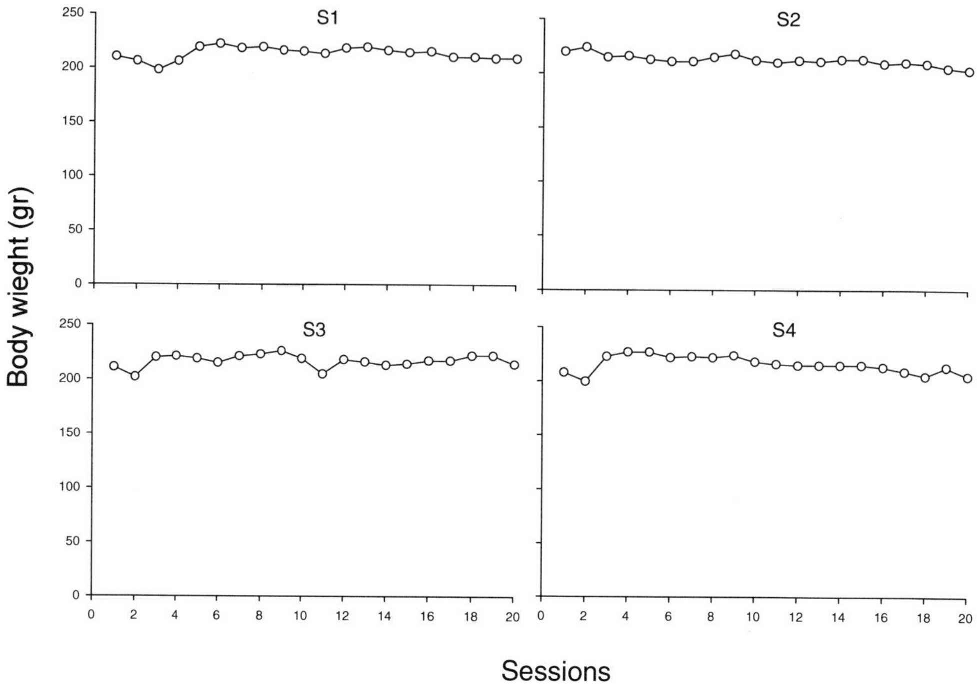

Figure 4. Body weight per session for each rat.

Discussion

The main objective of this study was to obtain a baseline of the natural eating, drinking and running patterns in the rat. In the current study the rats exhibited several eating and drinking episodes along the light-dark cycle. However, there are some inconsistencies with the results reported by Díaz and Bruner (2007) and Richter (1927) about the subjects maintaining night patterns of feeding and activity. Although the subjects of the present experiment showed a relative stability in their eating and drinking patterns, the activity in the running wheels was higher during the light cycle than the dark cycle, specifically towards the end of the study.

Likewise, the results show an interactive pattern among the three activities that the subjects could make. For example, when the activity was higher during the dark cycle, also the food intake and water consumption was higher during this same cycle; complementary, when the activity was higher during the light cycle, also the food intake and water consumption was higher during this cycle. On the other hand, the body weight, the water consumption and food intake were stable during the whole study, only the activity in the running wheels increased along sessions. This finding is in agreement with those studies than have reported increased activity in the running wheel as the sessions pass, however those studies reported these results under conditions with food restriction (Cano, Gutiérrez and Pellón, 2006). These results highlight the fact that the subjects increase their activity under unrestricted food and water conditions.

In order to know how the activity in the wheel influences on the development of the activity-based anorexia, it is necessary to know how much the rat runs when they have free access to the food. The results of the present study showed that the subjects had less activity than subjects that have been exposed to activity-based anorexia procedures (Cano, Gutiérrez and Pellón, 2006).

Flores, Zárate and Mateos (2011) exposed three groups of rats to an activity-based anorexia procedure. The first group was pre-exposed to the restricted schedule of food (1h a day) until rats reached 80% of their body weights. The second group was also food deprived at 80% of their body weights and then it was recovered to 100%, and finally the third group began the experiment at 100% of their body weight without pre-exposure to food deprivation.

Their results showed that the subjects that began the experiment at 80% of their body weight had a higher activity in the running-wheel. When comparing our data with the results reported by Flores et al. (2011) it is observed that although the activity in the wheel was higher in their groups, the difference is not significant between the two groups at 100% and the subjects of the present study.

We can conclude two things: a) the activity that the rats exhibit when they have free access to the running wheel and free access to food, seems to be similar to that shown by the subjects under activity-based anorexia procedures; and b) the inverse relationship between increased activity in the running-wheel and body weight loss does not always occur. Future explorations are necessary to complete the study presented here in order to know the effects of access to food duration on body weight loss and the subjects' activity.

REFERENCES

Belke, T. W. (1996). The effect of a change in body weigth on running and responding reinforced by the opportunity to run. *The Psychological Record, 46*, 421-433.

Boakes, R. A. (2007). Self-Starvation in the Rat: Running versus Eating. *The Spanish Journal of Psychology, 10,* 251-257.

Cano, C., Gutiérrez, M., and Pellón, R. (2006). Preexposición al programa de comida y desarrollo de anorexia basada en actividad en ratas. *International Journal of Psychology and Psychological Therapy, 6*, 273-286.

Díaz, F., and Bruner, C. A. (2007). Comer y beber en ratas con libre acceso a la comida y al agua. *Acta Comportamentalia, 15*, 111-130.

Dwyer, D.M., and Boakes, R.A. (1997). Activity-based anorexia in rats as a failure to adapt to a feeding schedule. *Behavioral Neuroscience, 111,* 195-205.

Flores, C., Zárate, L. F., and Mateos, L. R. (2011). Efecto de la pre-exposición a la restricción de alimento sobre el desarrollo de anorexia. Trabajo presentado en el Congreso de la Sociedad Mexicana de Psicología, *Revista Mexicana de Psicología, (número especial, memoria in extenso)*, 1283-1284.

Epling, W. F., and Pierce, W. D. (1988). Activity-based anorexia: A biobehavioral perspective. *International Journal of Eating Disorders, 7,* 475-485.

Lett, B. T., Grant, V. L., Smith, J. F., and Koh, M. T. (2001). Preadaptation to the feeding schedule does not eliminate activity-based anorexia in rats. *The Quarterly Journal of Experimental Psychology, 54B,* 193-199.

López, A., and Martínez, H. (2004). Cambios del patrón alimentario como efecto de la privación de agua o alimento en ratas en crecimiento. *International Journal of Psychology and Psychological Therapy, 4,* 93-104.

Pérez, A., Magalhäes, P., and Pellón, R. (2010). The effects of food presentation at regular or irregular times on the development of activity-based anorexia in rats. *Behavioural Processes, 84,* 541-545.

Richter, C.P. (1927). Animal Behavior and internal drives. *Quaterly Review of Biology, 2,* 307-343.

Routtenberg, A., and Kuznesof, A. W. (1967). "Self-starvation" of rats living in activity wheels on a restricted feeding schedule. *Journal of Comparative and Physiological Psychology, 64,* 414-421.

In: Recent Hispanic Psychological Research ... ISBN: 978-1-62948-919-3
Editors: C. H. Garcia Cadena, A. Lopez-Espinoza et al. © 2014 Nova Science Publishers, Inc.

Chapter 7

Evaluating Body Weight and Food Intake in Two Sizes Home Box in Rats

Alma Gabriela Martínez Moreno*[*], *Diana Merced Venancio López*, *Antonio López-Espinoza* and *Carmen Livier García Flores
Center of Research on Feeding Behavior and Nutrition (CICAN)
CUSur – Universidad de Guadalajara, México

Abstract

The experimental evidence shows that modification of the physical space has effects on behavior; among the most evident are the alterations in body weight and food intake. With the purpose of determining the effect of space modifications on body weight and food intake, eight male rats from the same litter were used and two groups of four subjects each were formed. They remained in free food and water access conditions. During 40 days their body weight, food, and water intake was registered daily by group. The experiment was divided into two phases with duration of 20 days each. During the first phase group 1 was placed in a 16x28x18 size box and group 2 in a 20x38.5x23.5 size box. At the end of the first phase, group 1 was moved into the box that group 2 was in and group 2 was moved to the box group 1 was in. The obtained results did not show significant changes between the groups in spite of the space modifications and the concentration of subjects.

Keywords: Space modification, body weight, food intake, rats

---

[*] Supported by 101314 CONACyT. First autor is the technnical responsable of proyect. All authors contributed to the implementation of the study. First author designed and wrote this document. Address for correspondence: Dra. Alma Gabriela Martínez Moreno, Center of Research on Feeding Behavior and Nutrition. South University Center. Universidad de Guadalajara, Prolongación Colón s/n, Edificio X-3, Zapotlán el Grande, Jalisco, México. Web: www.cusur.udg.mx/cican/ email: alma.martinez@cusur.udg.mx.

INTRODUCTION

The behavior of animals is linked to the concept of space. This assertion is visible: the behavior is carried out by a subject, at a particular moment and place (Rifá, 1988). The experimental evidence reveals that the modification of the physical space has effects over behavior (Cáseres, Jiménez, Ara, Huamán and Huamán, 2004; González, Castro and Berea, 1981; Hernández, Ángeles, Zapata, Montaño and Gómez, 2006; López and Escalante, 1982; Polanco and López, 1984; Serio, 1999; Southiwick, 1971). This modification includes the expansion or reduction of the physical dimensions in which the subjects are in, as well as the reduction of the physical space from the density, which is the physical measurement expressed by the number of subjects per unit in the area (Santoyo and Anguera, 1992).

One of the most evident consequences in the reduction of physical space is the delay in the growth of the animals and the decrease in their food intake (Hernández, Ángeles, Zapata, Montaño and Gómez, 2006). Also, in human beings, evident behavioral changes are observed due to the reduction of space. Today, large cities more and more have smaller housing spaces which cause inappropriate behaviors, such as crime, violence, felonies and even sexual aberrations (Lagemann, 1967).

Borders are a way to demarcate the reduction of space. Southiwick (1971), Minteguiaga and Corte (2005), as well as the Animal Behavior Society (2008) point out that the restricted space in some animal species is the cause of displaying uncommon behaviors and conducts when presented with freedom or an adequate space fit to their needs.

In 1981, González, Castro and Berea carried out an investigation with broilers in which the subjects were distributed into three groups with a different number of subjects per square meter (densities), in order to find the adequate density for the young and an increase in meat production per bird. The results showed that with the increase in density the body weight decreased. Food intake decreased due to the reduction of movements and the loss of heat.

In another investigation carried out with chickens to study productivity by used surface area, four groups were formed with a different number of subjects per square meter of floor. The tendency to decrease food intake was observed as the density of birds per square meter of floor increased. The body weight was also reduced, and as the density increased, so did the meat production (López and Escalante, 1982).

Polanco y López (1984) carried out an investigation to determine the effect of density on growth and feeding using 14, 16, 18, 20, 22 and 24 birds/m^2. The obtained results demonstrated that food intake did not show changes among the various densities. However, they observed a tendency to decrease the live weight (meat) when the space per bird was reduced; this was more evident in males than in females and it was attributed to the greater volume reached by the males, because they have a greater body weight, for which they have a greater vital space requirement than of females which are lighter.

Meanwhile, Hernández et al. (2006) carried out an investigation in which they evaluated the productive variables and stress indicators in three groups of pigs as a result of a reduction of the floor, due to the increase of pigs per pen. In the observed results it was found that food intake and weight gain decreased when increasing the density, even though the stress indicators were not related or underwent change between densities.

In another investigation white-tailed deer in captivity were observed. The first group had four specimens in a land of 1500 m^2, without any disruptive events that disturbed or altered the usual behavior of the animals. The second group had eleven specimens on a piece of land of 1875m^2; this enclosure was characterized by an intense human disturbance. The results produced that in the second group, the time spent on their eating behavior was greater than the first. This is ascribed to the customary close relationship with human beings and the difficulty that would be presented in a situation of entire independence that would have repercussions over its feeding possibilities (Serio, 1999).

The effect of space over the productive parameters has also been researched in guinea pigs. An investigation carried out with this specie in five different vital spaces with five different quantities of animals found that a reduced vital space generated inconveniences for feeding, movement, rest, and reproductive levels. When guinea pigs were exposed to a greater vital space, higher weight gain, less alfalfa intake, and a lesser number of scars was obtained, which indicated a lower number of fights (Cáseres et al., 2004).

This way the previous experimental evidence suggests that space has an effect on body weight, food intake, and reproductive levels. As a result, a reduction or expansion of space could modify the feeding behavior. In lab animals, the home boxes have a standard size which is supposedly adequate for the size of the animals (16x28x18cm). However, some experiments require housing a group of animals, a situation where density is increased. Therefore, the objective of the current investigation is to determine the effect of space modification over body weight and food intake in rats through changes in the physical dimension of the home box and density.

METHOD

Subjects

Nine-Thirty day old male naive Wistar rats (of the same litter) from the colony housed at University Center of Health Sciences of University of Guadalajara were used. All procedures of this study were realized according to ethical guidelines for research with animals of The Official Mexican Norm (NOM-062-ZOO-1999).

Apparatus and Materials

Three transparent plastic home boxes were used, (16x28x18 [2) and 20x38.5x23.5), each one with a metal grille on the top and two compartments used as a feeder and a drinking trough. The boxes had a floor covering of sawdust which was removed daily. Food with standard nutrients for lab animals was used (3% fats, 7% ashes, 1% calcium, 23% protein, 6% fiber, 49% NFE (nitrogen-free extract), 0.6% phosphorus, and 12% humidity). The liquid was provided in graduated troughs of 270 ml, unique for laboratory rats, they had anti-spill nozzles designed to prevent gas entry.

Procedure

Two groups of four subjects each, with similar weights were formed to achieve homogenous groups. One control subject was housed alone. All the subjects were members of the same litter. Each of the four subjects that were formed into groups was identified with a register number, birth date, and a mark at the base of the tail. They remained in free food and water access conditions.

The measurement that was carried out was of the total amount of food and water intake by group. The body weight of each subject was registered to calculate the total body weight by group. The experiment was divided into two phases, each phase with duration of 20 days. During the first 20 days of the experiment, group 1 was placed in house box with 16x28x18 and group 2 in house box with 20x38.5x23.5, at the end of the 20 days, group 1 was changed into the box where group 2 was, and group 2 into the box of group 1. The subject housed individually remained in the same home box for the 40 days.

RESULTS

The Figure 1 shows body weight, food intake, and calorie intake. The axis of the abscissas shows the number of days of the experiment, and the ordinate the body weight, food intake, and calorie intake. The daily register of group 1 is represented with black circles and group 2 with white circles. Figure 2 shows body weight, food intake, and calorie intake of control subject.

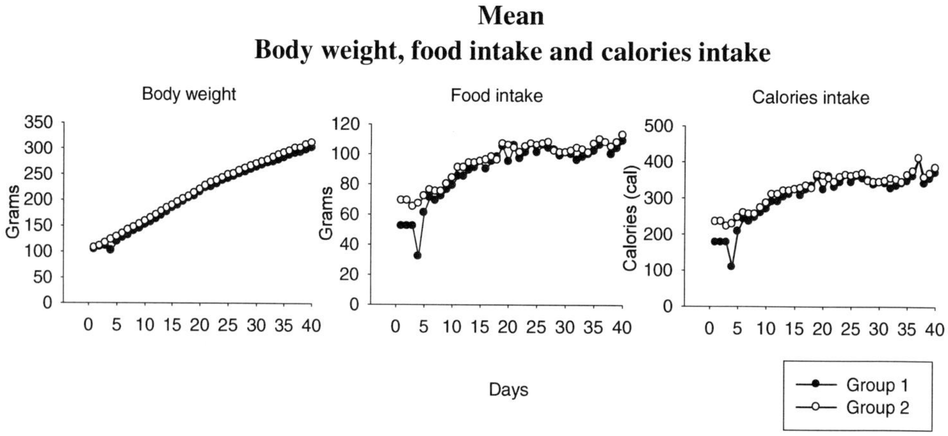

Figure 1. Shows body weight (left panel), total food intake (central panel), and total calorie intake (right panel) of groups 1 and 2 during the 40 days of this experiment. No significant differences were found between the data of the groups in the three measurement variables (p>.05).

The left panel of the Figure 1 shows the average body weight registered during both phases of the experiment. In general, no significant differences were observed among the groups from the statistical *t* test for independent samples (p>0.05). All of them showed a gradual increase of body weight in accordance to its normal growth pattern. In particular, on day 4 of the experiment a decrease in body weight was observed in group 1, which began the experiment in house box 6x28x18.

The central panel of the Figure 1 shows the obtained results from food intake. The total consumption obtained is demonstrated by the four subjects of each group, because there was no register of the individual consumption of each subject. A decrease in consumption is observed in group 1 during the first days of the experiment which seems to correspond to the decrease of body weight. No significant differences were observed between the groups ($p>0.05$).

Finally, the right panel shows the measurement of the consumed calories. Also, the total calorie intake by group is shown. As in the central panel, the caloric intake is practically the same amongst the groups, with the exception of the first few days of the experiment in group 1. Figure 2 shows same results of group 2 in control subject, who stayed alone in house box with 16x28x18.

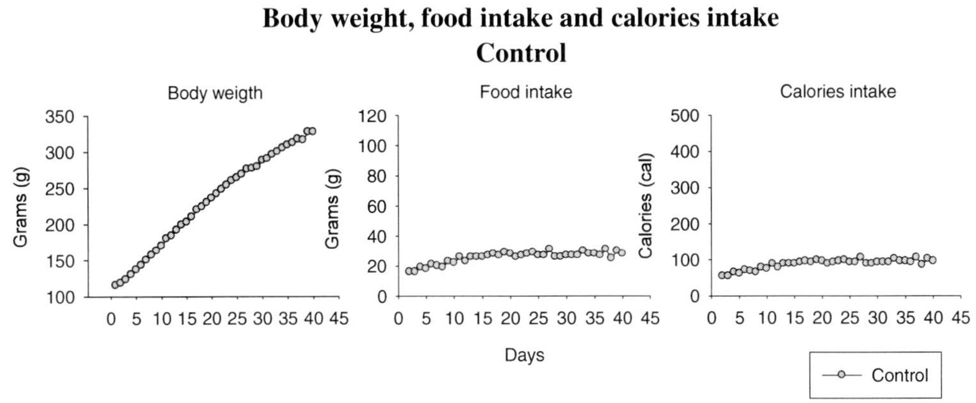

Figure 2. Shows the body weight (left panel), food intake (central panel), and calorie intake (right panel) of control subject.

DISCUSSION

The results showed that there are no significant differences in body weight and in caloric and food intake in the spaces used during the 40 days in which the experiment was carried out. The performed comparison between group 1 and group 2 did not show relevant changes in food intake when carrying out the space modification in the two phases. These findings coincide with those of López and Polanco (1984) where they report that there is no notable change in food intake within the different densities used in this investigation.

González, Castro and Berea (1981), as well as López and Escalante (1982), reported that the less space the subjects have, a decrease in body weight and food intake is observed. The results in this investigation do not show such changes which seems to indicate that the space was enough for the subjects and it does not alter its growth or diet.

In turn, Cáseres et al. (2004) suggested that with a larger space per subject, a greater weight gain is obtained and aggressive behaviors are avoided. In this case, the registered body weight of the subjects in group 1 and 2 did not present any changes when the space was larger. This means that those experiments require manipulating the groups by locating them in the same environment will not be affected by the reduction of space or by the density if the conditions from the present experiment are repeated. It seems that four subjects occupying a standard home box does not alter their growth or food intake, at least not during 40 consecutive days. The same happened in the larger box. It is possible that by increasing the subject density in both of the boxes used could generate differential results. However, it is a fact that by using spaces that become smaller each time in laboratories, it would seem to have no effect on the subject's behavior.

This affirmation allows extending these results to the explanation of certain elicited behaviors by the reduced space. Various investigations point out that feeling enclosed due to housing spaces becoming smaller each time, affect mainly aggressive, sexual, and feeding behaviors. Possibly these results are not only due to the modification of the physical space but to the stress generated by the enclosure. In the case of these experimental subjects, their environment was habitual, in other words, no changes were made to their eating or resting routine, which can indicate that the reduction of their physical space was not synonymous of a stressful stimulus. Nevertheless, the previous could be certain from physiological signs being presented during states of anxiety. This way it would be possible to state if the manipulated subjects presented signs of anxiety from the space modification and density by number of subjects. This procedure would allow new conclusions to be drawn about the relation between the reduction of physical space as a stressful stimulus and changes in their feeding, sexual and aggressive behaviors.

References

Animal Behavior Society. (2008). Guide to programs in animal behavior. *Washington: American Society of Zoologist.*

Cáeseres, F., Jiménez, R., Ara, M., Huamán, H., and Huamán, A. (2004). Evaluación del espacio vital de cuyes criados en pozas. *Revista de Investigaciones Veterinarias del Perú.* 15 (2), 100-112.

Gonzalez, E., Castro, O. and Berea, G. (1981). Disminución del espacio vital en pollos de engorde criados en piso. *Revista Cubana de Ciencia Avícola.* 8 (2), 125-140.

Hernandez, M. G., Ángeles, M. D., Zapata, L., Montaño, M., and Gómez, S. (2006). Efectos de la densidad por corral sobre la producción y las concentraciones sanguíneas de metabolitos y cortisol en cerdos en crecimiento y finalización. *Veterinaria México.* 37 (1), 59-77.

Lagemann, K. J. (1967). ¿Cuánto espacio vital necesita el hombre?. *Selecciones. 324,* 39.

López, S., and Escalante, A. (1982). Comportamiento del pollo de engorde B-6 en dependencia de la densidad de cría x m^2 de superficie de piso. *Revista Cubana de Ciencia Avícola.* 9 (2), 153-159.

Minteguiaga, M., and Corte, S. (2005). Propuesta de enriquecimiento ambiental para un ejemplar de Babuino Papio papio en cautiverio. *Revista de Etología.* 7 (1), 15-23.

Polanco, G., and López, S. (1984). Crecimiento de pollos de engorde criados en piso con diferentes densidades. *Revista Cubana de Ciencia Avícola.* 11 (1-2), 67-76.

Rifá, B. H. (1988). El espacio en la conducta animal. *Anuario de Psicología.* 39 (2), 191-200.

Santoyo, C., and Anguera, M. (1992). El hacinamiento como contexto: Estrategias metodológicas para su análisis. *Psicothema.* 4 (2), 551-569.

Serio, J. C. (1999). Conducta en cautiverio de dos grupos de venado cola blanca (Odocoileus virginianus) con diferente grado de exposición al humano. *Veterinaria de México.* 30 (4), 323-328.

Southwick, C. H. (1971). The biology and psychology of crowding in man and animals. *The Ohio Journal of Science.* 71 (2), 65-72.

In: Recent Hispanic Psychological Research … ISBN: 978-1-62948-919-3
Editors: C. H. Garcia Cadena, A. Lopez-Espinoza et al.

Chapter 8

EFFECTS OF A VARIETY OF FOODS ON FEEDING BEHAVIOR IN RATS

Antonio López-Espinoza**, *Alma G. Martínez*, *Virginia Aguilera*, *Alma Galindo*, *Asucena Cárdenas-Villalvazo*, *Elia H. Valdés*, *Ana Patricia Zepeda and Cristina Espinoza

Center of Research on Feeding Behavior and Nutrition (CICAN)
Cusur -Universidad De Guadalajara, México

ABSTRACT

Purpose of this study was to evaluate effects on water and food intake when exposed to a variety of foods. 12 Wistar rats were used, six females and 6 males. Three groups were created: Norm-Caloric Group, Hypo-Caloric Group, and Hyper-Caloric Group, each were assigned two females and two males. Experiment was divided in 7 phases. Phases 1, 3, 5, and 7 lasted 10 days. In these phases the norm-caloric group was exposed to a norm-caloric diet, the hypo-caloric group to a hypo-caloric diet, and the hyper-caloric group to a hyper-caloric diet. Phases 2, 4, and 6 lasted three days, and all subjects were exposed to three diets simultaneously (Variety of foods). Results showed that subjects in norm-caloric and hypo-caloric groups, and also females of the hyper-caloric group, increased their food intake during the exposure periods to the variety of foods, regardless of the type of diet they previously received. However, hyper-caloric group maintained its intake. Evidence shows that when exposed to a variety of foods the rats did not regulate their food or calorie intake.

Keywords: Diets, variety, calories, feeding behavior, rats

* This research was financed by the project CB 156821of CONACyT. Address for correspondence: Dr. Antonio López-Espinoza. Center of Research on Feeding Behavior and Nutrition (CICAN) CUSur, Universidad de Guadalajara, Av. Enrique Arreola Silva No. 883, Edificio X-3, Colonia Centro C.P. 49000. Ciudad Guzmán, municipio de Zapotlán el Grande, Jalisco, México. E-mail: Antonio López-Espinoza e-mail: antonio.lopez@cusur.udg.mx

INTRODUCTION

It has been reported that the organisms are capable of regulating their caloric intake and body weight when exposed to a variety of foods with different flavors or energy content (Martínez and López-Espinoza, 2007; Martínez, López-Espinoza and Martínez, 2006; Naim, Brand, Kare and Carpenter, 1985). It has also been shown in several reports that in presence of a palatable variety of foods, organisms do not regulate their caloric intake, thus demonstrating a tendency to consume a higher quantity of calories of those which are normally consumed, and gaining body weight (Armitage, Hervey, Rolls, Rowe and Tobin, 1983; Barber, Viña, Viña and Cabo, 1985; Ramírez, 1987; Raynor and Epstein, 2001). It has been suggested that characteristics of the diet, such as flavor (Treit, Spetch and Deutsch, 1983; Galindo and López-Espinoza, 2006; Johnson and Vickers, 1993) or its nutritional value (Naim et al., 1985) are factors that can determine the amount of food consumed.

Cafeteria diets have been applied to study the effects of palatability, energy or nutritional content of foods on feeding behavior (Armitage et al., 1983; Barber et al., 1985; Galef, 1991; Rothwell and Stock, 1988). However, it has been suggested that these types of diets are not a suitable tool because of the difficulty in controlling the amounts of macronutrients consumed by the experimental subjects (Moore, 1987). Naim et al., (1985) used alternative diets to those of cafeteria diets to facilitate the control over the consumed macronutrients. They designed a variety of diets with different sensory characteristics and nutritional value, and they presented them to the experimental subjects simulating a cafeteria diet. This way it was possible to control the amounts of food consumed by each subject.

López-Espinoza, et al. (2011) used a variety of diets with diverse nutritional characteristics: norm-caloric, hypo-caloric, and hyper-caloric. The characteristics of these diets allowed researching the effects of exposure to a variety of foods, controlling the macronutrient quantities found in each type of diet. Purpose of this study was to evaluate effects of exposure to a variety of foods on feeding behavior of rats, after a food deprivation period. Results showed that during the exposure to a variety of foods after a food deprivation period, rats consumed a higher quantity of food and calories. These results allow questioning the role of deprivation as a precursory component of excessive food consumption. In other words, it is necessary to evaluate if the exposure to a variety of foods by itself produced the large food consumptions, or if the intake was large due to food deprivation.

López-Espinoza and Martínez (2001, 2004) reported that after a food deprivation period organisms presented *post-deprivation effects*: binge eating, binge drinking, and the recovery of lost body weight during deprivation. According to this, it is probable that in López-Espinoza, et al. (2011) study the large food intakes registered during periods of exposure to a variety of foods were due to food deprivation and not to the availability of a variety of foods with different sensory and nutritional characteristics.

On the other hand, it could be argued that large food intakes were due to food deprivation, as well as the exposure of a variety of foods. Rolls (1990) pointed out that the exposure to a variety of foods with different sensory characteristics increased the food intake in organisms. Rolls (1990) stated that in presence of a variety of foods, organisms consume a higher quantity of food due to a phenomenon he called *sensory-specific satiety*. The *sensory-specific satiety* refers to a decrease in liking that organism presents to a certain food it had been consuming. Organism will appear to be satiated from a certain type of food, but will consume those it had not tasted, only in situations where a variety of foods with different sensory characteristics is available (Hetherington and Rolls, 1992; Johnson and Vickers, 1993; Rolls, 1990).

To clarify the acquired results in experiment reported by López-Espinoza, et al. (2011) and according to the data reported by López-Espinoza and Martínez (2001, 2004) and Rolls (1990), we considered it is appropriate to carry out this study in which a variety of foods will be used, without deprivation periods. This way we will evaluate if the sole exposure of a variety of foods produces by itself large food intakes in experimental subjects.

METHOD

Subjects

Twelve Wistar rats, six females and six males, experimentally naive and three months old at the beginning of the experiment.

Materials and Equipment

Twelve individual home boxes were used, measuring 13cm high by 27cm wide and 38cm long, with a metal grille on the top, with three dividers used for feeders and one for a drinking trough. The bottom of the box was maintained covered with sawdust, which was removed and substituted every four days. For the registering of food intake and body weight, an electronic precision weight was used. Three types of diets from the commercial brand Science Diet of Hill's Pet Nutrition, Inc. were the food provided (Table 1). The beverage provided was water placed in 200ml graduated troughs.

Table 1. Nutritional Characteristics of the diets

Diet Type	Cal/kg	Protein Percentage	Fat de Percentage	Percentage of Carbohydrates
Norm-Caloric Diet	3705	23.00 %	14.3 %	47.00 %
Hyper-Caloric Diet	4619	27.60 %	25.2 %	32.70 %
Hypo-Caloric Diet	2997	22.20 %	8.1 %	43.00 %

Procedure

Subjects were identified with a number, birth date, and body weight at the beginning of the experiment. They were placed in individual home boxes, which remained in the vivarium with a light-dark cycle of 12x12 hours, with an average temperature of 22°C. Body weight, as well as the water and food intake, was registered daily at 9:30am. To calculate the calories obtained from the food, the number of calories that a gram of each type of food has was multiplied by the grams consumed daily by the animal. Water provided zero calories.

Three experimental groups were formed; each one had two females and two males. The subjects H1, H2, M1, and M2 were assigned to the Norm-Caloric Group, the subjects H3, H4,

M3, and M4 to the Hypo-Caloric Group, and the subjects H5, H6, M5, and M6 to the Hyper-Caloric Group. Subjects were randomly assigned to the groups.

The experiment was divided into 7 phases. Phases 1, 3, 5, and 7, had duration of ten days each. In these phases, 50g of norm-caloric diet was provided to the Norm-Caloric Group, 50g of the hypo-caloric diet was provided to the Hypo-Caloric Group, and 50g of the hyper-caloric diet was provided to the Hyper-Caloric Group. As for the beverage, 200ml of water were provided for all the subjects. Phases 2, 4, and 6 had duration of five days each one. During these phases, all subjects were exposed to the norm-caloric, hypo-caloric, and hyper-caloric diets at the same time (variety of foods). Distribution of the food in the dividers was carried out at random. As for the beverage, 200ml of water were provided for all subjects (Table 2).

Table 2. Experimental Design

	Phases	1	2	3	4	5	6	7
Groups	Norm-Caloric	Norm	Variety	Norm	Variety	Norm	Variety	Norm
	Hypo-Caloric	Hypo	Variety	Hypo	Variety	Hypo	Variety	Hypo
	Hyper-Caloric	Hyper	Variety	Hyper	Variety	Hyper	Variety	Hyper
	Days	10	5	10	5	10	5	10

RESULTS

Figure 1 shows standard deviation of the data of body weight of all the subjects. The top panels show the data from the Norm-Caloric Group, the middle ones the Hypo-Caloric Group, and the lower ones the Hyper-Caloric Group. Columns to the left represent the females and the columns to the right the males. Continuous line indicates phases in which norm-caloric, hypo-caloric, or hyper-caloric diets were provided, correspondingly to Norm-Caloric Group, Hypo-Caloric Group and Hyper-Caloric Group. Black circles represent days of exposure to the variety of foods.

Figure 2 shows the averages of food consumption during each phase. Top panels show data from the Norm-Caloric Group, middle ones Hypo-Caloric Group, and lower ones Hyper-Caloric Group. Left columns represent females and right columns males. Gray bars represent norm-caloric diet, white ones hypo-caloric diet, and black ones hyper-caloric diet. In the boxes located on the top of each graph, the averages of food consumption in grams are showed.

The left side of each box shows the averages of food consumption during the phases of exposure to only one type of food and to the variety of foods. The right side of the box shows the averages of each type of food consumed during the phases of exposure to the variety of foods.

It can be observed that subjects showed a tendency to consume a greater quantity of food during the exposure phases to variety of foods. However, subjects in Hypo-Caloric Group consumed a lesser quantity of food during exposure phases to variety of foods. In addition, it is possible to observe that females and males from the Hypo-Caloric Group consumed greater quantities of food then the other groups, during exposure phases to only one type of diet. Females from Hypo-Caloric Group consumed an average of 11.9g during exposure phases to only one type of diet, contrary to females from Norm-Caloric (10.1g) and Hyper-Caloric (8.5g) Groups.

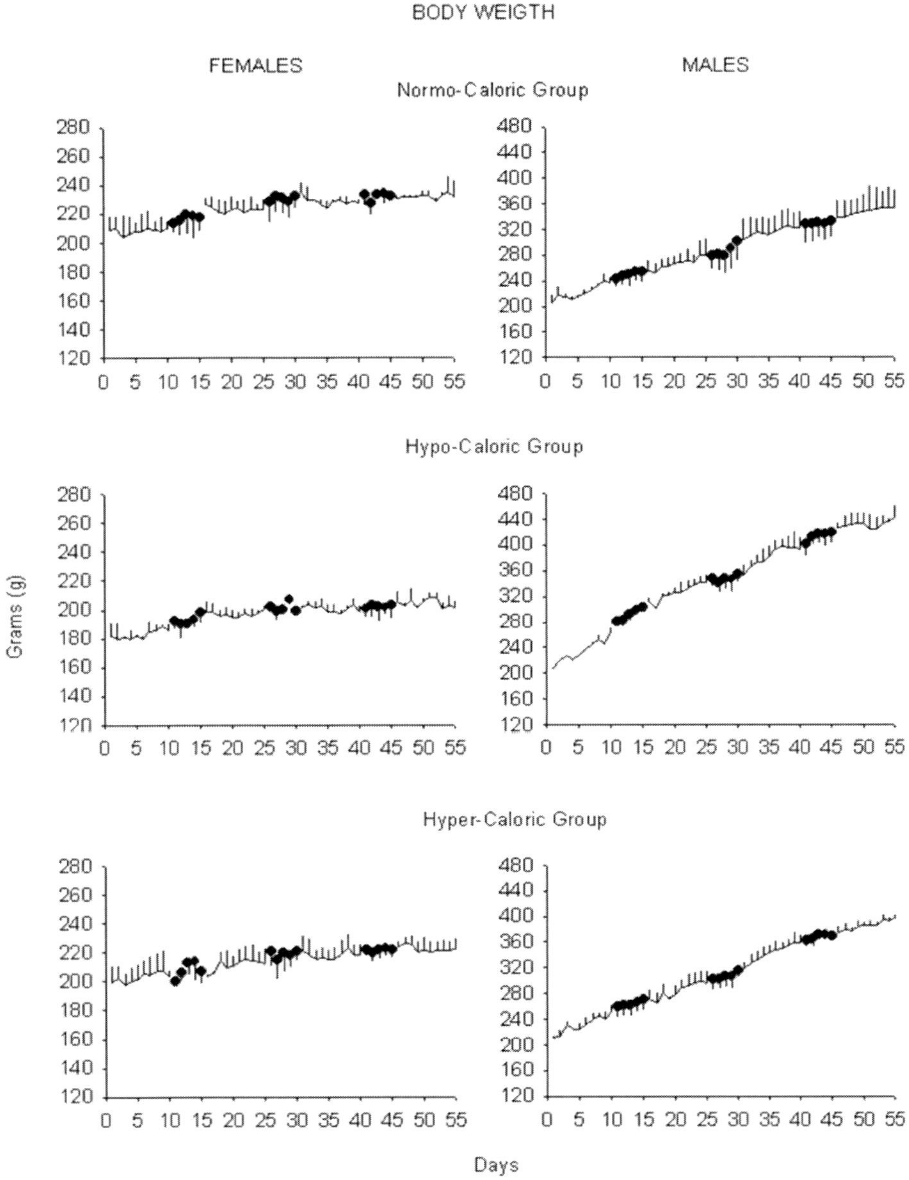

Figure 1. Standard deviation of body weight in females and males from Norm-Caloric, Hypo-Caloric and Hyper-Caloric Groups. Continuous line indicates phases in which only one type of diet was provided, circles represent days of exposure to the variety of foods.

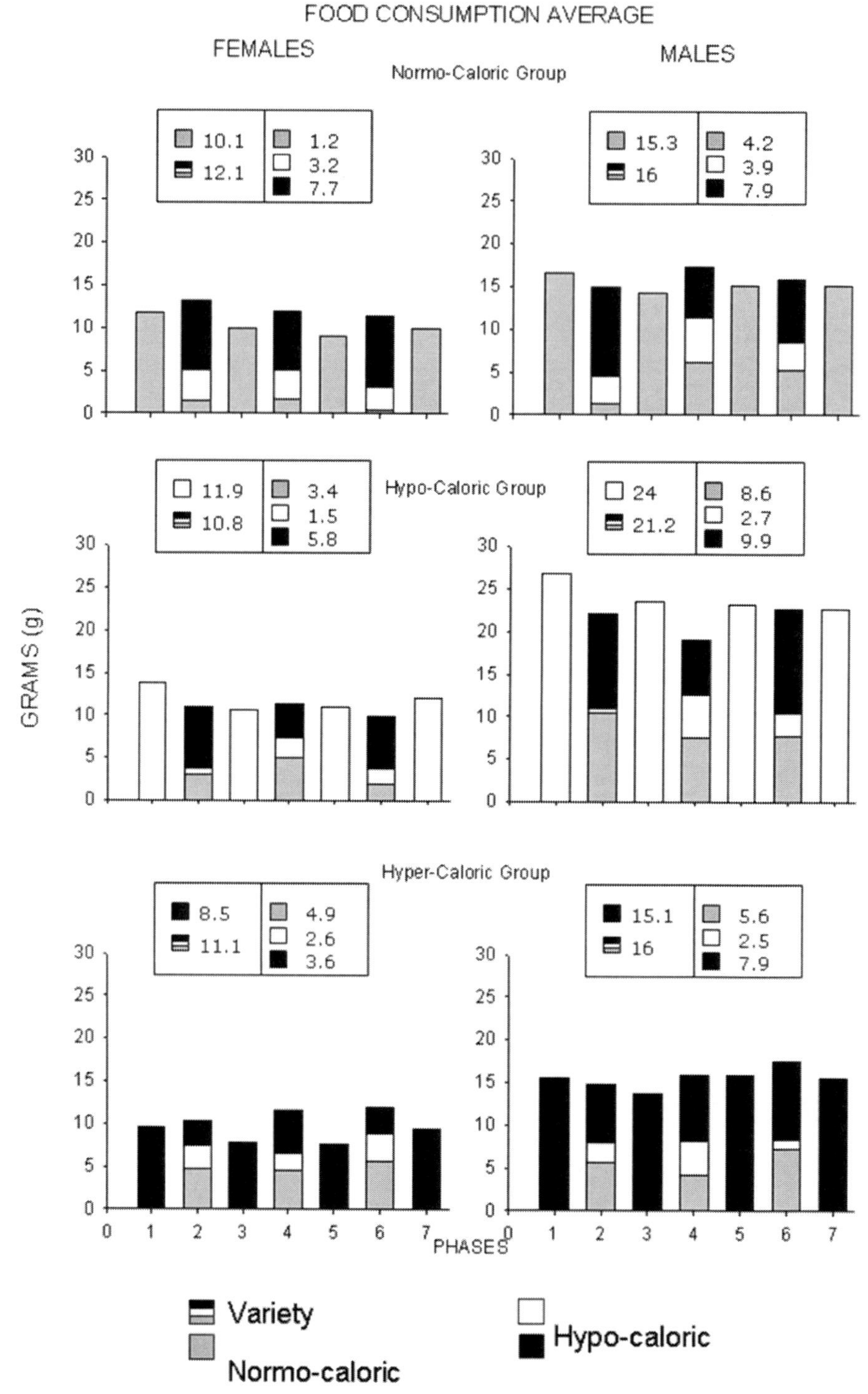

Figure 2. Averages of food consumption by females and males from Norm-Caloric, Hypo-Caloric and Hyper-Caloric Groups. Single tone bars represent phases in which only one type of diet was presented. Three toned bars show phases of exposure to variety of foods. Grey bars point out norm-caloric diet, white bars hypo-caloric diet and black bars hyper-caloric diet.

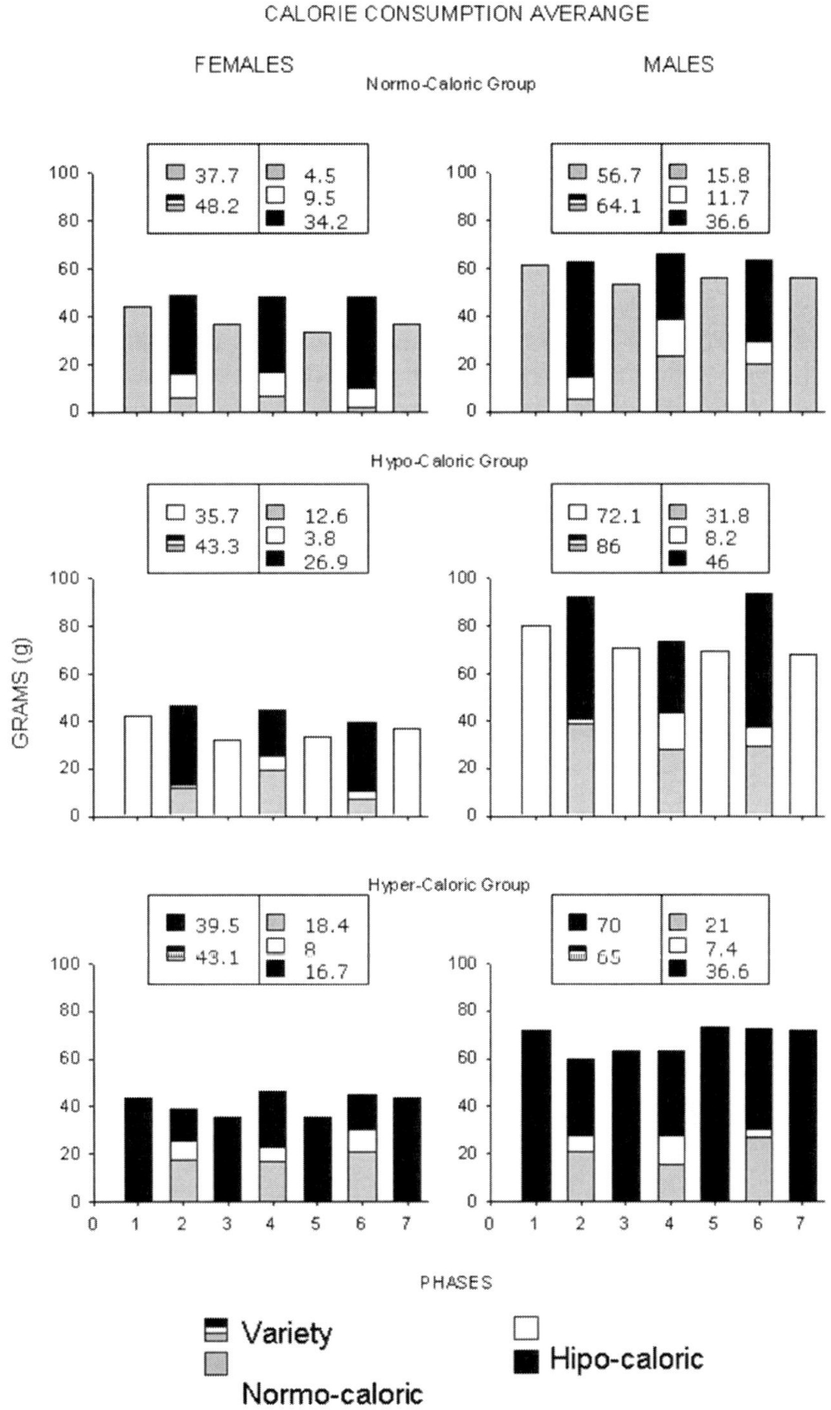

Figure 3. Averages of calorie intake in females and males from Norm-Caloric, Hypo-Caloric and Hyper-Caloric Groups. Single tone bars represent phases in which only one type of diet was presented. Three toned bars show phases of exposure to variety of foods. Grey bars point out calories from norm-caloric diet, white bars calories acquired from hypo-caloric diet and black bars calories from hyper-caloric diet.

On the other hand, males from Hypo-Caloric Group consumed an average of 24g, in comparison to males from the Norm-Caloric Group (15.3g) and males from the Hyper-Caloric Group (15.1g). Meanwhile, differences were observed in consumption of each type of diet during exposure phases to the variety of foods. During these phases, subjects in all groups showed a tendency to consume a higher quantity of hyper-caloric diet and a lesser quantity of hypo-caloric diet.

Figure 3 shows averages of consumed calories during each phase. The top panels show data for Norm-Caloric Group, central panels Hypo-Caloric Group, and bottom panels Hyper-Caloric Group. Left columns represent females and right ones males. Grey bars represent norm-caloric diet, white ones hypo-caloric diet, and black ones hyper-caloric diet. In boxes located on top part of each graph, averages of consumed calories are shown. Left side of each box shows averages of calories consumed during phases of exposure to only one type of food and to variety of foods. Right side of the box shows averages of consumed calories derived from each type of food during exposure phases to variety of foods. It is possible to observe that with the exception of the males from Hyper-Caloric Group, all subjects consumed a higher quantity of calories during phases of exposure to the variety of foods. However, difference between consumed calories during exposure phases to only one type of food and exposure phases to the variety of foods is not very noticeable, with exception of males from the Hypo-Caloric Group, that during phases of exposure to only one type of food, in wich they consumed an average of 72.1 calories, whereas during phases of exposure to variety of foods, they consumed an average of 86 calories.

Discussion

Results showed that subjects: 1) maintained a stable body weight throughout all experiment; 2) with exception of males from Hypo-Caloric Group, all other groups showed an increase in their food intake during exposure phases to the variety of foods; and 3) with exception of males from the Hyper-Caloric Group, the other groups increased their calorie intake during exposure phases to variety of foods.

Although, in general, food and calorie intake during exposure phases to variety of foods were greater than those registered during exposure phases to only one type of food, difference between both intakes is minimal, with exception of data from males in Hypo-Caloric Group. This could indicate that the subjects regulated the consumption of different types of food during exposure periods to variety of foods, consuming quantities of food and calories slightly greater than the ones they had been consuming.

Rothwell and Stock (1979) stated that regulation of caloric intake of the rats is result of a precise control in the consumption and use of energy. Keesey (1986) named this phenomenon *set point*. He pointed out that adult mammals show a tendency to preserve a stable body weight regardless of changes in type of diet and availability of food. From this, we can suggest that in our experiment, subjects regulated their food and calorie intake during periods of exposure to variety of foods, due to the fact that they did not show large increases in food and calorie intake, and did not increase their body weight.

Various authors confirmed that organisms exposed to a variety of foods showed a tendency to increase food consumption and their body weight (Armitage et al., 1983; Barber et al., 1985; McCrory, Fuss, McCallum, Yao, Vinken, Hays and Roberts, 1999; Ramírez,

1987; Raynor and Epstein, 2001). From this, we were expecting, as a result in our experiment, that experimental subjects would increase their food intake and body weight. The acquired results indicate that type of diet used probably did not favor food intake in large proportions during exposure periods to a variety of foods. In the study of Naim et al., (1985) diets were used in which the amounts of macronutrients contained in each type of food were controlled. Results showed that those subjects that were exposed to a variety of foods (with different sensory characteristics, but equal in nutritional value) consumed the same amounts of food than that of subjects exposed to a balanced diet. Naim et al., (1985) reached the conclusion that variety in the sensory characteristics such as color and flavor of foods is not a factor to favor a greater food intake. On the other hand, they pointed out that exposure to a variety of diets with different nutritional value can provoke subjects to consume large amounts of food and increase their body weight.

Even though diets offered in our study had, besides different flavors, different nutritional value, it is probable that differences in fat, carbohydrates, and proteins were not stressed enough so that subjects consumed greater quantities of food during exposure phases to variety of foods. Then again, even though subjects did not consume great amounts of food, they showed a tendency to consume *a little more* food during exposure to variety, in comparison with phases in which only one type of food was provided. This may be due to phenomenon of *specific sensory satiation*, in which an animal will stop consuming food it had been consuming, but will consume those it had not tried when a variety of foods is available with different characteristics (Hetherington and Rolls, 1992; Rolls, 1990).

On the other hand, the history of exposure to a determined diet could have influenced in consumption of different types of diet during exposure to variety of foods. During these phases, subjects consumed different amounts of each type of diet. A tendency to consume a higher amount of hyper-caloric diet (with exception of females from Hyper-Caloric Group) and a lesser amount of hypo-caloric diet was observed.

Particularly, females from Hypo-Caloric Group consumed a minimal amount of hypo-caloric diet (1.5g on average), this in comparison to consumptions of females in Norm-Caloric Group (3.2g) and females from Hyper-Caloric Group (2.6g). Furthermore, differences between food and calorie intake during exposure periods to variety of foods were shown. Particularly, subjects in Hypo-Caloric Group consumed a lesser amount of food but a greater amount of calories, during exposure phases to variety of foods. On the other hand, males from Hyper-Caloric Group consumed a greater quantity of food, but a lesser amount of calories, during exposure phases to variety of foods.

Warwick and Synowski (1999), Warwick, Synowski and Bell (1999) and Warwick, Synowski, Rice and Smart (2003) stated that diets with a higher content of fat are consumed in a greater proportion rather than diets with a high carbohydrate content, despite of caloric density in food. The hyper-caloric diet used in this experiment had a high content in fat (25.2%) in comparison to norm-caloric (14.3%) and hypo-caloric (8.1%) diets. This could explain why the hyper-caloric diet was consumed in greater quantities then other diets during exposure periods to a variety of foods. However, Bensaïd et al., (2002) pointed out that foods with high protein content have an effect of a higher satiety than that of carbohydrates; thus, more protein a food has, effect of produced satiety will be greater. Hypo-caloric diet contained a higher percentage of proteins (27.6%) in comparison to other diets. This could account for the decrease in food intake by subjects in Hypo-Caloric Group during exposure periods to a variety of foods. Furthermore, it is likely that large food intakes registered by

Hypo-Caloric Group during exposure phases to only one type of diet (in this case, hypo-caloric) are due to needs the subjects had to compensate for the amounts of protein required (White, Porter and Martin, 2000).

Lastly, we can confirm that, in our experiment, subjects did not consume great quantities of food during exposure period to a variety of foods, regardless of type of diet the subjects had been consuming. This may indicate that in study carried out by López-Espinoza, et al. (2011) large food consumptions during exposure to a variety of diets were due to food deprivation and not so much to presence of a variety of foods. The aforementioned points out the need to carry out other studies in which diets should be used with more stressed nutritional differences, and with different sensory characteristics (flavor, color), without exposing the experimental subjects to food deprivation during the post-deprivation period.

REFERENCES

Armitage, G., Hervey, G. R., Rolls, B. J., Rowe, E. A. and Tobin, G. (1983). The effects of supplementation of the diet with highly palatable foods upon energy balance in the rat. *Journal of Physiology, 342*, 229-251.

Barber, T., Viña, J. R., Viña, J. and Cabo, J. (1985). Decreased urea synthesis in cafeteria-diet-induced obesity in the rat. *Biochemical Journal, 230*, 675-681.

Bensaïd, A., Tomé, D., Gietzen, D., Even, P., Morens, C., Gausseres, N. and Fromentin, G. (2002). Protein is more potent than carbohydrate for reducing appetite in rats. *Physiology and Behavior, 75*, 577-582.

Galindo, A. and López-Espinoza, A. (2006). Efectos del sabor y del contenido calórico del agua sobre la conducta alimentaria durante un período de privación de comida en ratas albinas. *Revista Mexicana de Análisis de la Conducta, 32*, 95-109.

Hetherington, M. M. and Rolls, B. J. (1992). Sensory-specific satiety: theoretical frameworks and central characteristics. In E. D. Capaldi (Ed). *Why we eat, What we eat.* USA: American Psychological Association, 267-290.

Johnson, J. and Vickers, Z. (1993). Effects of flavor and macronutrient composition of food servings on liking, hunger and subsequent intake. *Appetite, 21*, 25-39.

Keesey, R. E. (1986). A set-point theory of obesity. In K. D. Brownell and J. P. Foreyt (Eds.), *Handbook of eating disorders.* (pp. 63-87) New York: Basic Books., Publishers.

López-Espinoza, A., Galindo, K., Martínez A. G., Franco, F., Aguilera, V., Cárdenas-Villalvazo, A., Valdés, E., Magaña, C. and Santoyo, F. (2011). Effects of variety of foods on feeding behavior during post-deprivation period. *International Journal of Hispanic Psychology. 4, (3)*

López-Espinoza, A. and Martínez, H. (2001). Efectos de dos programas de privación parcial sobre el peso corporal y el consumo total de agua y comida en ratas. *Acta Comportamentalia, 9*, 5-17.

López-Espinoza, A. and Martínez, H. (2004). Cambios en el patrón alimentario como efecto de la privación de agua o alimento en ratas en crecimiento. *International Journal of Psychology and Psychological Therapy, 4*, 93-104.

Martínez, A. G. and López-Espinoza, A. (2007). Efectos post-privación con dos alternativas energéticas en ratas. *Revista Mexicana de Análisis de la Conducta, 33*, 1, 43-59.

Martínez, A. G., López-Espinoza, A. and Martínez, H. (2006). Efectos de modificar el contenido energético del agua sobre el peso corporal, consumo de agua, alimento y calorías en ratas. *Universitas Psychology, 5*, 12, 361-370.

McCrory, M. A., Fuss, P. J., McCallum, J. E., Yao, M., Vinken, A. G., Hays, N. P. and Roberts, S. B. (1999). Dietary variety within food groups: association with energy intake and body fatness in men and women. *American Journal of Clinical Nutrition, 69*, 440-447.

Moore, B. J. (1987). The cafeteria diet-an inappropriate tool for studies of thermogenesis. *Journal of Nutrition, 117*, 227-231.

Naim, M., Brand, J. G., Kare, M. R. and Carpenter, R. G. (1985). Energy intake, weight gain and fat deposition in rats fed flavored, nutritionally controlled diets in a multichoice ("Cafetería") design. *Journal of Nutrition, 115,* 1447-1458.

Ramírez, I. (1987). Feeding a liquid diet increases energy intake, weight gain and body fat in rats. *Journal of Nutrition,117*, 2127-2134.

Raynor, H. A. and Epstein, L. H. (2001). Dietary variety, energy regulation, and obesity. *Psychological Bulletin, 127*, 3, 325-341.

Rolls (1990). The role of sensory-specific satiety in food intake and food selection. In E. D. Capaldi, and T. L. Powley (Eds.). *Taste, experience and feeding: Development and learning*. USA: American Psychological Association, 197-209.

Rothwell, N. J. and Stock, M. J. (1979). Regulation of energy balance in two models of reversible obesity in the rat. *Journal of Comparative and Physiological Psychology, 93*, 6, 1024-1034.

Rothwell, N. J. and Stock, M. J. (1988). The cafeteria diet as a tool for studies of thermogenesis. *Journal of Nutrition, 118*, 925-928.

Treit, D., Spetch, M. L. and Deutsch, J. A. (1983). Variety in the flavor of food enhances eating in the rat: a controlled demonstration. *Physiology and Behavior, 30*, 207-211.

Warwick, Z. S. and Synowski, S. J. (1999). Effect of food deprivation and maintenance diet composition on fat preference and acceptance in rats. *Physiology and Behavior, 68,* 235-239.

Warwick, Z. S., Synowski, S. J. and Bell, K. R. (1999). Dietary fat content affects energy intake and weight gain independent of diet caloric density in rats. *Physiology and Behavior, 77,* 85-90.G.

Warwick, Z. S., Synowski, S. J., Rice, K. D. and Smart, A. B. (2003). Independent effects of diet palatability and fat content on bout size and daily intake in rats. *Physiology and Behavior, 80,* 253-258.

White, B. D., Porter, M. H. and Martin, R. J. (2000). Protein selection, food intake, and body composition in response to the amount of dietary protein. *Physiology and Behavior, 69*, 383-389.

In: Recent Hispanic Psychological Research … ISBN: 978-1-62948-919-3
Editors: C. H. Garcia Cadena, A. Lopez-Espinoza et al.

Chapter 9

TOURISM ECOLOGIES, ALCOHOL VENUES, AND HIV: MAPPING SPATIAL RISK*

Vincent Guilamo-Ramos*†, *Mark Padilla, Leah Meisterlin, Katharine McCarthy and Kevin Lotz
Silver School of Social Work, and Center for Latino Adolescent and Family Health
New York University, US
University of Michigan School of Public Health
Center for Latino Adolescent and Family Health
New York University, US

ABSTRACT

Tourism areas are increasingly characterized as environments of increased HIV risk. Alcohol venues located in tourism areas have been implicated in facilitating HIV transmission; however few studies have spatially characterized alcohol venues and their potential relationship with elevated HIV risk. The limited attention to how HIV transmission is facilitated by social and spatial aspects of alcohol venues warrants further attention. We systematically assessed the social, spatial and behavioral characteristics of alcohol venues in a Dominican tourism town. A venue-based survey was completed for 135 alcohol venues located within the targeted area. Additionally, we employed geographic information systems (GIS) to spatially describe the venues in relation to HIV risk factors.

Results suggest the Sosúa tourism area is characterized by: 1) a high concentration of alcohol venues; 2) widespread population mixing between risk groups; 3) spatial co-occurrence of alcohol venues, sexual commerce, and drug transactions, and 4) low availability of HIV prevention services.

Our results suggest alcohol venues should be targeted for HIV prevention efforts in Dominican tourism areas. Data underscore the importance of context in shaping individual risk behavior. HIV prevention interventions and policies should consider the broader social dynamics of alcohol venues and target such venues for structural interventions.

---

* This research was supported by National Institute on Alcohol Abuse and Alcoholism (Grant No. R21AA018078).

† Corresponding author: Silver School of Social Work, New York University. 1 Washington Square North. New York, NY 10003-6654 (R321). E-Mail: vincent.ramos@nyu.edu.

Keywords: Tourism Ecologies, HIV Risk, Alcohol Venues, Spatial Risk

INTRODUCTION

The Caribbean has the world's highest regional HIV/AIDS prevalence outside of Sub-Saharan Africa, with 1.0% (0.9%-1.1%) of the adult general population living with the disease (UNAIDS, 2010). Despite the disproportionate concentration of disease burden in the region, the Caribbean has not received adequate public health attention in the global response to HIV/AIDS (Editorial, 2008). The primary mode of HIV transmission in the Caribbean is via sexual behavior, fueled, in part, by well-established risk factors including sexual commerce, sex between men, and drug use (UNAIDS, 2010).

While a recent report suggests that the HIV prevalence in the Caribbean is declining (Halperin, de Moya, Perez-Then, Papas, and García Callejas, 2009), findings from across the region indicate that HIV rates remain unacceptably high among at-risk populations engaging in these behaviors. Rates of HIV infection among female sex workers in the region, for example, have been documented as 9% in Jamaica and 27% in Guyana. HIV infection levels among men who have sex with men are estimated to be as high as 20% in Trinidad and Tobago, where one in four men who have sex with men also regularly engage in sex with women, and 32% in Jamaica. Furthermore, in Bermuda and Puerto Rico, injection drug use has contributed substantially to the HIV epidemic, accounting for 40% of new infections among men in Puerto Rico and 27% among women (UNAIDS, 2010). One underlying factor unique to the Caribbean and related to each of these drivers of the epidemic is tourism. Tourism areas of the Caribbean have been previously described as distinct risk ecologies facilitating HIV transmission (Padilla, Guilamo-Ramos, and Godbole, 2012), yet remain understudied by the HIV prevention science literature. One country particularly noted for its booming tourism economy and which, together with Haiti on the island of Hispaniola, accounts for 70% of the disease burden in the region, is the Dominican Republic (UNAIDS, 2010).

The Dominican Republic is an internationally known tourism destination (Brennan, 2004; León, 2007). The Caribbean Tourism Organization (CTO) estimates that 4,117,598 tourists entered the Dominican Republic in 2012, more than any other Caribbean country in 2012 (CTO, 2012). The majority of these visitors stem from countries with high rates of infection such as the United States (30%), Canada (16%), Germany, (4%), the United Kingdom (4%), and other European countries (20%) (CTO, 2011; UNAIDS, 2010). These data are worrisome as regional mapping of HIV prevalence in the Dominican Republic demonstrates that regions with the greatest tourism development are most heavily impacted by HIV (CESDEM, 2003). This variation in disease burden may be due, in part, to the presence of high-prevalence most at-risk populations (MARPs) such as female sex workers (4.8%), men who have sex with men —MSM (6.1%), injection drug users (8.0%) and Haitian sugar cane workers (4.7%) which tend to cluster via geographic location (Padilla, Guilamo-Ramos, Bouris, and Reyes, 2010; UNAIDS, 2010). Research on HIV risk in tourism areas has also documented a high frequency of risky sexual exchanges between tourists and locals engaged both formally (i.e., hotel and resort employees) and informally (i.e., sex workers) in the tourism industry, which has significant implications for the spread of HIV (Forsythe, Hasbun, Butler de Lister, 1998; Kerrigan, Ellen, Moreno, Rosario, Katz, Celentano et al., 2003; Padilla, 2007; Padilla et al.,

2010; Padilla, Guilamo-Ramos et al., 2012; Padilla, Reyes, Connolly, Natsui, Puello, and Chapman, 2011). The transcontinental linkage between the Dominican Republic and other high HIV prevalence countries in conjunction with sexual exchanges between tourists and locals suggests population mixing may be an important factor facilitating HIV transmission in the Caribbean that warrants further attention.

A defining feature of tourism implicated in facilitating risk behavior is the wide availability and high consumption of alcohol (Padilla, Guilamo-Ramos, and Godbole, 2012). The ubiquitous presence of alcohol in Caribbean tourism areas stems largely from the heavy investments of transnational alcohol companies in Caribbean tourism markets (Parry, 2000; Room and Jernigan, 2000). Related to the increase in the availability of alcohol is the recorded rise in alcohol consumption in Caribbean countries. In the Dominican Republic, for example, the estimated liters of pure alcohol consumed per person aged 15 and older increased from 1.18 liters to 6.11 liters between 1961 and 2005. Of those aged 15 and older who drink alcohol, males consume an estimated 12.54 liters of pure alcohol per year and women an estimated 8.13 liters per year (WHO, 2011). The expanded presence of alcohol and alcohol venues in Caribbean tourism areas has important implications for HIV risk, as there is a strong documented association between alcohol consumption and HIV infection (Baliunas, Rehm, Irving, and Shuper, 2010).

Alcohol consumption influences HIV risk through behavioral pathways such as increased behavioral disinhibition which leads to sexual risk-taking (Abbey, Parkhill, Buck, and Saenz, 2007; Curtin and Fairchild, 2003) and reduced patient adherence to antiretroviral medication (Hendershot, Stoner, Pantalone, and Simoni, 1999). Alcohol may also influence biological pathways such as the immune response, which can not only impair the body's defenses to HIV infection (Hahn, Woolf-King, and Muyindike, 2011; Pandrea, Happel, Amedee, Bagby, and Nelson, 2010) but may also accelerate disease progression.

Despite the established link between alcohol use and HIV risk as well as the demonstrated availability and consumption of alcohol in Caribbean tourism areas, less understood is how the overall context of alcohol venues contributes to HIV risk. Some evidence evaluating alcohol serving establishments in South Africa (Kalichman, Simbayi, Vermaak, Jooste, and Cain, 2008), Southern India (Go, Solomon, Srikrishnan, Sivaram, Johnson, Sripaipan et al., 2007), and Zimbabwe (Fritz, Woelk, Bassett, McFarland, Routh, Tobaiwa et al., 2002) suggest a higher prevalence of HIV risk behaviors in alcohol settings. These behaviors are often facilitated by alcohol business norms and practices, such as providing private rooms for customers to engage in commercial and transactional sex (Fritz et al., 2002; Morojele, Kachieng'a, Mokoko, Nkoko, Parry, Nkowane et al., 2006). However, more evidence is needed to explore how the spatial and behavioral dimensions of alcohol venues influence HIV risk behavior in Caribbean tourism areas. The dearth of research in this area limits the ability to effectively design prevention interventions in tourism areas classified as having disproportionate disease burden. Given the vast numbers of tourists converging in alcohol venues of Caribbean tourism areas annually, the lack of attention to tourism areas as unique ecologies of risk has global public health implications for both the local population as well as foreign nationals returning to their country of origin.

The purpose of the current study was to characterize the social and spatial dimensions of alcohol venues with the overall aim of describing the HIV risk ecology of a Dominican tourism town. In order to achieve this aim, we used anethnographic mapping approach consisting of both geographic analysis and a survey of venue key informants to systematically characterize the spatial, social and behavioral characteristics of alcohol venues of Sosúa, Dominican Republic.

METHOD

Contexts and Scenarios

Phase 1 of the 2-phase research strategy used an ethnographic mapping process which involved canvassing Sosúa to document the locations of alcohol venues. Using a printed reference map, each street of the town was canvassed, yielding a final count of 135 venues. These venues included all alcohol-serving businesses such as bars, cabanas, nightclubs, discos, and *colmadones* (liquor stores where liquor could be consumed on site).

At each venue, latitude and longitude coordinates were recorded using handheld global positioning system (GPS) devices. The coordinates were compiled into a single database for later geographic information systems (GIS) analysis. Using ESRI's ArcGIS software, the database was visualized by plotting the GPS coordinates. Given the relatively small area of Sosúa and the point-level data (each venue is described by a point on the map), simple descriptive spatial statistics were used to measure the geographic distribution of the venues with the software's built-in tools.

To understand the spatial organization of alcohol venues in Sosúa, directional distribution (standard deviational) ellipses were calculated around the venues' mean center. Much like traditional statistics, the mean center describes the mean latitude and longitude coordinates calculated from the locations of all recorded venues. The directional distribution describes a spatial equivalent to the standard deviation about the mean for the data points.

Procedures and Assessment

After spatially mapping the alcohol venues using the GIS activities of phase 1, a research team member visited each venue and conducted one hour of participant observation to record the characteristics of the type of venue (i.e., bar, hotel nightclub, etc.), peak business days and times, and to identify an ideal key informant.

The key informant was a designated staff person of the venue who served as a point person to complete a brief, cross-sectional survey related to characteristics of the venue's clientele, the types of social interactions, including transactional exchanges, and the presence of HIV prevention services. These indicators were derived and adapted from a recent rapid assessment tool developed to identify areas where HIV transmission is most likely to occur and to direct local AIDS prevention and care efforts (MEASURE Evaluation, 2005).

These data enabled the generation of a comprehensive map of alcohol venues in Sosúa, geocoded with on-going HIV risk activities, such as drug activity, commercial and transactional sex, and where most at-risk populations such as MSM, Haitians, and sex workers were likely to converge. Informed consent was obtained from all key informants prior to participation and participants were offered 350 pesos, approximately U.S. $10 dollars. Institutional approval was obtained prior to conducting the study.

RESULTS

Descriptive Statistics

Spatial analysis of alcohol venues in Sosúa reveal a high density of alcohol venues concentrated within a small geographic area. Specifically, analysis of the directional distribution (standard deviational) ellipses around the venues' mean center in Figure 1 reflects that the majority of venues (92 of 135 venues; 68%) are concentrated within 0.86 square kilometers of the first directional ellipse. The second distribution contains 132 venues within 3.69 square kilometers and finally, all but one venue was contained within the third distribution. Overlaying the spatial organization of alcohol venues with the geography of the town of Sosúa, the vast majority of venues concentrated along the linear strip in the first ellipse are situated along the central beach. In terms of the Sosúa community, the beach and adjacent area to the north is the tourist region known as El Batey. Distinct from this area and to the south of the central area of the beach is the Sosúa community of Charamicos, where the local population primarily resides. Taken together, these data reflect a dense number of alcohol venues within the small area of Sosúa and particularly clustered along the central beach strip in the tourist area of El Batey.

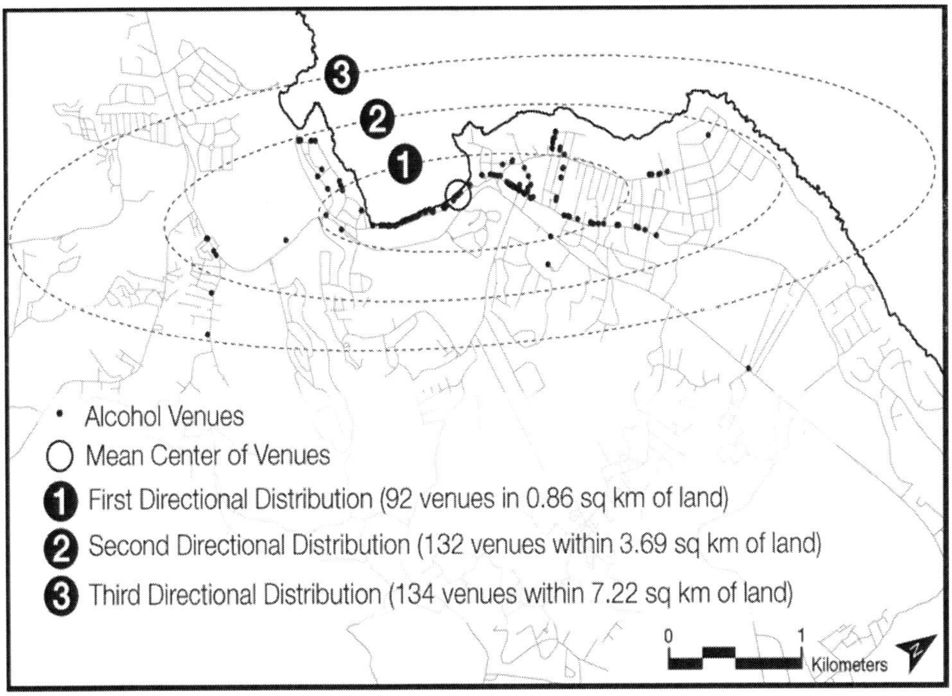

Figure 1. Distribution of Alcohol Venues in Sosúa, Dominican Republic.

Alcohol Venue Clientele

Central to HIV transmission dynamics are the types of populations who are interacting and their respective HIV risk. Figure 2 describes the distribution of five categories of Sosúa alcohol venue customers: tourists, sex workers (i.e. chicas, sankies, and bugarrones), people who buy drugs, gay men and Haitians.

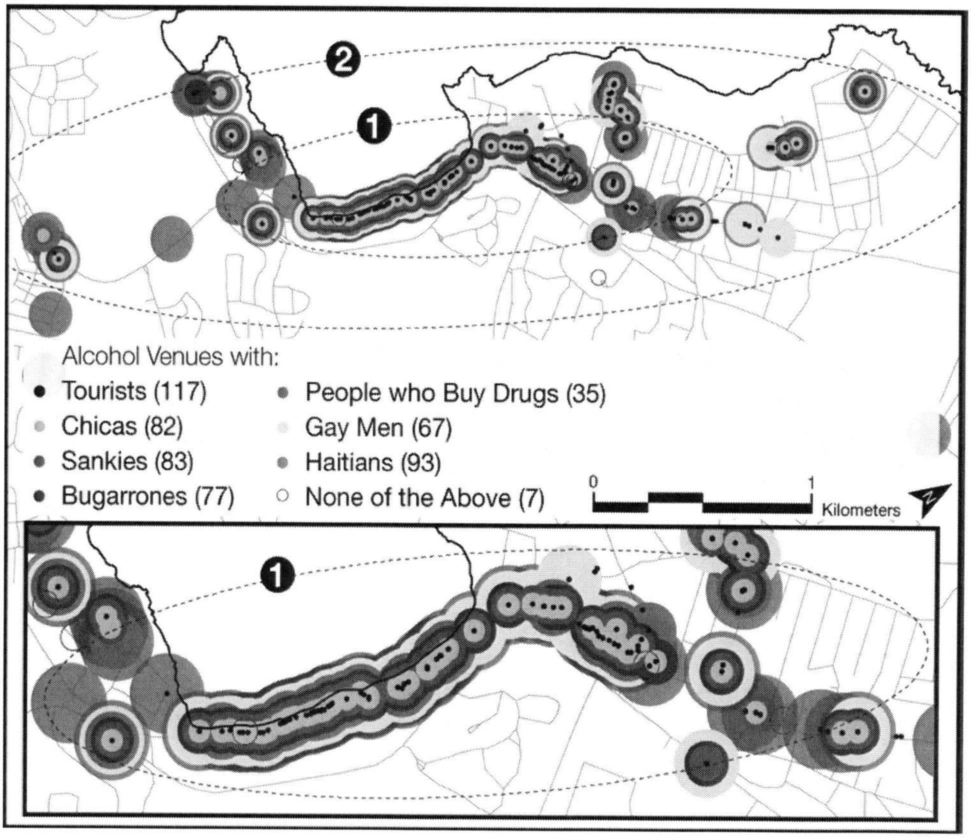

Figure 2. High Prevalence Population Mixing in Alcohol Venues.

The most common types of venue clientele are tourists, sex workers, and Haitians. Specifically, the vast majority of alcohol venues (117 of 135 venues; 87%) are frequented by tourists and more than half of venues are frequented by at least one type of sex worker, either female sex workers —chicas (82; 61%), male sex workers who have sex primarily with women —sankies (83; 61%), or male sex workers who have sex primarily with men —bugarrones (77; 57%). Haitians also visit a large number of venues (93; 69%) and largely mix with both tourists and sex workers. To a lesser degree, people who buy drugs also visit alcohol venues (35; 26%). As previously noted, sex workers, men who have sex with men, drug users, and Haitians in the Dominican Republic experience elevated rates of HIV infection (UNAIDS, 2010). Taken together, these data demonstrate that alcohol venues in Sosúa —particularly those situated along the beach in the tourist region of El Batey— are the locus of population mixing among high-risk groups. These data highlight the potential for HIV transmission as highly HIV burdened local populations come into contact with tourists. In contrast, only 7 of the 135 alcohol venues in Sosúa are characterized as not having any of the above risk groups, suggesting these venues cater to local patrons. These venues are also largely located in the local residential community of Charamicos, further supporting their characterization as local venues. These data suggest a dichotomy of alcohol venues in Sosúa:

those characterized by high risk population mixing in the tourism area of El Batey, and those frequented predominately by locals in the local community of Charamicos.

Alcohol Venue High Risk Interactions: Tourists and People Who Buy Sex

In addition to describing population mixing among alcohol venue clientele, we describe the nature of high risk group interaction. One major driver of the Dominican HIV epidemic is risky sexual exchanges, such as commercial and transactional sex. Figure 3 provides data related to the degree and type of population in demand for commercial and transactional sex by describing the spatial correspondence between tourists and people who buy sex in Sosúa alcohol venues. Seventy-four (55%) of the alcohol venues in Sosúa are locations where people buy sex, suggesting these venues may have either formal or informal sex work available on site. Notably, 73 of venues with customers who buy sex (99%) are also venues frequented by tourists. The high degree of overlap between people who buy sex and tourists demonstrates that tourists frequent venues where sex sells and suggests that individuals who buy sex are often tourists. This correlation further supports the characterization of tourism areas of the Dominican Republic as international destinations for sex tourism and hence high risk ecologies for HIV transmission.

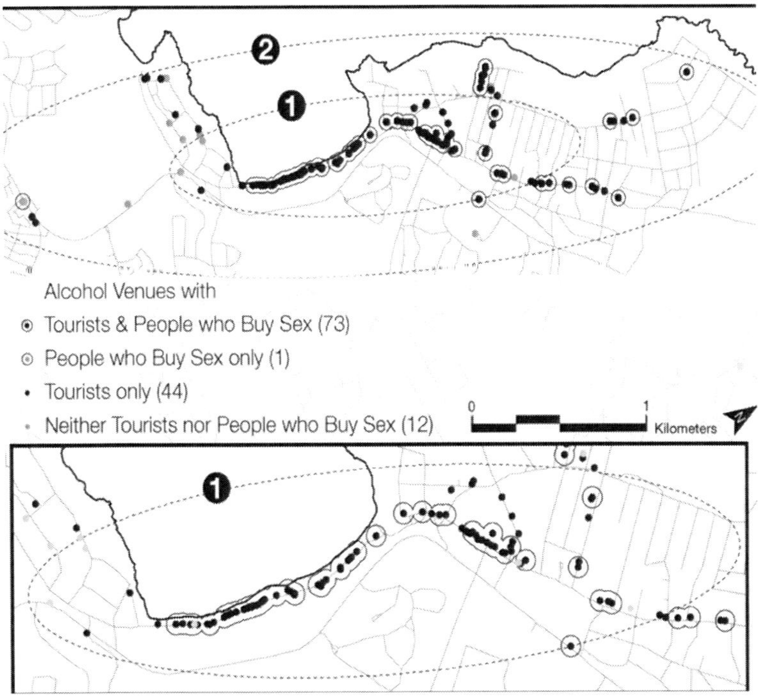

Figure 3. Tourists and People who Buy Sex in Alcohol Venues of Sosúa.

Alcohol Venue High Risk Interactions: People Who Buy Drugs and People Who Buy Sex

In addition to the correspondence between sexual commerce and tourism, we also describe the simultaneous engagement in sex and drug-related transactions in Sosúa alcohol venues (Figure 4). Our data reveal that following alcohol sales, sexual commerce is the main transaction in Sosúa, occurring in 71 (53%) venues. A substantial number of alcohol venues (27; 38%) where patrons can buy sex are also venues where patrons can buy both illicit drugs as well as sex. These data demonstrate that although sex-related transactions are most common, sexual commerce spatially corresponds to drug-related transactions. A notable exception to this trend is alcohol venues where drug exchanges are the primary transaction. Specifically, the 8 venues where patrons can buy drugs only are predominately located in the local community of Charamicos. Moreover, sexual commerce was documented in only one alcohol venue located in Charamicos. This contrasts greatly with the tourism area of El Batey where all places where drugs are available for purchase are also locations where sex is available for purchase.

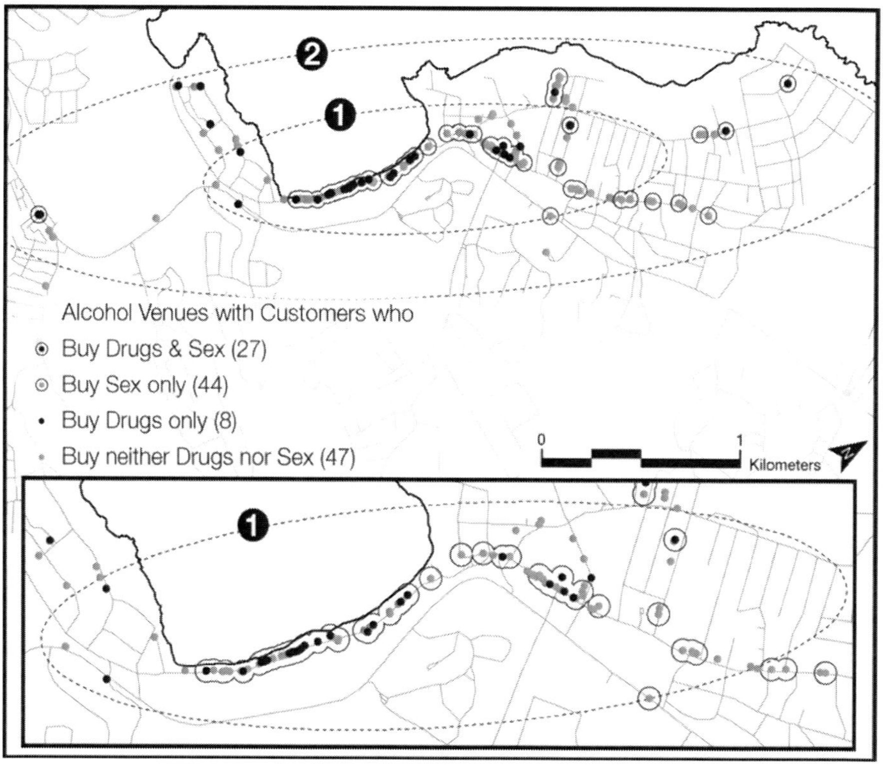

Figure 4. People who Buy Drugs and Sex in Alcohol Venues of Sosúa.

HIV Prevention Activities in Alcohol Venues

Another key indicator of HIV risk is the availability of HIV prevention activities in venues, described in Figure 5. More than half of Sosúa alcohol venues (69; 51%) have sex work available on site; the majority of which (60; 87%) do not have condoms available on the premise. Nine venues with sexual commerce on site (13%) did have condoms available for customers. All but one of these venues was located in El Batey. Interestingly, a greater number of venues with no documented sexual commerce had condom availability (16; 26%) compared to venues with on-going sex work. A small number, 6 venues, offered HIV prevention activities on site. For the purposes of this study, HIV prevention activities were defined broadly to include any form of risk education, health check-ups for sex workers, available HIV testing or referrals, or condom availability, for free or purchase. Of these venues, one had no documented sex work. Overall, these data reveal that HIV prevention resources are not directed to areas of need and the vast majority of alcohol venues with on-going sex work have no available prevention services.

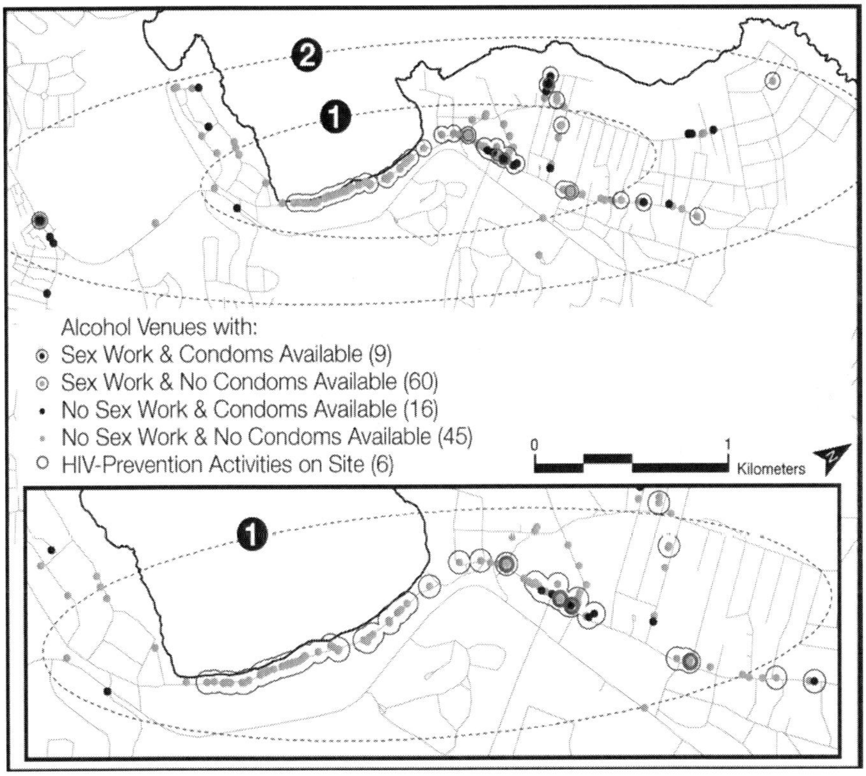

Figure 5. Sex work and HIV-Prevention Activities in Alcohol Venues of Sosúa.

DISCUSSION

The overall aim of the current study was to describe the ecological context of alcohol venues in a Caribbean tourism town. We focus on key indicators of HIV transmission: population mixing among high risk groups, transactional exchanges between high risk groups, and the availability of HIV prevention services. Our data demonstrate that alcohol venues in tourism areas are unique contexts facilitative of HIV transmission. Specifically, we document a high density of alcohol venues within a small geographic area. These venues are characterized not only by a heavy concentration of population mixing among most at-risk groups, but also a high degree of high risk interactions among venue clientele. The most common high risk interaction in Sosúa, apart from the sale of alcohol, is transactional sexual exchanges, which occur in more than half of Sosúa venues. Venues characterized by customers looking to buy sex are predominately located in the tourist community of El Batey and are heavily frequented by tourists. Most worrisome is the relative lack of HIV preventative services at alcohol venues with customers seeking to engage in sexual exchanges.

Our data also reveal a distinct spatial dichotomy between the presence of high risk groups, risky transactions, and HIV prevention services among alcohol venues by community geography. Specifically, high rates of population mixing and sexual commerce characterize alcohol venues in the tourism region of El Batey. In contrast, the setting of Charamicos has a less dense concentration of alcohol venues and several venues are not frequented by any high risk group. Furthermore, venues in Charamicos in general do not have sexual commerce, but do have on-going drug transactions. These data highlight the importance of environmental context, as drinking in each setting exposes individuals to different risks. Therefore, it is the alcohol environment in which an individual is embedded that influences to which risks an individual is exposed. For example, locals in Charamicos are more likely to be exposed to risks associated with drug-related transactions while tourists in El Batey are more likely to be exposed to unprotected sexual exchanges. Local policymakers and public health practitioners should utilize knowledge of where high rates of unprotected transactional sex or drug exchanges are likely to occur to prioritize the availability of condoms and other HIV prevention services at venues where resources are most needed.

A notable limitation to the current study is that our data result from preliminary work that is solely descriptive in nature. As such, we make no formal classifications of high or low risk alcohol venues and we do not examine the relationship between the alcohol environment and health outcomes. Additional work is needed to categorize and cluster types of venues frequented by high risk groups or characterized by high risk behaviors to determine where these factors overlap as "hot spots" facilitative of HIV transmission. Furthermore, we are limited in our ability to make statements about venues with on-site drug exchanges, as we only collected data on venue patrons seeking to buy drugs and thus can only infer that these transactions are likely to take place in venues. Additionally, we collected no data on types of drugs bought or methods of use and as such cannot make inferences about the presence or absence of injection-drug users in alcohol venues. However, our data do highlight that context matters. Specifically, we show that the contextual environment of alcohol venues links individuals with risk factors for HIV transmission by providing opportunities for population mixing and risky interactions with high risk groups. These data suggest that alcohol-based HIV prevention efforts that are limited to the level of the individual are inadequate. Future HIV prevention interventions and policies should account for the social and contextual environment that shapes individual behavior.

In sum, we describe how the ecological context of alcohol venues in a tourism town potentially facilitates HIV risk behavior. Most notably, we observe a relative lack of available condoms or HIV prevention services in alcohol venues with on-going sexual exchanges and which are heavily frequented by tourists, suggesting local policymakers should prioritize condom availability in venues characterized by sexual commerce. While previous findings established in the literature have found such interventions to increase condom use among female sex workers in the Dominican Republic can be efficacious in reducing sexual risk behavior (Kerrigan et al., 2003), a prior review of HIV prevention efforts in Caribbean tourism areas found a relative lack of long-term HIV prevention programs in the region. The absence of sustainable prevention programs constitutes a major barrier to addressing the relationship between tourism and HIV in the Caribbean (Padilla, Reyes et al., 2011).

Based on our findings highlighting the importance of addressing the alcohol environment in which an individual is embedded, we advocate for the adoption of multi-level interventions encompassing not only individual level behavior but also the structure of the venue itself and the social dynamics of the larger community to enhance the sustainability and long-term impact of HIV prevention interventions targeting alcohol environments (Scribner, Theall, Simonsen, and Robinson, 2010). For example, Padilla, Reyes et al., highlight neighborhood level societal norms among tourism officials who view HIV prevention efforts as potentially harmful to the industry due to the perception that tourists may find such programs alarming and avoid vacationing in a known environment of risk, as an obstacle to long-term implementation of HIV prevention programs (Padilla, Reyes et al., 2011). To address this barrier, HIV interventions to increase the availability of condoms could be implemented in conjunction with venue employee and tourism management education about the potential benefits of the policy on the tourism industry, thus reframing societal norms related to alcohol and HIV in tourism areas to engender a beneficial view of HIV prevention for the tourism industry. Such an image could be achieved, for example, by educating managers on the potential for economic gain if tourists' perception of alcohol venues as "safe" led to an increased number of customers. Ultimately, we suggest that intervention programs designed to increase condom availability in tourism venues should be integrated with long-term policy approaches that address not only individual behavior, but the social and environmental context of alcohol venues in order to enhance program efficacy as well as long-term sustainable impact of prevention programming.

CONCLUSION

Lack of knowledge on the role of alcohol venues in HIV transmission hampers the effectiveness of prevention interventions, potentially escalating the HIV epidemic in high risk areas. Our data suggest that alcohol venues may be appropriate targets for HIV prevention efforts in tourism areas, as these are locations where HIV transmission risk factors converge and an at-risk audience can be reached. Specifically, we document the spatial locations of alcohol venues where at-risk behavior is likely to occur. While future research is needed to formally categorize the risk typology of alcohol venues in Sosúa to better inform HIV prevention policies and interventions, our findings are of utility to local policymakers and prevention scientists to direct local HIV prevention efforts to areas of need. In order to enhance prevention program sustainability and long-term impact, future prevention programs should address the social and environmental context of alcohol venues in addition to individual level behavior.

REFERENCES

[Editorial] (2008). HIV/AIDS in Latin America and the Caribbean. *The Lancet, 372 (9635),* 263.

Abbey, A., Parkhill, M.R., Buck, P.O., and Saenz, C. (2007). Condom use with a casual partner: What distinguishes college student's use when intoxicated? *Psychology of Addictive Behaviors, 21,* 76-83.

Baliunas, D., Rehm, Jr. I.H., and Shuper, P. (2010). Alcohol consumption and risk of incident human immunodeficiency virus infection: a meta-analysis. *International Journal of Public Health, 55,* 159-166.

Brennan, D. (2004). *What's love got to do with it?: transnational desires and sex tourism in the Dominican Republic.* Durham, NC: Duke University Press.

Caribbean Tourism Organization (CTO) (2012). *Latest statistics 2012.* En Internet: http://www.onecaribbean.org/content/files/JAN28Lattab12.pdf. [Accessed 15/ March/ 2013].

Caribbean Tourism Organization (CTO) (2011). *Latest tourism statistics: Dominican Republic.* En Internet: www.onecaribbean.org/statistics/tourismstats. [Accessed 15/March/ 2012].

Centro de Estudios Sociales y Demográficos (CESDEM) [República Dominicana] 2002. República Dominicana: Encuesta demográfica y de salud (ENDESA 2002). Informe Preliminar Sobre VIH/SIDA. Santo Domingo, República Dominicana: CESDEM.

Curtin, J.J. and Fairchild, B.A. (2003). Alcohol and cognitive control: Implications for regulation of behavior during response conflict. *Journal of Abnormal Psychology, 112,* 424-436.

Forsythe, S., Hasbun, J. and Butler de Lister, M. (1998). Protecting paradise: tourism and AIDS in the Dominican Republic. *Health Policy Planning, 13,* 277-286.

Fritz, K.E., Woelk, G.B., Bassett, M.T., McFarland, W.C., Routh, J.A., Tobaiwa, O., et al. (2002). The association between alcohol use, sexual risk behavior, and HIV infection among men attending beerhalls in Harare, Zimbabwe. *AIDS and Behavior, 6,* 221-228.

Go, V.F., Solomon, S., Srikrishnan, A.K., Sivaram, S., Johnson, S.C., Sripaipan, T., et al. (1999). HIV rates and risk behaviors are low in the general population of males in South India, but high in alcohol venues: results from 2 probability surveys. *Journal of Acquired Immune Deficiency Syndromes, 46,* 491-497.

Hahn, J.A., Woolf-King, S.E., and Muyindike, W. (2011). Adding fuel to the fire: Alcohol's effect on the HIV epidemic in Sub-Saharan Africa. *Current HIV/AIDS Reports, 8,* 172-180.

Halperin, D.T., de Moya, E.A., Pérez-Then, E., Papas, G., and Garcia Callejas, J.M. (2009). Understanding the HIV in the Dominican Republic: a prevention success story in the Caribbean? *Journal of Acquired Immune Deficiency Syndromes, 51 (Suppl.),* S52-S59.

Hendershot, C.S., Stoner, S.A., Pantalone, D.W., and Simoni, J.M. (1999). Alcohol use and antiretroviral adherence: review and meta-analysis. *Journal of Acquired Immune Deficiency Syndromes, 52,* 180-206.

Kalichman, S.C., Simbayi, L.C., Vermaak, R., Jooste, S., and Cain, D. (2008). HIV/AIDS risk among men and women drink at informal alcohol serving establishments (Shebeens) in Cape Town, South Africa. *Preventive Science, 9,* 55-62.

Kerrigan, D., Ellen, J.M., Moreno, L., Rosario, S., Katz, J., Celentano, D.D., et al. (2003). Environmental-structural factors significantly associated with consistent condom use among female sex workers in the Dominican Republic. *AIDS, 17,* 415-423.

León, Y.M. (2007). The impact of tourism on rural livelihoods in the Dominican Republic's coastal areas. *Journal of Development Studies, 43,* 340-359.

MEASURE Evaluation (2005). *Priorities for local AIDS control efforts (PLACE): A manual for implementing the PLACE Method.* U.S. Agency for International Development: United States.

Morojele, N.K., Kachieng'a, M.A., Mokoko, E., Nkoko, M.A., Parry, C.D., Nkowane, A.M., et al. (2006). Alcohol use and sexual behavior among risky drinkers and bar and shebeen patrons in Gauteng province, South Africa. *Social Science and Medicine, 62,* 217-227.

Padilla, M.B. (2007). *Caribbean pleasure industry: Tourism, sexuality, and AIDS in the Dominican Republic.* Chicago, IL: The Chicago University Press.

Padilla, M.B., Guilamo-Ramos, V., and Godbole, R. (2012). A syndemic analysis of alcohol use and sexual risk behavior among tourism employees in Sosua, Dominican Republic. *Qualitative Health Research, 21,* 89-102.

Padilla, M.B., Guilamo-Ramos, V., Bouris, A., and Reyes, A.M. (2010). HIV/AIDS and tourism in the Caribbean: an ecological system perspective. *American Journal of Public Health, 100,* 70-77.

Padilla, M.B., Reyes, A.M., Connolly, M., Natsui, S., Puello, A., and Chapman, H. (2011). Examining the policy climate for HIV prevention in the Caribbean tourism sector: a qualitative study of policy makers in the Dominican Republic. *Health Policy Planning,* [Epub ahead of print].

Pandrea, I., Happel, K.I., Amedee, A.M., Bagby, G.J., and Nelson, S. (2010). Alcohol's role in HIV transmission and disease progression. *Alcohol Research and Health, 33,* 203-218.

Parry, C.D.H. (2000). Alcohol problems in developing countries: challenges for the new millennium. *Suchtmed, 2,* 216-220.

Room, R. and Jernigan, D. (2000). The ambiguous role of alcohol in economic and social development. *Addiction, 95,* 523-535.

Scribner, R., Theall, K.P., Simonsen, N., and Robinson, W. (2010). HIV risk and the alcohol environment. *Alcohol Research and Health, 33,* 179-183.

UNAIDS (2010). *UNAIDS Report on Global AIDS Epidemic.* Geneva: World Health Organization.

WHO (2011). *Global status Report on Alcohol and Drugs.* Geneva: World Health Organization.

(Manuscript received on 30 April 2012. Accepted for publication on 26 June 2012)

In: Recent Hispanic Psychological Research … ISBN: 978-1-62948-919-3
Editors: C. H. Garcia Cadena, A. Lopez-Espinoza et al.

Chapter 10

A REVIEW OF SCHOOL HIV/AIDS PREVENTION PROGRAMS IN SPAIN*

José P. Espada[†], Alexandra Morales, Mireia Orgilés, José A. Piqueras, and José Luis Carballo
Miguel Hernández University
Elche (Alicante), Spain

ABSTRACT

Preventive interventions for HIV/AIDS within a school context have increased in the last few years, although no recent data on the quality and impact of these actions are available. In this paper we aimed to describe and assess school HIV/AIDS prevention programs administered in Spain from 1995 to 2010, which have been evaluated. Preventive interventions for HIV/AIDS and sexual health programs targeting adolescents in schools lasting more than 1 hour. We evaluated the quality and impact of programs following quality criteria associated with successful interventions. Fourteen controlled studies were identified, of which 4 were high quality (28%), 3 intermediate-high quality (21%), 4 intermediate-low quality (28%) and 3 low quality (21%). No progressive evolution in the quality of interventions was observed. Evaluative deficiencies and lack of follow-up on the intervention effects in the medium to long term do not allow for learning about their impact upon adolescents. We discuss the strengths and weaknesses of prevention programs and propose measures for the future.

Keywords: Prevention, HIV/AIDS, Adolescents, Effectiveness, Evaluation, Evidence-Based Programs

---

* This research was supported by the Foundation for AIDS Research and Prevention in Spain (REF. FIPSE 360971/10) and the VALi+d Program of Ministrythe Department of Culture, Education and Science of the Generalitat Valenciana (Spain)

† Address for correspondence: José P. Espada. Universidad Miguel Hernández. Departamento de Psicología de la Salud. Avenida de la Universidad s/n. 03202 Elche (Alicante), España. E-mail: jpespada@umh.es.

INTRODUCTION

HIV/AIDS has a significant impact on the young population. In 2009, around 890,000 new infections were estimated in persons between 15 and 24 years of age (UNICEF, 2009). Adolescents are more vulnerable to the transmission of sexually transmitted diseases (STDs) and unwanted pregnancies, and therefore require special attention in the form of preventive actions (UNAIDS, 2010). Activities promoting sexual health education have increased in schools in recent decades because of their educational contexts and their facilitating access to youth.

The main objective of school HIV/AIDS prevention programs is to reduce or eliminate high-risky sexual behaviors. A recent international review of programs promoting adolescent health indicates evolution in the preventive model (Petergal, Oliva, and Hernando, 2010). It has shifted from a risk-based perspective to one focused on promoting skills and healthy development of youth. The first sex education programs managed to increase knowledge about the HIV virus, transmission routes and AIDS as a disease. However, experimental studies show that transmitting information is not enough to prevent sexual risk behaviors (DiClemente, 1992; Moreno-Iribas, Irisiarri, Elizalde, Urtiaga, Sola, Fernández et al., 2004). Thus, other variables involved in sexual behavior have been added to the HIV/AIDS prevention equation, such as attitudes towards the disease and condoms, intention of using protective measures, perceived self-efficacy, condom use and communication skills, especially negotiating healthy sexuality with a partner. These factors are indicators of the intervention's effectiveness so much that they are considered predictors for healthy sexuality (Lameiras, Failde, Bimbela, and Alfaro, 2008; Sheeram, Abraham, and Orbell, 1999; Villamarín and Juárez, 2002).

The effectiveness of programs to prevent unwanted pregnancies and sexually transmitted diseases is frequently questioned. Data indicate that interventions improve knowledge and promote a positive attitude towards condom use among adolescents. However, programs that include skills training have proven most effective (DiCenso, Guyatt, William, and Griffith, 2002; UNAIDS, 2006). The impact of preventive measures is often unknown because of the poor evaluation method in the studies. The success of interventions is associated with programs based on theoretical models of behavior modification to distribute the contents into a minimum of four or more sessions and to have a participatory methodology (Fernández, Juárez, and Díez, 1999; Grunseit, 1999; Oakley, Fullerton, and Holland, 1995).

In Spain, the promotion of healthy sexuality among young people represents 87% of the public funding allocated for HIV/AIDS prevention (Plan Nacional del Sida, 2009). Despite existing resources, not all teenagers receive sexual health education in their respective schools. Today, almost all the Spanish autonomous communities implement HIV/AIDS prevention programs at high schools; however, most of these actions are loosely evaluated and their effects are not always known (León, Lozano, and Paricio, 2009). It is estimated that more than half of the program evaluations are poor in quality, and that interventions have a 27% and 41% high and intermediate quality, respectively (Juárez and Díez, 1999). These findings indicate the need to improve the quality of the programs and design evaluations that report on the effects deriving from the interventions. Although some reviews exist (Fernández, Juárez, and Díez, 1999), recent data on the effectiveness of school-based HIV/AIDS prevention programs targeting Spanish adolescents have not been published.

The purpose of this work is to describe and assess AIDS prevention programs implemented in Spanish schools from 1995 to 2010, which have been objects of evaluation. The quality of the programs is analyzed depending upon whether they are based on a theoretical model, they devote a minimum time of intervention, develop skills beyond knowledge and attitudes, as well as the methodology employed. The intervention assessment analyzes the type of evaluation (process or outcome), if a comparison group exists, the data availability and follow-up of their effects. Finally, the key points involved in the effectiveness of preventive measures are described and the transfer of research results assessed.

METHOD

The information sources used in the search for studies were computerized scientific databases, previous reviews, entities promoting sex education, organizers of autonomous AIDS plans, and researchers. The keywords used during the literature search were *prevention programs, intervention, HIV/AIDS, adolescents, youth, sex education, school evaluation* and their Spanish translations. The databases used were Pubmed, CSIC-ISOC, Medline, Scopus, Science direct and PSICODOC. Table 1 describes the inclusion criteria for the studies reviewed.

Table 1. Inclusion criteria of Spanish school HIV prevention programs

1. HIV preventive interventions and sexual health education programs.
2. Directed at adolescents within a school context.
3. Duration of 60 minutes (1 session).
4. Controlled studies published from 1995 to 2010.
5. Programs administered in Spain.
6. Availability of the data from the intervention evaluations.

A comprehensive database was created, starting from the descriptive card for each selected study that met the inclusion criteria. The description includes the names of the authors, year of publication, the number of participants and its location, contents and number of intervention sessions, methodology, assessment tools, type of design with or without a control group, and the results. When the program components were not specified (knowledge, attitudes and skills), they were inferred from the contents description and the work method. We assessed the theoretical model criteria when this issue is reflected in the program information.

Coinciding with the previous reviews (Fernandez, Juárez, and Díez, 1999), we have analyzed the programs in terms of their own quality criteria of the intervention and evaluation. Added were two quality parameters, evaluation of results/impact and follow-up time. The first allows learning the short-term intervention effects, and the second, the effects in the medium and long term. In order to obtain a larger number of studies, the sample size criterion was disregarded.

The fact that not all the studies include analysis of the sample loss during follow-up is noteworthy. Although, some interventions implemented by trained peers have been successful (Díez, Fernández, Riera, Soria, Villamarín, Juárez et al., 2002; Siegel, Aten, and Enaharo,

2001; UNAIDS, 2006), recent studies report better results when the program is implemented by experts (Morales, Espada, Orgilés, Secades-Vila, and Remor, under review; Espada, Remor, Lloret, Ballester, and Secades, 2010). Therefore, the facilitator variable was not considered a quality criterion.

Table 2 shows the quality criteria based on the analysis of interventions and assessments of the studies reviewed. The quality was assessed on three levels: intervention, evaluation, and overall. The quality classification has four categories: no quality if no criteria are met, low if one is met, intermediate-low if two are met, intermediate-high if 3 are met, and high if 4 criteria are met. The overall quality assessment is the sum of the quality of the intervention and the quality of the assessment summation. The scores range between 0 and 8. The studies were considered high quality when they obtained a total of 7 or 8 points, intermediate-high quality with 5 or 6, intermediate-low quality with 3 or 4, low quality with 1 or 2, and zero if no criteria are met.

Table 2. Quality criteria for the studies: Intervention and evaluation

Intervention Criteria	Evaluation Criteria
1. Theoretical reference model.	1. Outcome or impact assessment.
2. Four or more sessions.	2. Control group.
3. Contents: knowledge, attitudes and skills.	3. Pre/post design.
4. Participatory methodology.	4. Medium/long term follow-up.

RESULTS

Program Features

The review included 14 controlled studies whose main characteristics and valuation are listed in tables 3 and 4, respectively. Descriptive studies that did not provide data from the results were not included. The main objectives of the programs were to provide information and raise awareness about HIV/AIDS, its ways of transmission and its effects on health, improve attitudes toward safer sexual behaviors, and prevent further STD transmissions. The purposes are achieved by providing information, and training in the skills of communication, negotiation, and problem solving. The sample sizes vary, ranging between 50 and 1575 participants. The large-scale studies assume greater statistical reliability and validity; however, these experiments lose individuality because the same program is applied without addressing the specific needs of the group (Prado, Schwartz, Pattatucci-Aragón, Clatts, Pantin, Fernández et al., 2006). Regarding the facilitators, 10 of the 14 interventions were implemented by experts in sexual education and HIV/AIDS prevention. In three cases, peer groups participated in running the intervention (Díez, Fernández, Riera, Soria, Villamarín, Juárez et al., 2002; Prats, 1997), while the rest were directed by highly trained teachers. Research, like that from Callejas, Fernández, Méndez, León, Fábrega, Villarín et al. (2005) and Prats (1997), combined all three facilitator types. In terms of geographical diversity, Catalonia is a major focal point for Spanish HIV prevention, as 6 of the 14 (42%) applications were implemented in this region.

Intervention Quality

In the evaluation of the intervention, 6 of the 14 studies met the four criteria, and so they were rated high quality. Of the remainder, 3 were rated intermediate-low quality, 3 were low quality, and 2 were of no quality.

Table 3. Controlled studies included in the review of school-based prevention programs in Spain (1995-2010)

#	Author (s) and publication year	Sample age range, number, and location	Theoretical basis and intervention duration	Facilitator and methodology	Results
1	Prats (1997) SIDA: SABER AYUDA	14-18 N= 50 Valladolid	- - - Activities for half an academic year	Experts, teachers and peers Interdisciplinary Participatory Group dynamics. Discussion and reflection. Individual and team work.	+ Knowledge + Attitude
2	Cerdà, Díez, and Juárez (1996) PRESSEC	N= 1215 Barcelona	HBM TSC TPA PRECEDE model ASE model	Teachers Participatory	+ Knowledge + Attitude + Intentions + Behavior
3	Fernández et al. (2000) AULASIDA	12-19 N= 1575 Valencian Community	- - - 1 colloquium talk and participatory activities: exhibition posters, interactive games and educational material.	Experts Participatory and interactive	+ Knowledge + Attitude
4	Díez et al. (2000) PRESSEC	15-17 N= 1215 Barcelona	HBM SCT TPA PRECEDE model ASE model 7 sessions	Teachers	+ Knowledge + Attitude + Intentions + Behavior

Table 3. (Continued)

#	Author (s) and publication year	Sample age range, number, and location	Theoretical basis and intervention duration	Facilitator and methodology	Results
5	Díez et al. (2002) PARLEM CLAR	16-18 N= 442 Barcelona	SCTM 2 sessions (4 or 5 hours total)	Teachers and peers Participatory	+ Knowledge + Attitude + Intentions + Behavior
6	Usieto and Sastre (2002)	12-15 N= 1697 Cantabria	- - - - - -	Experts	+ Knowledge + Attitude
7	Rebull et al. (2003)	14-17 N= 805 Tarragona	HBM 1 session (60-90 min).	Experts Informative	+ Knowledge
1	Callejas et al. (2005)	15-16 N=238 Toledo	- - - Advertising Competition + 2 sessions (50min/1).	Experts, teachers and peers Participatory	+ Knowledge + Attitude + Skills (correct condom use)
2	Carreras et al. (2006) AGARIMOS	12-16 N= 212 Galicia	- - - 28 sessions	Experts Participatory and interactive activity	+ Knowledge + Attitude
3	Espada (2007) COMPASS	14-18 N= 1200 Alicante, Castellón, Madrid Murcia and Oviedo.	SLT TPA IMB model 5 sessions	Experts and peers Participatory	+ Knowledge + Attitude + Skills + Behaviors (condom use).
11	SIDA STUDI (2008) by Calciati et al. (2011) PREVENIR PARA DISFRUTAR	Mean age: 15.22 N= 628 Catalonia	ASE model HBM TRA TSE 3 sessions of 2 hours	Experts	+ Knowledge - Perception of control + Attitudes
4	Hernández-Martínez et al. (2009)	16-17 N= 481 Albacete	- - - 5 sessions	Experts Theoretical and practical	+ Knowledge + Attitude + Behavioral (condom use)

#	Author (s) and publication year	Sample age range, number, and location	Theoretical basis and intervention duration	Facilitator and methodology	Results
13	SIDA STUDI (2009) by Marqués et al. (2011) PREVENIR PARA DISFRUTAR	14-22 N= 524 Catalonia	ASE model HBM TAR TSE 3 sessions of 2 hours	Experts	+ Knowledge
5	SIDA STUDI (2010) PREVENIR PARA DISFRUTAR	14-19 N= 527 Not specified	ASE model. HBM TRA TSE 3 sessions of 2 hours	Experts	+ Knowledge + Skills (correct condom use)

+ Significant increase after intervention.
- Significant decrease after intervention.

More than half of the programs (57%) are based on theoretical models of behavioral change. Among them are the Theory of Reasoned Action (Ajzen and Fishbein, 1980), the Health Belief Model (Glanz, Lewis, and Rimer, 1990), Social Cognitive Theory, formerly known as Theory of Social Learning (Bandura, 1977, 1986), the PRECEDE model (Green and Kreuter, 1991), the Information-Motivation-Behavioral Skills Model (Fisher, Fisher, Bryan, and Misovich, 2002) and the ASE model (Vries, Dijkstra, and Kuhlman, 1988), which is based on the first three.

The intervention duration is equal to or greater than four sessions or 4 hours in 8 studies (57%). It is noteworthy that the Prats program (1997) is multidisciplinary, having a transversal methodology and integrating the activities into the courses of the academic curriculum. Knowledge and attitudes are worked on as much as skills in 7 of the 14 studies reviewed. After the intervention, all of them reported an increase in knowledge, 11 (78.6%) reported more favorable attitudes toward condom use and the disease, and half of them showed behavioral changes and improved skills on how to use condoms. These data should be treated cautiously because several studies infer behavioral improvements beginning with the increase in knowledge, improved attitudes toward safe sex, better perceived self-efficacy and intentions to use condoms. The participatory method is that most frequent (71.4%).

Quality Assessment

Only 2 of the 14 studies are rated high in quality in the evaluation of preventive intervention. Another 4 of them are rated intermediate-high in quality, 6 are intermediate-low in quality, 1 is low in quality and 1 is of no quality.

Table 4. The intervention and evaluation quality of school programs for HIV prevention in Spain (1995-2010)

		Intervention quality					Assessment quality					Overall quality
	Author (s)	Theoretical basis	Duration (≥4) (+4 h)	Contents: knowledge, attitudes, and skills	Participatory methodology	Intervention quality	Type: Outcomes	Control group	Pre- and post-test	Follow-up and 3rd evaluation	Quality assessment	
1	Prats (1997)				*	1					0	1
2	Cerdà, Díez, and Juárez (1996)	*	*	*	*	4	*	*	*		3	7
3	Fernández et al. (2000)					0	*		*		2	2
4	Díez et al. (2000)	*	*	*	*	4	*	*	*		3	7
5	Díez et al. (2002)	*	*	*	*	4	*	*	*Post: 4 months		3	7
6	Usieto and Sastre (2002)					0	*		*Post: after 2 months		1	1
7	Rebull et al. (2003)	*			*	2	*		*Post: after 6 months		2	4
8	Callejas et al. (2005)			*	*	2	*		*6 months		2	4
9	Carreras et al. (2006)		*			1	*	*	*		3	4
10	Espada (2007)	*	*	*	*	4	*	*	*	*12 months	4	8
11	SIDA STUDI (2008) by Calciati et al. (2011)	*	*	*	*	4	*		*		2	6
12	Hernández-Martínez et al. (2009)		*		*	2	*	*	*	*6 months	4	6
13	SIDA STUDI (2009) by Marqués et al. (2009)	*				1	*		*		2	3
14	SIDA STUDI (2010)	*	*	*	*	4	*		*		2	6

Intervention/Quality Assessment: High (4 points), intermediate-high (3 points), intermediate-low (2 points), low (1 point) and zero (0 points). Overall Quality: High (7 and 8 points), intermediate-high (5 and 6 points), intermediate-low (3 and 4 points) and low (1 and 2 points) and zero (0 points).

Ninety-two percent of the investigations carried out an outcome assessment, which allows determining the effectiveness of the preventive action. However, less than half (42.8%) include a comparison or control group in the design in order to attribute the results to the intervention when significant differences exist. With the exception of the *SIDA: Saber Ayuda* program (Prats, 1997), all of them reported a pre- and post-evaluation. However, only a small group specifies the sample losses attributed to the follow-up. Although, the most programs evaluate the effects in the last session, some planned the assessment at two months (Usieto and Sastre, 2002), four months (Díez et al., 2002) and six months (Callejas et al., 2005; Rebull, Reverte, Piñas, Orti, González, and Contreras, 2003) from the intervention. Regarding the follow-up of the effects achieved, only 2 studies performed a third evaluation at six months (Hernández-Martínez, 2009) and one year later (Espada, 2007).

Overall Quality

Of the four high-quality studies, only one meets the 8 criteria (Espada, 2007). This investigation of multicentre character consisted in the validation of COMPAS, an HIV/AIDS prevention program based on developing skills. Adolescents are trained in social skills, problem solving and self-control as well as transmitting information with duration of 5 sessions (Espada, Orgilés, Morales, Ballester, and Huedo-Medina, 2012). The quality criterion that it shares with another study (Hernández-Martínez, García-Serrano, Simón, Coy, García-Fernández, Liante et al., 2009), but which differentiates it from the other three high-quality studies (Cerdà, Díez, and Juárez, 1996; Díez et al., 2000, Díez et al., 2002), is the follow-up time. The researchers evaluated on a third occasion one year after application.

Three of the 14 studies are intermediate-high quality (Hernández-Martínez et al., 2009; Calciati, Pasarín, Juárez, Ariza, Díez, and Artazcoz, 2011; SIDA STUDI, 2010) and 4 are intermediate-low quality (Marqués, Juárez, Pasarín, Díez, Ariza, and Ramos, 2011; Callejas et al., 2005; Carreras, Lameiras, Foltz, Núñez, and Rodríguez, 2006; Rebull et al., 2003). Three studies were rated low quality by meeting one (Prats, 1997; Usieto and Sastre, 2002) or two criteria (Fernández, Molina, Ramírez, Pérez, Castilla, Marrodán et al., 2000).

Discussion

From an evolutive perspective of the programs, no progressive improvement has been observed in the quality of school-based HIV prevention interventions in Spain over the past 15 years. The programs rated as high quality have improved knowledge, attitudes, intention to use condoms, perceived self-efficacy and sexual behaviors. They are based on theoretical models of behavior modification; they form skills, in addition to attitudes and knowledge in at least 4 sessions/hours and employ a participatory methodology. With respect to valuation, these works include evaluation of results, control group, assess before and after intervention, and additionally one has a follow-up one year following the intervention (Espada, 2007). Although most studies reviewed have deficits in the intervention design, half of them are not based on a theoretical model nor do they form skills, and they are short interventions.

Overall, the assessments of the reviewed studies are characterized by not including a control group in their design and by not re-evaluating in the medium to long term.

Notwithstanding, the well-controlled studies conducted outcome assessments and compared the effects of the intervention with the prior baseline.

This systematic review reports the evolution of Spanish HIV prevention programs that had been implemented during the last 15 years. On the one hand, we describe the characteristics of the programs and highlight its strengths. On the other hand, we evaluate them in terms of quality criteria based on the effectiveness of interventions and identify areas for improvement the effectiveness that should be taken into account in the design and implementation of scholar sex education programs in Spain. This work also has some limitations that should be explained. It is possible that the scientific literature results have not been comprehensive enough, and this is an attributable feature to the reviews. Although, bias in the availability of information might have influenced the selection of studies, different sources for knowledge were used. On the other hand, there is variability in the content and methodology of the interventions, an issue that hinders the comparative analysis. The selection and quality criteria delimited inclusion and facilitated the assessment of the studies. The parameters that were used have proven more effective in school-based interventions; however, others such as motivation, participant profiles, the relationship established with the facilitator and the group atmosphere can contribute positively. On the other hand, this study shows the evolution of Spanish programs for HIV/AIDS prevention and examines the weaknesses in order to learn what is and what we can be done.

The transfer of research means the implementation of programs previously evaluated and the consideration of quality criteria in the interventions by the agencies responsible for HIV prevention. In Spain, associations and NGOs attend to much of the demand for sexual health education in the school environment. Their main funding source is public. An analysis of 38 organizations working on HIV prevention reports that only 14% assess the impact of their actions, 40% do not consider young people in designing the intervention, and only 3 out of 10 evaluate the previous intervention. In addition to the lack of evaluations, their impact is unknown because of the absence of dissemination of the results (León, Lozano, and Paricio, 2008). Consequently, the lack of evaluation constitutes an important limitation because it does not allow learning the qualities of successful interventions and improving those that are being applied.

Another limitation in school HIV/AIDS prevention programs in Spain that may be affecting the objective is the age of their participants. Despite greater efficiency in early applications (Fernández et al., 2000; Rebull et al., 2003), samples from the reviewed studies reach 18 years of age. Both the delay as well as the absence of sexual health education in schools can be explained by political and ideological matters. Information about sexuality has been popularly associated with the early onset of intimate relationships and promiscuous behavior. On the contrary, studies show that besides not lowering the age of first intercourse (Basen-Engquist and Parcel, 1992; Visser and van Bilsen, 1991), it also increases condom use and delays the age when teenagers are well informed about sexuality (Usieto and Sastre, 2002). Paradoxically, various programs promoting abstinence actually managed to increase sexual behavior (Christopher and Roosa, 1990; Jacobs and Wolf, 1995; Oakley et al., 1995), and so they proved to be ineffective.

According to the results from the Spanish Ministry of Education and Science and the Ministry of Health (MEPSYD and MSC, 2008), the lack of continuity is a feature of most studies reviewed. School preventive interventions are usually an isolated experience, specific and inadequate for the intended purpose. Undoubtedly, the main limitation of HIV prevention in Spain is the evaluation. In the best cases, the effect is assessed with two measurements, before and after the intervention, but without medium or long term follow-up. Behavioral changes can appear some months after intervention with knowledge and attitudes softening over time, making reevaluation necessary.

In conclusion, to improve the quality of HIV/AIDS preventive interventions within the school context, the results of controlled studies should be taken into account for when designing programs. Besides, it is essential to evaluate the effects of interventions to determine whether the targets are met. Using a rigorous evaluation method allows for feedback and adapts programs to the target population. If preventing sexual risk behaviors in adolescents is intended, the tendency must be to reduce the number of targeted interventions that transmit information and integrate sex education in school curricula, implementing programs based on skills development and empirically validated.

References

Ajzen, I. and Fishbein, M. (1980). *Understanding attitudes and predicting social behaviour.* Englewood Cliffs, NJ: Prentice Hall.

Bandura, A. (1977). Self-efficacy: toward a unifying theory of behavior change. *Psychological Review, 84*, 191-215.

Bandura, A. (1986). *Social foundations of thought and action.* Englewood Cliffs, NJ: Prentice-Hall.

Basen-Engquist, K. and Parcel, G.S. (1992). Attitudes, norms, and self-efficacy: a model of adolescents HIV-related sexual risk behavior. *Health Education Quarterly, 19,* 263-277.

Calciati, E., Pasarín, M.I., Juárez, O., Ariza, C., Díez, E., and Artazcoz, L. (2011). Programes preventius en centres d'educació secundària de Barcelona. Avaluació curs 2008-09. Barcelona: Agència de Salut Pública de Barcelona. In Internet: www.aspd.cat [Retrieved 10 May 2011].

Callejas, S., Fernández, B., Méndez, P., León, M.T., Fábrega, C., Villarín, A., et al. (2005). Intervención educativa para la prevención de embarazos no deseados y enfermedades de transmisión sexual en adolescentes de la ciudad de Toledo. *Revista Española de Salud Pública, 79*, 581-589.

Carreras, M.V., Lameiras, M., Foltz, M.L., Núñez, A. M., and Rodríguez, Y. (2006). Evaluación de un programa de educación sexual con estudiantes de educación secundaria obligatoria. *International Journal of Clinical and Health Psychology, 7*, 739-751.

Cerdà, N., Díez, E., and Juárez, O. (1996). *Prevenció de la sida a l'escola secundària. Programa PRESSEC. Disseny i avaluació preventiva.* Barcelona: Diputació de Barcelona. Servei de Salut Pública i Consum.

Christopher, F.S. and Roosa, M.W. (1990). An evaluation of an adolescent pregnancy prevention program: is "just say no" enough? *Family Relations, 39*, 68-72.

DiCenso, A., Guyatt, G., William, A., and Griffith, L. (2002). Interventions to reduce unintended pregnancies among adolescents: systematic review of randomized controlled trials. *British Medical Journal, 324*, 1426-1434.

DiClemente, R. (1992). *Adolescents and AIDS: a generation in jeopardy.* Newbury Park, CA: Sage Publications.

Díez, E., Juárez, O., Nebot, M., Cerdà, N., and Villalbí, J.R. (2000). Effects on attitudes, knowledge, intentions and behaviour of an HIV prevention programme targeting secondary school adolescents. *Promotion and Education, 3,* 17-22.

Díez, E., Fernández, S., Riera, C., Soria, M., Villamarín, F., Juárez, O., et al. (2002, July). Randomised trial of Parlem Clar (Straight Talk), a high school HIV prevention program. XIV International Conference on AIDS. Barcelona, Spain.

Espada, J. P. (2007). *Programa COMPASS. Programa educativo sobre el sida.* Documento no publicado. In Internet: http://aitanainvestigacion.umh.es [Retrieved 12 May 2011].

Espada, J.P., Huedo-Medina, T.B., Orgilés, M, Ballester, R., Secades, R., Remor, E., et al. (under review). Short-term evaluation of a school-based intervention to prevent sexual risk behaviors.

Espada, J.P., Orgilés, M., Morales, A., Ballester, R. and Huedo-Medina, T.B. (2012). Effectiveness of a school HIV/AIDS prevention program for Spanish adolescents. *AIDS Education and Prevention, 6*, 500-513.

Espada, J.P., Orgilés, M., Huedo, T.B., Ballester, R., Remor, E., Secades, R., et al. (2009, November). Evaluation of a peer-implemented intervention to prevent sexual risk behaviors among adolescents. 42nd Annual Convention of the Association for Behavioral and Cognitive Therapies (ABCT). New York, NY.

Espada, J.P., Remor, E., Lloret, D., Ballester, R., and Secades, R. (2010, August). Long-term evaluation of two modalities of a program for HIV prevention with adolescents: peers and experts. International Congress of behavioral Medicine. Washington, DC.

Fernández, S., Juárez, O., and Díez, E. (1999). Prevención del sida en la escuela secundaria: recopilación y valoración de programas. *Revista Española de Salud Pública*, *73*, 687-696.

Fernández, C., Molina, R., Ramírez, C., Pérez, E., Castilla, J., Marrodán, J., et al. (2000). Cambios en las actitudes y conocimientos de los adolescentes sobre la infección por VIH tras la intervención escolar de AULASIDA, 1996-1997. *Revista Española de Salud Pública, 74*, 163-176.

Fisher, J.D., Fisher, W.A., Bryan, A.D., and Misovich, S.J. (2002). Information-Motivation-Behavioral Skills model-based HIV risk behavior change intervention for inner-city high school youth. *Health Psychology, 21*, 177-186.

Glanz, K., Lewis, F., and Rimer, B. (1990). *Health behavior and health education. Theory, research and practice*. San Francisco, CA: Jossey-Bass Publishers.

Green, L.W. and Kreuter, M. (1991). *Health promotion planning. An educational and environmental approach* (2nd ed.). Mayfield, IL: Publishing Company.

Grunseit, A. (1997). *Impact of HIV and sexual health education on the sexual behaviour of young people: a review update.* Geneva: WHO/UNAIDS.

Hernández-Martínez, A., García-Serrano, I., Simón, M., Coy, R., García-Fernández, A.M., Liante, et al. (2009). Efectividad de un programa de educación sexual en adolescentes acerca de la adquisición de conocimientos y cambios de actitud antes el empleo de métodos anticonceptivos. *Enfermería Clínica, 19*, 121-128.

Jacobs, C.D. and Wolf, E.M. (1995). School sexuality education and adolescent risk-taking behavior. *The Journal of School Health, 65*, 91-95.

Juárez, O. and Díez, E. (1999). Prevención del SIDA en adolescentes escolarizados: una revisión sistemática de la efectividad de las intervenciones. *Gaceta Sanitaria, 13*, 150-162.

Lameiras, M., Failde, J.M., Bimbela, J.L., and Alfaro, N. (2008). Uso del preservativo masculino en las relaciones con coito vaginal de jóvenes españoles entre catorce y veinticuatro años. *Diversitas-Perspectivas en Psicología, 4*, 401-415.

León, M.J., Lozano, J., and Paricio, D. (2008). Jóvenes y VIH/sida: mejorando las intervenciones de prevención. Barcelona: SIDA STUDI. In Internet: www.sidastudi.org/Ddigitals/DD6867.pdf [Retrieved 10 May 2011].

León, M.J., Lozano, J., and Paricio, D. (2009). Diagnóstico de intervenciones grupales de las ONG/sida para la prevención del VIH/sida entre jóvenes escolarizados. En II Encuentro FIFPSE sobre investigación social en VIH/sida (pp. 188-198). San Sebastián, España: FIFPSE.

Marqués, M., Juárez, O., Pasarín, M.I., Díez, E., Ariza, C., and Ramos, P. (2011). Programes preventius en centres d'educació secundària de Barcelona. Avaluació curs 2009-2010. Barcelona: Agència de Salut Pública de Barcelona. (In Internet www.aspd.cat [Retrieved 13 April 2011].

Morales, A., Espada, J.P., Orgilés, M., Secades-Vila, R., and Remor, E. (under review). Contribution of the Type of Applicator to the Effectiveness of a Sexual Risk Behavior Prevention Program in Adolescents. Evaluation and Program Planning.

MEPSYD and MSC (2008). Criterios de calidad para el desarrollo de proyectos y actuaciones de promoción y educación para la salud en el sistema educativo. Guía para las administraciones educativas y sanitarias. In Internet: www.educacion.es/cide/espanol /publicaciones/materiales/salud/inn2008ga/inn2008ga.pdf [Retrieved 10 April 2011].

Moreno-Iribas, C., Irisarri, F., Elizalde, L., Urtiaga, M., Sola, J., Fernández, C., et al. (2004). Progresos en el control de la infección por el VIH y el sida en Navarra, 1985- 2003. *Anales del Sistema Sanitario de Navarra, 27*, 221-231.

Oakley, A., Fullerton, D., and Holland, J. (1995). Behavioural interventions for HIV/AIDS prevention. *AIDS, 9,* 479-486.

Oakley, A., Fullerton, D., Holland, J., Arnold, S., France-Dawson, M., Kelley, P., et al. (1995). Sexual health education interventions for young people: a methodological review. *British Medical Journal, 310*, 158-162.

Petergal, M.A., Oliva, A., and Hernando, A. (2010). Los programas escolares como promotores del desarrollo positivo adolescente. *Cultura y Educación, 22*, 53-66.

Plan Nacional sobre el Sida (2009). ICAP 2008. Informe del cuestionario de actividades de prevención del VIH en las comunidades autónomas. Año 2008. In Internet: www.msc.es/en/ciudadanos/enfLesiones/enfTransmisibles/sida/docs/ICAP2008/ICAP2008.pdf [Retrieved 9 May 2011].

Prats, J. (1997). Aplicaciones didácticas del programa "Sida: saber ayuda". In Internet: www.ddhhrosario.gob.ar/wpcontent/uploads/2010/pdf/19488_es_sidacastella.pdf [Retrieved 10 April 2011]

Prado, G., Schwartz, S.J., Pattatucci-Aragón, A., Clatts, M., Pantin, H., Fernández, M., et al. (2006). The prevention of HIV transmission in Hispanic adolescents. *Drug and Alcohol Dependence, 84 (Suppl.)*, S43-S53.

Rebull, J., Reverté, M., Piñas, I., Ortí, A., González, L.I., and Contreras, E. (2003). Evaluación pre-post de una actividad preventiva de la infección por VIH dirigida a los adolescentes de las comarcas del sur de Tarragona. *Revista Española de Salud Pública, 77*, 373-382.

Sheeran, P., Abraham, C., and Orbell, S. (1999). Psychosocial correlates of heterosexual condom use. A meta-analysis. *Psychological Bulletin, 125*, 1, 90-132.

SIDA STUDI (2010). Resultados evaluación de la acción educativa "Prevenir para disfrutar" curso 2009-2010. In Internet: www.sidastudi.org/resources/doc/100623-resultados_ evaluacion_educativa-542617673126563861.pdf. [Retrieved 10 April 2011]

Siegel, D.M., Aten, M.J., and Enaharo, M. (2001). Long-term effects of a middle school-and high school-based human immunodeficiency virus sexual risk prevention intervention. *Archives of Pediatrics and Adolescent Medicine, 155*, 1117-1126.

UNAIDS (2006). *Linking EDUCAIDS with other on-going initiatives. An overview of opportunities. An assessment of challenges.* Geneva: UNESCO. In Internet: www. educaids. org/ [Retrieved 10 April 2011].

UNAIDS (2010). Podemos empoderar a los jóvenes para que se protejan del VIH. In Internet: unaids.org/en/media/unaids/contentassets/documents/unaidspublication/2010/2010-12-16_JC1830_young_people_es.pdf [Retrieved 10 May 2011].

UNICEF (2009). Prevenir la infección entre los adolescentes y los jóvenes. In Internet: www.unicef.org/spanish/aids/index_orphans.html [Retrieved 15 April 2011].

Usieto, R. and Sastre, J. (2002). La información y educación sobre el SIDA como estrategia de prevención en los jóvenes. Una experiencia concreta entre los adolescentes escolarizados de Cantabria. *Revista Española de Drogodependencias, 27*, 445-465.

Villamarín, F. and Juárez, O. (2002). Predictores psicológicos del comportamiento sexual seguro en la prevención de la infección por el VIH. *Revista de Psicología de la Salud, 14*, 81-104.

Vries, H. de, Dijkstra, M., and Kuhlman, P. (1988). Self-efficacy: the third factor besides attitude and subjective norm as a predictor of behavioural intentions. *Health Education Research, 3*, 273-282.

Visser, A.P. and Van Bilsen, P. (1991). Effectiveness of sex education provided to adolescents. *Patient Education Counselling, 23*, 147-160.

(Manuscript received on 23 June 2011. Revised version accepted for publication on 18 July 2011)

In: Recent Hispanic Psychological Research ... ISBN: 978-1-62948-919-3
Editors: C. H. Garcia Cadena, A. Lopez-Espinoza et al.

Chapter 11

THE BEST THING IS TO FEEL HIS WARM SEMEN*

Patricia Noboa-Ortega and Irma Serrano-Garcia
Universidad de Puerto Rico
Recinto de Río Piedras, Puerto Rico

ABSTRACT

The main purpose of this study was to examine how women's constructions about sexual pleasure configure high-risk behaviors during sexual encounters. Results emerge from a qualitative study. Using the technique of discourse analysis stemming from a *post-*structuralist perspective we analyze women's discourses during sexual encounters. Finally, we point out the scope of this work for psychology, some conclusions to be drawn from this research and recommendations for future research and interventions for HIV /AIDS.

Keywords: HIV/AIDS Prevention, Discourse Analysis, Sexual Encounter

INTRODUCTION

Without doubt, "The best thing is to feel his warm semen" is a suggestive and provocative title, whose authorship is from a participant who shared her experience and understanding from sexual encounters with her couple in a study carried out at the University of Puerto Rico (Recinto de Río Piedras) between 2004 and 2005. For us, it was appropriate to use it as a title, since it clearly illustrates the work we present now. We describe and analyze the results around constructions from a group of women about sexual intercourse with their couples, and how such relations, based on their upbringing experience from catholic and protestant speech, finally facilitated risky HIV infection sexual practices were carried out.

* Mail address: Avenida Los Filtros # 300, Apartamento 1323. Guaynabo (00971); Puerto Rico. E-Mail: pnoboa@ipsi.uprrp.edu.

Why this Research?

For a start, it is interesting to explore constructions about sexual intercourse for different reasons. First, since HIV infection rate continues growing in women population. In effect, at the end of May 2011, a total of 42,715 accumulated HIV/Aids cases were notified in Puerto Rico; 11 027 out of them were women. From this group, 63% (n = 6 954) reported to be infected by sexual transmission, specifically, by heterosexual relations (Health Statistics Office, 2011).

Second, there is an obvious lack of work in psychology field —and more accentuated in HIV/aids— that explore such constructions, bonds and relations women establish from Judeo-Christian speeches (Protestant and Catholic). Some of the works about HIV risk infection and religious tradition in psychology field review subjects about Marianism and virginity (Marin, 2003; Markes, Cantero, and Simoni, 1998; Ortiz-Torres, Serrano-Garcia, and Torres-Bugos, 2000; Wood and Price, 1997; Yeakley and Gant, 1997); homophobia (Toro-Alfonso, 2000) and women's roles (Fernández, 1995; Galarza, 1998; Mayo and Resnick, 1996; Weiss, Whelan, and Rao-Gupta, 2000; Wood and Price, 1997). In other works regarding these kinds, there have been related different and risky sexual behaviors with determined religious values; at theoretical level, however, it has not been possible to get deeper concerning how this religious discourse, when assigning it or adopting it as reference in active sexual life, configures and produces significant bonds with sexual intercourse.

Third, it seems to us that once bonds established by speeches and their formation constitutive role are understood, it is possible to prepare theoretical and prevention models, taking into account those complex processes. Therefore, conceptual model serving as a base of this research was social constructionism. This model was chosen because it allowed how women built multiple meanings about sexual intercourse. Moreover, as model emphasizes on historicity of those constructions, it provided us some coordinates to formulate and to address questions proposed in in-deep interviews. It should be clarified that processes linked to build women's subjectivity surpass the goals of this article, so results from this research objective are not included. Below, we explain some of its basic premises.

Theoretical Model: Social Constructionism

The core of this theoretical perspective is to examine and explain how people describe and explain the world and reality in which they live. These ways of understanding reality are the result from an historical process (Gergen and Gergen, 2003). Reality comes from an activity developed by individuals and interchange process with the other; meaning, we, the subject, are essential to form the vision of reality (Ibáñez, 1994). Some representatives of constructionist perspective accentuate language function (speeches are attached herein), by underlying acquisition process as a fundamental means to form subjectivities (Berger and Luckmann, 1986; Ibáñez, 1994). These subjectivities are understood as *psique* constitution, that is, as those forms to understand oneself and to understand social environment. Each individual is formed by those modes of understanding oneself and his context in the framework of his life. Subjectivity is organized by processes and configurations, which are interpenetrated permanently that are in constant development and very linked to subject's simultaneous insertion in other similarly complex system: society. To assume this proposal in our research allowed us to understand that women are being formed through their life, which stamps an incomplete character to subjectivity construction processes. Each woman's subjectivity is expressed and resetting simultaneously in view of their social life.

To Gonzalez-Rey (1997), this subjectivity constitutes a moment of each one of the subject's construction acts. In other words, at a subjective level, historical and current matters are configurated in dynamic states expressed by human beings in different ways. This subjectivity is being set from multiple matrixes (*i.e.,* sexuality, gender, work processes, social class and religion), that in turn is being formed and transformed from coherent and antagonistic discourses (Gillies, 1999; Vargas, 1994). From this framework, subject is seen as "discourses subject" characterized by incoherence, contradiction, absence of a defining center and lack of uniqueness. Diversity of social discourses and inherent contradictions to dialectics of social processes make possible the appearance of *dis*-oriented subjects. That configuration concept allows representing subjectivity in a dynamic, contradictory and irregular way, by forming part of current complex system of subject's integration to his social space (González-Rey 1997). This proposal suggested us to approach our research to women subjectivity topic, recognizing to face the impossibility of establishing predictive lines and/or categories which define them in categories like heterosexuality, which we certainly assumed in this research in a provisional manner.

Sexual Intercourse and HIV Infection Risk

As it was stated at the beginning of this work, most of the Puerto Rican women reported to have been infected through heterosexual contact. We refer to sexual intercourse as that mutual experience between man and woman body that included multiple sexual practices, such as *masturbation* (*i.e.,* to stimulate genitals with the hand, to caress the penis, to put fingers inside the vagina or inside the anus, or to stimulate the clitoris); *oral sex* (*i.e.,* to put mouth or tongue in genitals or in breasts; to suck penis, testicles, clitoris, vagina, anus, nipples and breasts); *penetrative sex* (*i.e.,* to penetrate the penis partially or completely in the vagina or anus, with or without condom, having or not having ejaculation), and *non penetrative sex* (*i.e.,* to caress penis, anus, vagina or breasts (Muñoz-Laboy, 2004; page. 33).

What happens between man and woman, meaning, selection of sexual practices during sexual intercourse used to occur around five basic axes: 1) Social standards linked to sexuality; 2) Social standards linked to gender; 3) Maximization of pleasure during sexual intercourse; 4) Emotional closeness derived from sexual intercourse, and 5) Construction of risk out of couple's context. These axes, as detailed below, have been also identified in preventive literature as HIV risk factors. Let's see each axis and its relation to infection risk about the problem object of our study.

Social standards related to sexuality: It has been proposed in preventive works that sexual practices performed during sexual intercourse is consequence of social standards related to sexuality (Simon and Gagnon, 1999). These standards are transmitted and perpetuated formal institutions like Church and school. Catholic Church, through priests' sermon and talks, promotes penetrative sex (penis-vagina) is only for reproduction and it is, par excellence, the natural practice. Young are granted, then by being kept virgin before marrying, in such a way anal penetration and masturbation are identified as *no*-natural and "sinful" practices. In turn, by the interaction existing in the confessional, where it is determined under which framework such sexual practices shall be carried out —like marriage. In confessionals, Church officials find out about sexual life of their parishioners, trying in this way, to regulate desire and sexual practices; in other words, avoidance of feelings is overwhelmed, by promoting what Foucault (1988) called discursive practices, moving from what is "permitted" to what is "prohibited".

From the foregoing, the obligatory question we propose is: How these regulations can promote risky situations during sexual intercourse? For example, in researches performed in Puerto Rico with university young, it was revealed that many women preferred to practice anal sex as strategy to preserve virginity (Cunningham, Rivera, Bothwell- Toro, and Domenech-Miller, 1996, Cunnigham, Diaz-Esteve, Gonzalez-Santiago and Rodriguez-Sanchez, 1994). This strategy does not sacrifice the pleasure from one or from the other; but it is a high risky sexual practice to contract HIV, since, as it can be seen, the surrounding skin of the anus has many capillaries, it is very thin and sensitive, so it is easy HIV enters into body's bloodstream of the woman who is being penetrated. (CDC, 2011).

As a second axis, there are social standards related to gender: codes structuring and organizing women and men relations are established by them. These include since how they approach (*i.e.*, sometime, man is the one taking the initiative to invite a girl going out, and the woman responds) until how sexual intercourse is given (*i.e.,* sometime, man is the one suggesting and insisting in certain sexual practices, but woman says yes or no). One of the ways of thinking that has been promoted by Christian speech has been characterized by dichotomies and oppositions. These oppositional categories fall in both women and men, like for example, the good or bad women, the pure or the "hooker"; the respectable housewife and the prostitute, the other. These figures of differentiation influence the patterns and forms in which women establish their relation with men, their gender construction, and in consequence, how they behave during such sexual intercourse. Promotion and value of characteristics associated with naivety, sacrifice and satisfaction for their couple could provoke HIV risk. For example, women, in order to please their couple, could perform risky practices. As it was mentioned, these topics about Marianism, virginity and risk have been examined in prevention field.

Naivety related to gender standards promotes as well the risk during sexual intercourse. The *Real Spanish Academy* defines naivety as *out of malice*. Here it is related as well as *lack of knowledge*, resulting in *ignorance*. It seems to us that if woman ascribes such naivety as desirable, could understand it is not necessary to know about her physiology and reproductive system, so it will be difficult to recognize symptomatologies associated with different sexually transmitted diseases —STD (in her body and in her sexual couple's) during sexual intercourse. Moreover, to ascribe such naivety limits her possibilities to negotiate with her couple safe sexual practices.

This sexual negotiation with the couple not only requires sexual practices knowledge that could eroticize both man and woman, but to feel comfortable regarding sexual practices, to feel comfortable with her body and sexuality (Noboa-Ortega, 2006). Anyway, women need at least to move away from naivety and to transgress those Church guidelines, by executing their assertiveness, particularly when their couples suggest them sexual risky practices, or men resist practicing the ones suggested by women.

It seems to us that it is there where seduction and eroticization become indispensable resources for protection and pleasure. Third axis deals with maximizing the pleasure during sexual intercourse, process which is ruled as well. There is, both in Puerto Rico and United States of North America, an industry in the media addressed to "educate" about what sexual practices must be effectuated, and how to maximize the pleasure, both in men and women. This legitimation and perpetuation of sexual practices have the effect of establishing the limits between what is permitted and appropriate, as well as what is inappropriate and prohibited (Carrillo, 2002).

Men and women take over those rules regarding maximization of pleasure during sexual intercourse, by choosing the most pleasant ones, such as masturbation or oral sex (Muñoz-Laboy, 2004). In ethnographic researches in the United States of North America, it has been documented how meanings linked to sexual practices are mediated by selecting the places where intercourse occurs. For example, to masturbate in the movies or on the beach, as well as to have a sexual intercourse in a public toilette, influence excitement level and pleasure experienced by women and men (Muñoz-Laboy, 2004; Parker 2001). Nonetheless, risk to be coped when performing such action and the possibility to be seized (a) by the law makes sexual practice more exciting to both. That is a transgressive sexual practice, meaning, it infringes the rules about what is permitted. Similarly, concerning maximization of pleasure, there is the construction that sexual desire is "uncontrollable".

Presently, this construction is an obstacle to low risky sexual behaviors, like condom use, since it requires planning and stopping sexual intercourse to put the condom on (Marin, 1996; Marin and Gomez, 1997; Ortiz-Torres, 1995; Willig, 1999). Think about sexual desire as something uncontrollable positions women and men as vulnerable subjects of such desire; in other words, to be at the mercy of something higher. Consequently, to be in a vulnerable position in view of their own desire facilitates risky practices. Fourth axis has to do with emotional intimacy drawn from sexual intercourse.

In different researches, it has been identified that some sexual practices, like vaginal penetration, promote emotional intimacy during sexual intercourse (Seal and Ehrhardt, 2003). About this particular matter, it is stated that gay and heterosexual men consider penetrative practices - besides pleasant and erotic - as an intimate space. In consequence, they tend to reject behaviors threatening such notions and sensations, like condom use (Parker, 2001; Seal and Ehrhardt 2003).

Finally, to conceive risk out of the space of the relation constitutes the last axis. In a research accomplished by Willig (1999) in England, author identified how discursive constructions of marriage, confidence and sexual activity, both in women and men, positioned them under low risk sexual practices.

Among results worthy to be stood out, we have the following: 1) People constructed marriage and stable relations as sexually safe; married women were positioned out of HIV infection risk and other STD, and 2) Confidence construction was part of marriage discourse and included confidence as safety and symbolic practice. It was observed that the possibility to take protection measures was ignored when there is high confidence level in the relations. Confidence, as a symbolic practice, was showed by making love without protection, understood as a normal happening in a marital relation.

To suggest condom use in this confidence context could be construed as doubt and mistrust in couple. Lastly, it was clear that discourses —Christian and Protestant— set and constitute subjectivities as they rule and promote sexual practices chosen by men and women. However, both break that configurative and constitutive action, as they choose other sexual practices moved away from official discourses. In other words, rules are never entirely accomplished.

METHOD

This research was composed of two phases: 1) Participants recruiting and selection, and 2) Data collection by a pilot study, deep interviews accomplishment, interviews transcription, and finally its analysis.

First Phase: Participants Recruiting and Selection

10 women were interviewed, considering it is an appropriate and sufficient amount to obtain the required information (Castro, 2002). Selection criteria were the following: 1) To be older than 21 years; 2) To be familiar with catholic or protestant religion since childhood; 3) to have had at least one sexual intercourse during the last year previous to research; 4) to have had in the last two years a stable relation with a man; 5) To be considered heterosexual, and at last, 6) To be, all of them, Puerto Rican.

In August 2004, the first author recruited women from organizations working on HIV prevention in the Metropolitan area of the city of San Juan, or in programs offering services to seropositive women. Three page leaflets wit contact information about research was posted in the three organizations. From a résumé given to each organization, managers of the case and social workers provided pertinent information about research to women who meet selection requirements. When interested women called, the first author informed about objectives, procedures and risks of research. In turn, author examined, through a brief screening interview, the eligibility of potential participants. Author interviewed those who met and not met requirements, thanking all of them their availability and interest in the research.

Second Phase: Instrument, Interviews Procedure, Transcription and Analysis

Structure of in-deep interview guide was composed of three parts: 1) Introduction; 2) Socio-demographic data and religious background, and 3) meanings bonded with variables of the study, including sexual intercourse. Interviews were applied by the first author, who started the questions concerning childhood and concluded with adulthood. At the end, author thanked women their participation.

Before starting each interview, contents of Informed Consent Sheet were submitted and discussed. Interviews lasted approximately of 2.5 hours to 3 hours; a pilot interview was accomplished in order to improve interviews guide. Some modifications were effectuated, like, for example, sections order, in addition to specifically ask what kind of messages the participant has received from her family, friends, boyfriends, neighbors, Church officials, etc. As we stated at the beginning of the article, results regarding this aspect of the research are not included herein.

Interviews were accomplished in organizations where participants were recruited. To transcribe contents thereof, codes proposed by Gail Jefferson were used (cited in Wood and Kroger, 2000), according to Table 1. An identification number – oscillating from 001 to 010 - was assigned to each transcribed interviewed.

Table 1. Codes used for transcription

Codes	Description
[ ]	Brackets between statements when participant or Interviewer makes an interruption.
(.)	Pause(less than two seconds)
-	Participant did not end the idea
____	Emphasizing on words
CAPITAL LETTERS	Participant talked higher compared with what he was saying
°word°	Participant talked lower compared with with was saying
Ha-ha	Participant laughs
.hh	Participant breaths inside
Hh	Participant breaths outside
Word(hh)	Participant is laughing meanwhile he is talking
(word) (it refers to)	Person transcribing/adding words so reader understands what the person wants to say. Moreover, it may be an explanatory statement.
( )	Words are not understood
...	cassette is over or text is cut so reader can understand it.
S:i	Points indicate extension of the next sound or syllable
P	Participant
E	Interviewer
Repetitive symbols like: hhhh, (...)	They mean long periods in which participant breaths inside (hhh) or pause lasted more than two seconds (...)

Discourse Analysis

In this research context, participants discourse comes from conversations first author had with interviewed people. They were stories, explanations and constructions women shared during interview, which were used as source or resource for analysis. This is compatible with Potter and Wetherell (1988) discourse definition, understood as text reproduced by someone in a communication interaction context.

It was used analytical method developed by Parker (1992) so as to analyze discourse; it was used years ago by Hollway (1989) in his book *Subjectivity and Method in Psychology: Gender, Meaning, and Science*. This method emphasizes manners in which discourse subjects are determined. For that, it is suggested that in order to identify the discourse, it is necessary to indicate: 1) What is talking about (*i.e.,* women talks about sexual desire in sexual intercourse), and 2) How this construction determines subject (*i.e.,* desire as something uncontrollable). From this perspective, analytical emphasis is about how objects and subjects are constructed from existing discourses. This perspective was nourished by intellectual post-structuralist movement initiated in France, with works made by Foucault (1968, 1985, 1988,

1999) and others. Foucault methodological preparations deal with genealogy of power, knowledge and craziness, sexuality device and ethics of the subject.

At a methodological level, Gillies (1999) provided a framework to analyze the discourse composed according to the following process: 1) to identify linguistic constructions, which are achieved through multiple reading of transcriptions. Even though we recognize that under this methodology participants collaboration is granted to clarify, correct and extend transcription, the task could not be done since the first author moved to another country; 2) To organize references linked to constructions per topics, and to identify their similarities and contrasts (*i.e.*, sexual intercourse is to enjoy/feel pleasure, or to connect love and intimacy, and 3) To identify discursive meanings constructing analysis categories. After organizing them and identifying properly the analysis category, it is initially possible to construe the text in a way, and then to modify the category. As this is a hermeneutic exercise, reader is advised this can occur regularly.

For codification process, it used computers program, since it made possible to organize selected texts in a short time. Developed analysis categories came from research questions and participants discourse. The work to create general categories and subcategories was aimed to organize and to study in-deep each category and to facilitate analysis. For purposes of this article, general and subcategories related to results will be submitted. Diagram 1 shows categories and subcategories relation.

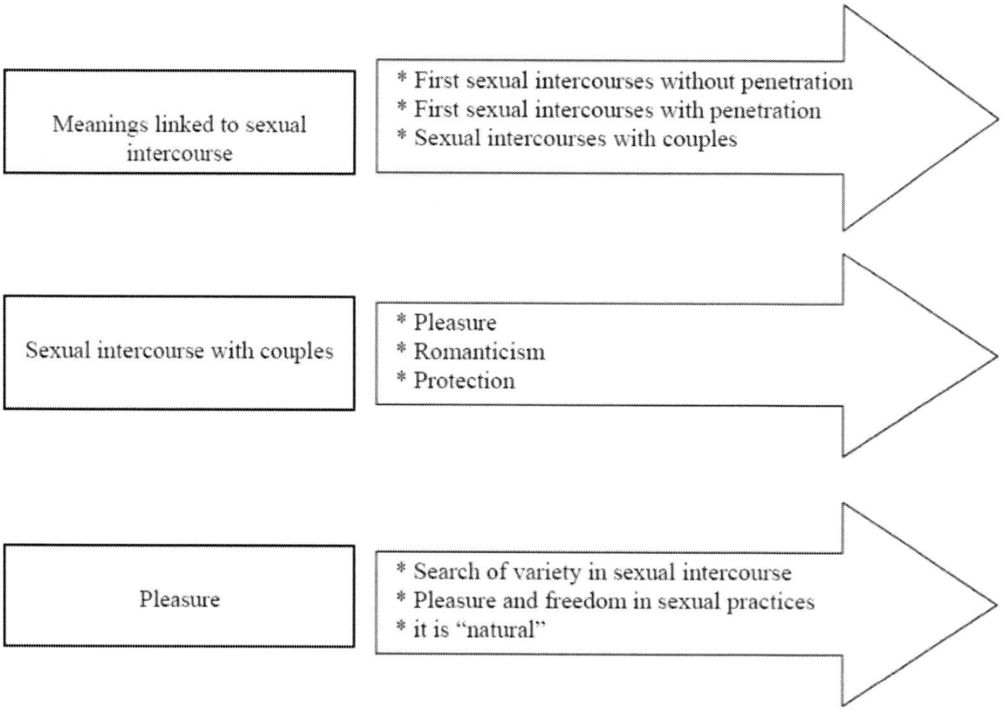

Diagram I. Relation between categories and subcategories to discourse analysis.

RESULTS

Participants' Description

Ten women recruited were between 24 to 29 years old. Most of them (n = 8) were born in the Metropolitan area of San Juan; same number of women who lived with their couples and siblings. All of them informed they have children, from nine months to 12 years old. Most of them (n = 8) had one or two children, but two of the participants informed to have five. About women marital status, four were legally married, three lived with their couples and three are divorced. Women who lived with someone or were married kept a 9 to 12 years couple relation. Almost half of the women had pursued their high school (n = 4); two of them had achieved master degree (n = 2); one in Social Work and other in Public health. Two women were finishing high school (n = 2).

Majority of the women were salaried employees; only two ones were not. Those working were social worker, sexual education program principal, woman services coordinator, recreative therapist and aerobics teacher, elevator operator and health teachers (n = 2), day-care worker and truck stack worker in a "pulguero" in the Metropolitan area of San Juan. Women religious formation had different origin. Religious formation origin was not limited to immediate home and to church, but it included geographical community where women were grown up and Catholic schools they attended, without discarding religious denomination they belonged to. Concerning religion formation, parents, together with grandmothers, aunts, neighbors and friends were part of. All the women (n = 10) grew up in homes where their mother or father were identified with a Catholic religious group. Nonetheless, grandmothers and/or neighbors belonging to Protestant religion of Pentecostal denomination[1] participated actively in their religious formation (n = 5).

Concerning HIV infection risk, some of the women did not use any protection. Those who were protected using condom (n = 5), did it to avoid pregnancy; one of them reported her couple had Hepatitis C and she was HIV positive, and the other, as she was working as health teacher, it was expected to be protected.

Constructions about Sexual Intercourse

What constructions did participants have about sexual intercourse with their couples? Participants constructed some of their sexual intercourses from pleasure discourse[2], the one that Hollway (1989) identifies as permissive discourse. Pleasure discourse approves sexual expression and places both men and women as desirable subjects. From this discourse it is expected women have and enjoy sexual intercourse. Subjects categorized in this discourse consider sexual intercourse as a natural one, expressed spontaneously. As we will see in Results section, some women share this natural and spontaneous idea, even though others, without rejecting it, put ahead their religious background, and when they define the act as a

[1] Under Pentecostal denomination, Spirit gifts are emphasized, speaking in tongues and divine healing. It also promotes emotionally and freely adoration, characterized by continuous praises to God. Under this denomination, Pentecostal Churches of the Assemblies of God are included (Silva-Gotay, 1997).

[2] It is important to remind the reader that we are only presenting pleasure discourse results. According to Diagram 1, there are discourses related to romantic and protecting aspects of the intercourse.

"profit" they move away from Church official precepts discourse; let's see in detail their constructions.

Search of Variety in Sexual Intercourse

Some participants granted privilege to variety of sexual practices, a playing environment during the intercourse and spontaneity of such sexual sharing; the opposite would be "boredom" and "monotony". For a participant, if a woman is going to be with her couple for a long time, the tip is "not getting bored". She declared it is needed to look for diversity and intensity in sexual practices, and intercourse in different places. In that sexual intercourse, both "have to" satisfy the other's desires.

> We are going to be together for a long time and we try then, of not getting bore. I satisfy all the things he wants and vice versa. It is avoided to fall in monotony, like many other couples do; they do not have sex except in their bedroom. (We)...do it wherever we want, so varied (at the beach, in the car...). Very good. It is like if I abandon myself... I do not think what I am doing. After that... both fall... It is very varied... We have three months it has not been like this.. TOO MUCH time... although we are *together* every day, but...we have practically done everything..., well, not anal, not yet... I imagine that maybe someday I will do it because...imagine...we have changed places, positions, the way we do it...savage, softly...with candle sperm..soft, tender...wildly (008).

In that search of pleasure in sexual intercourse, where variety is the core and it is privileged, there is a moment of great satisfaction: it is when both do "canto", implying, among other things, to do any sexual practice "they both want".

> I am a person that in order to be completely satisfied...needs to do "canto". EVERYTHING. All what we want to do, we do it. If you want dog positions, do it; if you want normal position, do it; if you want to be up, do it; if you want to do it in a chair, do it... At least, my husband and I like to change. If certain day we do not want to have sexual intercourse...well...we masturbate each other...we change it; if today we do not want to do it, we have oral sex; if not, then...we do a quickie (004).

Moreover, sexual practices variety, environment granted during sexual intercourse was a fun one, with acts *executed* producing pleasure. In the interview, this participant had variations in her discourse. In the previous text, her desire is subject to her couple's desire. In the following text, she placed herself in a different psychic space, implying that in addition to satisfy her couple, she is searching her orgasm, a fact meant for her total satisfaction.

> We play a lot… I become prostitute and I want he talks to me roughly; I want he treats me bad...He loves that...He likes I wear spectacles, I put on long skirts and...I will be his *teacher,* he loves that...Sometimes we plan with hand and we end making love...I love to play and *I love* to punish him in the meantime...PLAY. We play until we reach the ORGASMIC POINT. We get the climax. Total excitement is to finish both at the same time; to have a simultaneous orgasm. Total satisfaction. I feel satisfy. When I reach orgasm, I feel satisfy. (004).

Participants shared sexual practices generating them high pleasure, joy and exciment; they argued their reasons, placing in a control position, working their desire and comfort during sexual intercourse.

Enjoyment and Freedom Drawn from Some Sexual Practices

For this participant, penetrative practice when her partner ejaculates inside her, was the most eroticizing one. This act he qualified as erotizing was "so delicious". For her, couple's semen was hers; semen was her "profit".

> ...He has to finish because I get upset when he starts but he does not finish...Coming inside...It is war, it is warm. It is something like...When he comes, semen is *very warm*...It is something so, so delicious, *TOO MUCH.* It is as I say to you: "take these 10 thousand pesos only for you...All is for you. *That is, it is something for me*...and then, he, instead of letting me go, he holds me tighter as saying "you are mine". Baby, not at all...This is mine...It is something of mine. It is something I earned (007).

For each participant, less traditional positions were the most exciting one because were the ones they could not do often since they had children.

> I would say that the most exciting thing is not penetration, but.. to explore clitoris and less traditional positions....not laid; stand, in a chair. The most traditional is not what give us more satisfaction...because we have less chance to practice them...we have two children (006).

Oral sex was a freedom and pleasure act, especially when it is related to Church standards. Oral sex implied to beat Church; in other words, to resist its discourse and break the law. It is not casual law breaking was considered as a freedom act.

> I feel...free...Sensation of freedom to think pleasure is important for me...I related to Church beliefs that sexuality is for reproduction...For me, pleasure is important, and to have oral sex means, indeed, there is no reproduction...Then, for me...is a freedom sensation that I got over such bond, that connection...I learned that there must have pleasure...I won this; yes, I reached this...This is my intimate part, and ...nobody cares (006).

It seems to us interesting this participant had been the only one who had established a relation between sexual practices and Churches guidelines. This discursive reposition shows the varieties happening in women and men internal life. This information deserves to state the importance of avoiding to establish prediction lines. Other of the subcategories bonded with pleasure is related to the body. Body was seen as an own entity not bonded with women.

Body Leads Us

This participant classified her sexual encounters as natural, since it was nothing forced. She yielded completely the responsibility of the intercourse to her body: "body leads us to it", meaning there is a space where body's desire makes lose control.

> I think my sexuality with him is one hundred percent better than with other persons I have been...We do not have to ask if we want to do sex or not... The body itself leads us...Instead of asking, he knows when I want and I know when he wants...There is no need to say it, you know, there is *body language…* Sometime he kisses me and I feel *upset.* Sometime, if I see him sleeping, I get excited in some way...We do not use creams and objects. We do it naturally; we do it different....Every time some different happens...All is well quite, natural, daily; nothing is forced, all is fluid... (008).

In conclusion, it is important to stand out discursive emphasis. So as to get pleasure during sexual intercourse, the following conditions must be given: 1) Sexual practices must be naturally expressed; 2) Sexual practices must be varied and different; 3) Sexual practices must produce enjoyment and pleasure to both; 4) Sexual practices must lead to simultaneous orgasm; 5) Sexual intercourse must have a transgressive element (either in sexual practices or in places where they are carried out), and 6) There must be a playing environment during intercourse.

Sexual practices execution, as well as women's pleasure and enjoyment show two important items: First, physical and psychic relation during intercourse (*i.e.,* "he holds me" as if "I were his"; "to have oral sex makes feel free"). Second, women placed in a control position, looking for their sexual satisfaction. This position seems to us one of power faced with their couple and of pro-activity faced with their desire.

Discussion

How some of constructions clung to pleasure discourse positioned women to effectuate risky practices? How searching of sexual variety and obtaining unlimited enjoyment and pleasure position them in front of HIV and other STD risk? Deepen studies shall be accomplished, regarding women's bonds and relations established with pleasure discourse.

When looking for pleasure, sometime participants stood out condom use. Citation from participant saying the satisfaction she felt when semen was inside her is just mentioned. Definitely, this practice put her in HIV and other STD infection risk. The result is confirmed in other researches, in the sense that all items threatening pleasure and eroticism, as condom use is, must be cast away (Carrillo, 2002; Dowsett, 2000, Gogna and Ramos, 2000; Muñoz-Laboy, 2004). However, it is important to deepen in its construction. For that woman, couple's semen was hers; she earns it. Semen was seen as a reward for her actions during sexual intercourse. We ask, then, how this semen construction places her in face of condom resource. For us, condom separates her from the liquid she wants to possess.

It is not possible to ignore her discursive emphasis. Semen is a "warm" liquid, pleasant and delicious for her. Then, her couple's action of "throwing it, placed her as recipient of such liquid; he tighted her, and she construed such conduct as "I am yours". There is no doubt this participant's emphasis was absolutely physical when referring sexual intercourse. We think she was psychically placed in a in the forefront. This term refers in her discourse there was no distance between him, object of her desire, and her. Symbolically, there was no interruption, neither separation between those these two bodies.

It could be seen that abandoning herself to the moment provoked in some of participants not to think in any other thing. The fact they thought only in pleasure and satisfaction, not in the possibility of risk, could promote to discard condom use. Such as it was mentioned before, most of participants did not use protection. This does not mean that if they would have known they were in danger, they would have protected; that premise comes from a rational logic that evidently does not favor sexual intercourse. Undoubtedly, then, for many participants, HIV and STD is not part of the issues important for them when they have kept long couple's relations- from nine to twelve years. Consequently, it is understandable couples' confidentiality is constructed under another logic, like, for example, if her word matches with her actions, which has nothing to do with the possible someone's serologic status. As it was previously stated, women's discourses in couple were of confidentiality and safety in that relation space (Willing, 1999). In other words, risk was constructed out of that space. This correlation among high reliable levels and risk possibility discard has been confirmed in multiple studies accomplished both in the United States of North America and in Puerto Rico (Ekhrardt, Yingling, Zaqwadzki, and Martinez-Ramirez, 1992; Gomez and Marin, 1996; Green, Fulop, and Kocsis, 2000; Ramos-Irrizary, Serrano-Garcia, Hernandez-Cartagena, and Varas-Diaz, 1998; Seal, Wagner-Raphael, and Ehrhardt, 2000).

Sexual intercourse constructed by participants as something spontaneously expressed, in a "natural" manner and favoring practices variety could lead them to perform risky sexual behaviors. From this framework, sexual behaviors, like condom use when you have anal or vaginal sex, "*dental dam*" use when you have oral sex, could be considered as unattractive or non seducing ones. If emphases correlated with sexual intercourse and specially "to burst suddenly, with so called "savage", "explosive" penetration are analyzed carefully, it can be seen all of them as "violent" definitions alluding to the end and termination of a state, at least physical one. We ask ourselves: What is there after "burst suddenly" and explosions? What is taken? On the other hand, if oral sex experience is analyzed, which the other participant classifies it as "freedom", "intimate" act, where "nobody mess with me", are definitions that could put aside prevention discourse. Up to here, it is clear preventive discourse regulates affection, makes think about consequences; therefore, make us be subjected and subordinated, and even more, it is a controlling discourse, meaning, it is involved with other subjects' life.

As from the foregoing, the action logic from participant women is centered in sensations search. Skin has receptors allowing to send this stimulus to brain in order to organize and construe such sensorial experience which provokes excitement, then enjoyment and satisfaction (Pinel, 2007). Nonetheless, the meaning such woman gives to physical experience ("hot milk") correlating it to a psychic condition ("I earned it"), points to a new research line in prevention field. This work was only the beginning of exploration of subjective experience during sexual act.

In their discourses, some participants expressed the pleasure they felt when satisfying their couple, "if you want dog position, we will do it". We ask, how this construction places them in view of their couple anal sexual practices request —without protection?, such as one anticipated: "I imagine he will ask me that since we have made everything". Where are the roles of some of them in view of their couple's request? For some women, to satisfy their couple place them in a power and control space over sexual intercourse. They did not perform as passive servants of their couple's requests. There is no doubt results submitted prove satisfaction produced in the participants when responds to their couple's request. We would like to emphasize this point, since through some feminist works (Correa, Figueroa-Sarriera, López, and Roman, 1994), especially those prepared in the first stage, this result could be construed as actions of submission from women and not, as one of the participants proposed, as a "game" occurring during sexual intercourse.

Having said that, what if women want to use protection and men don't? According to results submitted, no discrepancies can be drawn from their couple's request and women's desire. However, in Noboa-Ortega (2005), there are data leading to how some of women tried to use protection and strategies they use for such purpose. Nonetheless, this is the biggest challenge in prevention, meaning, there must be analyzed what alternatives and skills are provided for women to seduce, eroticize and to keep a playful environment meanwhile they protect their sexual health. How to satisfy their couple, if such act eroticizes her, with limits, meaning, not be at the mercy of her couple's exclusive desire and to give up her need to use protection?

Without doubt, all research work has challenges, and we would like to share some of them. The first was starting this research by interviewing participants. Sometimes, some of them were "deviated" to this study interests. They insistently talked about things that were not pertinent to the first author. This let us see particular agendas participants had when being part of this research.

The second challenge was transcription process. Codes system used at this level of process specificity of transcription was unnecessary to analyze discourse from a *post*-structuralist perspective. Finally, another challenge was to categorize in order to deepen in analysis technique. Even though Potter and Wetherell (1988) observations were followed, initial categories were wide, the most possible inclusive ones. As texts were read and read again, categories were more and more being "narrowed ". However, to have included initially wide categories created confusion, especially when facing the lack of work regarding this initial phase during the analysis.

Lastly, undoubtedly, discrepancies in approaching in view of discourse analysis, besides exposition of existing tensions concerning how discourse is analyzed, made difficult to select texts that led finally the analysis.

Finally, below we present the contribution and scope of this work for psychology and the own environment of HIV prevention infection. We believe results show women have changed their traditional and ascetic roles drawn from social standards. This work proves women find their pleasure, by showing a high level of comfort with the idea of not escaping from irrationality during sexual intercourse.

Data reported herein reflex richness about how women live some aspects of their sexual intercourse. Up to now, we have not read a work at this detailed level about how women are distanced from culture precepts; they do not evaluate consequences of their acts and operate from more primary dimensions. These results suggest the need to review how women sexual activity is conceptualized in HIV and STD researches/intervention, particularly in psychology field. Moreover, this work invites us to think how we classified women and how we think during sexual intercourse, and respect with their couples, in developed prevention interventions.

We invite you to deepen in pleasure discourse and axes that are framed in sexual intercourse and its bond with HIV and STD risk. Likewise, to think about methods to be used so as to continue exploring this research topic. Some initial questions that could provoke future researches are: How women and men transgress standards bond with gender when they search pleasure? What actions do women and men carry out during sexual intercourse so as to maximize pleasure? We trust both questions provoke research works in benefit of more friendly models development in view of human complexity and contradiction.

REFERENCES

Berger, P. and Luckmann, T. (1986). *La construcción social de la realidad.* Buenos Aires, Argentina: Amorrortu Editores.

Castro, R. (2002). Uno de hombre con la mujer es como una corriente eléctrica: Subjetividad y sexualidad entre los hombres de Morelos. En F. Mercado, D. Gastaldo y C. Calderón (Eds.), *Investigación cualitativa en salud en Iberoamérica: Métodos, análisis y ética* (pp. 181-210). Guadalajara, México: Universidad de Guadalajara.

Carrillo, H. (2002). *The night is young: Sexuality in Mexico in the time of AIDS.* Chicago, IL: University of Chicago Press.

CDC (2011). HIV among women. En Internet: http://www.cdc.gov/hiv/topics/basic/ index.htm [Retirado el 15/noviembre /2011].

Correa, N., Figueroa-Sarriera, H., López, M.M. y Román, M. (1994). Las mujeres, son, son, son… implosión y recomposición de la categoría. En H. Figueroa-Sarriera, M.M. López y M. Román (Eds.), *Mas allá de la bella (in)diferencia: Revisión post-feminista y otras escrituras posibles* (pp. 34-50). San Juan, PR: Publicaciones Puertorriqueñas.

Cunnin8gham, I., Díaz-Esteve C., González-Santiago, M., and Rodríguez-Sánchez, M.H. (1994). University students and AIDS: Some findings from three surveys—1989, 1990, 1992.

Cunningham, I., Rivera-Viera, S., Bothwell-Toro, F. and Domenech-Miller, K. (1996). *Sexualidad y el VIH/SIDA; Módulos innovadores de enseñanza.* Río Piedras, P.R. Centro de Investigación y Educación de VIH/SIDA.

Dowsett, G. (2000). Bodyplay: Corporeality in a discursive silence. En R. Parker, R. María-Barbosa, and P. Aggleton (Eds.) *Framing the sexual subject: The politics of gender, sexuality, and power* (pp. 29-45). Los Angeles, CA: University of California.

Ekhrardt, A.A., Yingling, S., Zawadzki, R., and Martínez-Ramírez, M. (1992). Prevention of heterosexual transmission of HIV: Barriers for women. *AIDS Education and Prevention, 8*, 37-56.

Fernández, M.I. (1995). Latinas and AIDS: Challenges to HIV prevention efforts. En A. O'Leary and S. Jemmott (Eds.), *Women at risk: Issues in the primary prevention of AIDS* (pp. 159-174). New York, NY: Plenum.

Figueroa-Sarriera, H. and López, M. M. (1990, mayo). *El sujeto descentrado y algunas implicaciones para las ciencias sociales o ¿Dónde vives tú finalmente?* Ponencia presentada ante el Coloquio Sociologies IV en la Université Paul Valéry en Montpellier, Francia.

Foucault, M. (1968). *Las palabras y las cosas.* México: Siglo XXI.

Foucault, M. (1985). *Saber y verdad.* Madrid, España: Ediciones de la Piqueta.

Foucault, M. (1988). *The history of sexuality.* New York, NY: Vintage Books.

Foucault, M. (1999). *Estética, ética y hermeneútica.* Barcelona: España: Ediciones Paidós

Galarza, M. (1998). La negociación sexual: Desarrollo preliminar de una escala y resultados en una muestra de mujeres puertorriqueñas. Tesis de Maestría no publicada. San Juan, Puerto Rico: Departamento de Psicología de la Universidad de Puerto Rico.

Gergen, K.J. and Gergen, M. M. (2003). *Social construction: A reader.* London: Sage.

Gillies, V. (1999). An analysis of the discursive positions of women smokers: Implications for practical interventions. En C. Willig (Ed.), *Applied discourse analysis: Social and psychological interventions* (pp. 66-86). Buckingham, PA: Open University Press.

Gogna, M. and Ramos, S. (2000). Gender stereotypes and power relations: Unacknowledged risks for STDs in Argentina. En R. Parker, R. María-Barbosa, and P. Aggleton (Eds.), *Framing the sexual subject: The politics of gender, sexuality, and power* (pp. 29-45). Los Angeles, CA: University of California.

Gómez, C.A. and Marín, B. (1996). Gender, culture, and power: Barriers to HIV-prevention strategies for women. *Journal of Sex Research, 33*, 355-362.

Gónzalez-Rey, F. (1997). *Epistemología cualitativa y subjetividad.* São Paulo, Brasil: EDUC Editorial.

Green, J., Fulop, N., and Kocsis, A. (2000). Determinants of unsafe in women. *International Journal of STD and AIDS, 11*, 777-783.

Hollway, W. (1989). *Subjectivity and method in psychology: Gender, meaning, and science.* London: Sage.

Ibánez, T. (1994). *Psicología social construccionista: Selección de textos.* Guadalajara, México: Universidad de Guadalajara.

Marín, B.V. (1996). *Cultural issues in HIV prevention for Latinos: Should we try to change gender roles? Understanding HIV risk behaviour.* Newbury Park, CA: Sage.

Marín, B.V. and Gómez, C.A. (1997). Predictor of condom accessibility among Hispanics in San Francisco. *American Journal of Public Health,* 82, 532- 595.

Markes, G., Cantero, P.J., and Simoni, J.M. (1998). Is acculturation associated with sexual risk behaviours?: An investigation of HIV-positive Latino men and women. *AIDS Care, 10*, 283-295.

Mayo, Y.Q. and Resnick, R.P. (1996). The impact of machismo on Hispanic women. *Affilia: Journal of Women and Social Work, 11*, 257-278.

Muñoz-Laboy, M.A. (2004). Beyond 'MSM': Sexual desire among bisexually-active Latino men in New York City. *Sexualities, 7*, 55-80.

Oficina de Estadísticas de Salud (2011). *Estadísticas para el mes de mayo del 2011.* San Juan, Puerto Rico: Autor.

Ortiz-Torres, B. (1995, junio). Estrategias de prevención de VIH/SIDA entre mujeres: La interacción entre género, cultura y contexto social. Trabajo presentado en el *XXV Congreso Interamericano de Psicología*. San Juan, Puerto Rico.

Ortiz-Torres, B., Serrano-García, I., and Torres-Burgos, N. (2000). Subverting culture: Promoting HIV/AIDS prevention among Puerto Rican and Dominican women. *American Journal of Community Psychology, 28*, 859-881.

Noboa-Ortega, P. (2005). *Subjetividad femenina... significados sobre cuerpo, género, sexualidad y encuentro sexul en mujeres puertorriqueñas y sus vínculos con el VIH/SIDA*. Tesis Doctoral no publicada. Río Piedras, Puerto Rico: Departamento de Psicología de la Universidad de Puerto Rico.

Parker, I. (1992). *Discourse dynamics: Critical analysis for social and individual psychology.* Florence, KY: Taylor and Francis/Routledge.

Parker, R. (2001). Sexuality, culture, and power in HIV/AIDS research. *Annual Review of Anthropology, 30*, 163-179.

Pinel, J. (2007). *Mecanismos de la Percepción: Visión, Audición, Olfato, Piel. Biopsicología* (6ª edición). Madrid: Pearson/Addison-Wesley.

Ramos-Irrizary, L., Serrano-García, I., Hernández-Cartagena, M., and Varas-Díaz, N. (1998, August). Relationship stability and the risk of HIV/AIDS among Puerto Rican women. Paper presented at the *Annual Convention of the American Psychological Association*. San Francisco, California.

Seal, D.W. and Ehrhardt, A.A. (2003). Masculinity and urban men: Perceived scripts for courtship, romantic, and sexual interactions with women. *Culture, Health and Sexuality, 5*, 295-319.

Seal, D.W., Wagner-Raphael, L.I., and Ehrhardt, A.A. (2000). Sex, intimacy, and HIV: An ethnographic study of a Puerto Rican social group in New York City. *Journal of Psychology and Human Sexuality, 11*, 51-92.

Silva-Gotay, S. (1997). *Protestantismo y política en Puerto Rico 1989-1930: Hacia una historia del protestantismo evangélico en Puerto Rico*. Río Piedras, Puerto Rico: Editorial de la Universidad de Puerto Rico.

Simon, W. and Gagnon, J. (1999). *Culture, society and sexuality: A reader*. London: UCL Press.

Toro-Alfonso, J. (2000). Implicaciones psicosociales en la intervención para la prevención de la transmisión del virus de inmunodeficiencia humana (VIH) con hombres homosexuales en Puerto Rico: Un modelo para el Caribe. *Revista Interamericana de Psicología, 34*, 173-193.

Vargas, R. (1994). Los discursos biomédicos y la construcción del VIH/SIDA: Una mirada a través de una historia de vida y de la perspectiva de un médico primario. Tesis de Maestría no publicada. Río Piedras, Puerto Rico: Departamento de Psicología de la Universidad de Puerto Rico.

Weiss, E., Whelan, D., and Rao-Gupta, G. (2000). Gender, sexuality and HIV: Making a difference in the lives of young women in developing countries. *Sexual and Relationship Therapy, 15*, 233-245.

Wetherell, M. and Potter, J. (1988). Discourse analysis and the identification of interpretative repertoires. En C. Antaki (Ed.), *Analyzing everyday explanation: A casebook of methods*. (pp. 168-183). Thousand Oaks, CA: Sage.

Willig, C. (1999). *Applied discourse analysis: Social and psychological interventions*. Buckingham, PA: Open University Press.

Wood, L.A. and Kroger, R.O. (2000). *Doing discourse analysis: Methods for studying action in talk and text*. Thousand Oaks, CA: Sage.

Wood, M. L. and Price, P. (1997). Machismo and marianismo: Implications for HIV/AIDS risk reduction and education. *American Journal of Health Studies, 13*, 44-53.

Yeakley, A.M. and Gant, L. (1997). Cultural factors and program implications: HIV/AIDS interventions and condom use among Latinos. *Journal of Multicultural Social Work, 6*, 47-71.

(Manuscript received on 28 November 2011. Revised version accepted for publication on 27 March 2012)

In: Recent Hispanic Psychological Research … ISBN: 978-1-62948-919-3
Editors: C. H. Garcia Cadena, A. Lopez-Espinoza et al. © 2014 Nova Science Publishers, Inc.

Chapter 12

A Psychological Model for Adherence Behaviors among HIV-Positive Persons: Research and Perspectives

Juan José Sánchez-Sosa*, José Luis Ybarra Sagarduy and Julio Alfonso Piña López
Facultad de Psicología
Universidad Nacional Autónoma de México
Unidad de Trabajo Social y Ciencias para el Desarrollo Humano
Universidad Autónoma de Tamaulipas, México
Investigador Independiente
Hermosillo, México

Abstract

In this paper we summarize the central core of a psychological model for adherence behaviors (PMAB) in the context of HIV-positive persons. First, we justify the importance of a conceptual analysis approaching a formal model. Second, we describe recent developments based on the model and the implications for future research to improve both, our knowledge on mechanisms underlying adherence behaviors, as well as designing and implementing intervention programs for behavior change from a psychological point of view.

Keywords: Psychological Model, Adherence Behaviors, HIV-Positive Persons, Conceptual Analysis, Research

---

* Address for correspondence: Facultad de Psicología. Universidad Nacional Autónoma de México. Avenida Universidad No. 3004, Edificio "E", 20 Piso, Cubículo "H". Delegación Coyoacán. México, Distrito Federal, C.P. 04510 (México). E-mail: jujosaso@yahoo.com.mx.

INTRODUCTION

Although the domain of health psychology seems clearly defined (Marks, 2008), the formulation and empirical validation of applied theories or models in Latin-American countries remain two pending tasks for a vast majority of psychologists (Piña, 2011, 2012). As in other scientific contexts, theories and models are necessary if psychologists wish to attain articulated explanations and stronger predictions, as well as to provide a guide for designing and validating intervention programs for behavior change (Noar and Zimmerman, 2005; Weinstein, 2007).

By articulated explanations we mean those which help scholars and professionals organize the assumptions of a theory or model, e.g., what types of concepts include such assumptions and whether or not such concepts have actually been functionally and/or operationally defined (see Baranowski, 2005; Ogden, 2003). Furthermore, as has been suggested (Ribes, 2004a), psychologists also need to know how concepts must be define. Thus, as Ryle has pointed out, when an author does not define concepts correctly, it is very likely that he/she is engaging in a category-mistake:

> From a theoretical viewpoint interesting category-mistakes are those made by people who are perfectly competent to apply concepts, at least in the situations with which they are familiar, but are still liable in their abstract thinking to allocate those concepts to logical types to which they do not belong (Ryle, 1949; p.19).

Following Ryle's propositions, a category-mistake occurs when words or expressions used as concepts represent facts of a certain kind as if they belonged to one logical category, when they actually belong to another. In ordinary language the concept of personality is a good example which can be understood as a dispositional statement describing and synthesizing the unique, singular and idiosyncratic psychological history of behavior (as outcome of an individual's biography).

Table 1. Conceptual categories in psychology according to Ryle (1949): Some examples

Concepts	Categories	Theories and models [a]
Beliefs	Tendencies (at social level)	HBM / TAR / PBT / IMBC
Abilities and self-efficacy	Capacities (as possibilities)	HBM / TAR / PBT / SET / IMBC
Attitudes	Adverbial	TAR / /PBT/ IMBC
Motivation (or Motives)	Inclinations and Propensities	PMAB
Competencies (as knowledge and abilities)	Modals (as probabilities)	PMAB/ PMBH
Personality	Tendencies (at individual level)	PMAB / PMBH

[a] HBM (Health Beliefs Model), TAR (Theory of Reasoned Action), PBT (Planned Behavior Theory), SET (Self-Efficacy Theory), IMBC (Integrative Model for Behavior Change), PMT (Protection Motivation Theory), IMB (Information-Motivation-Behavioral Kills Model), PMAB (Psychological Model for Adherence Behaviors) and PMBH (Psychological Model of Biological Health).

In this particular case, a category-mistake is identified when an author defines personality as *broad stable traits or states* as it's basic units (*see* Ajzen, 1988; Eysenck, 1988), as if they were actual tendencies of behavior; in spite of the fact that both tendencies and state categories are dispositional statements, as shown in Table 1 between them there are differences which authors should keep in mind.[1]

Such differences become more evident because the scope of conceptual categories is limited to the "logical geography" of any concept, and in the sense there are logical boundaries delimiting how concepts function or are used (Moore, 2001). We also want to note that psychological concepts play different logical functions in theories or models, depending on the type of concepts that authors use in relation to psychological events as processes, states and/or results. In fact, many psychological concepts can be conceived as dispositional statements as per Ryle's propositions, which can be grouped as: 1) Collections of occurrences, either simultaneous or successive; 2) Statements about individuals having a certain capacity, tendency, propensity or liability, and 3) Serving more a predictive value than law statements, since the latter are explanatory in nature (Ribes, 2003).

The key value of the previous discussion is that a theory or model will be both conceptually and empirically pertinent to the extent to which their general assumptions are well grounded on research, as well as how their core concepts are used. Thus, in the case of health psychology, theories or models will be pertinent only after research results clearly demonstrate that they are capable of predicting a behavior related to prevention, to risk, to easing adjustment to a disease or, more specifically, adhering to medical treatment. Thus, we also concur with the proposal that using a theory or model implies that researchers "move" along a continuum which starts with the use of a frame of reference or a few concepts and eventually leads to developing and testing a new theory or model (Painter, Borba, Hynes, Mays, and Glanz, 2008). As a logical colophon we would add that just as every analysis of the health-disease continuum touches upon an individual's behavior, every analysis of the empirical pertinence and viability of a theory or model should always start from its conceptual analysis.

A Psychological Model for Adherence Behaviors among HIV-Positive Persons

There are many factors linked to adherence behaviors (Bosworth, 2010; Sánchez-Sosa, 2002). Most of these factors are traditionally defined in terms of mental or cognitive activities happening inside the body; such as factors related to concepts like knowledge, attitudes, beliefs, perceived benefits, perceived barriers, self-efficacy, autonomous motivation, cognitive function, mood state, etc. (Barclay, Hinkin, Castellon, Mason, Reinhard, Marion et al., 2007; Garvie, Flynn, Belzer, Britto, Hu, Graham et al., 2011; Kennedy, Goggin, and Nollen, 2004; Malcolm, Ng, Rosen, and Stone, 2003; Reynolds, 2003; Tarakeshar, Srikrishnan, Johnson, Vatsu, Solomon, Merson et al., 2007).

---

[1] Once the concept of personality is defined as "traits" or "states" (e.g., neuroticism, psychoticism, introversion, hostility, impulsivity, etc.), when a person is somehow designated on the basis of one or more such categories, it is automatically assumed he/she shares some specific characteristics, in the same sense that are shared by other persons. Therefore, personality as both individual way of behaving and as outcome of each person's biography is canceled (Ribes, 2009).

Many psychologists tend to assume that these cognitions involve trans-spatial processes that are immune to direct observation. These cognitions or activities are based on the provocative question: "What takes place between the stimulus and the response?"; all public actions or behaviors, however, are conceived as caused by an internal agency, reducing the explanation of behaviors to some type of efficient cause (Kantor, 1978). As Enç pointed out:

> Typically, most causal theories found in the literature have a common feature—they all involve a system that has the function of bringing about a result or a final product. The normal path that connects the input to the final product in one that subserves the function of the system. More specifically, when causal theories offer a causal analysis of a type of entity, the type of entity is the output produced by the system when and only when the system's producing that output is part of what counts as the system's executing its function (Enç, 2004; p. 155).

How can we avoid references for internal agencies as well as for a causal analysis in the study of psychological variables underlying adherence behaviors in the domain of health psychology? In the first place, it would be necessary to *re*-define what we mean by behavior. Following Ribes' proposition, behavior, as a psychological concept, is an abstraction of the movements, actions, and effects of a person's *saying*, *feeling* or *doing* something in context (Ribes, 2004b). Behavior, as a term whose origin came from ordinary language can be identified and described by words and expressions dealing with occurrences or episodes (how people do, or should, act and react), as well as with collections of occurrences as inclinations or propensities (e.g., motives), modals expressions (e.g., behavioral competencies) and tendencies to behave (e.g., personality). Because inclinations or propensities, modals, and tendencies categories play specific theoretical roles regarding the formulation of predictions, the application of theories or models should consist of using concepts in strict correspondence with the roles given to terms in each of the different definition approaches.

On the basis of this assumption, we recently developed a psychological model for adherence behaviors (PMAB) under a more comprehensive theoretical umbrella (Piña and Sánchez-Sosa, 2007). The proposal attempts to provide an account of the way in which stress-related situations, motives, behavioral competencies, and dispositional events (social and biological) combine to predict adherence behaviors (Figure 1). This model contrasts with others not only in the sense of proposing an interbehavioral approach derived from J. R. Kantor's work (Kantor, 1959), including a behavior theory (Ribes and López, 1985) and a personality theory (Ribes and Sánchez, 1990), but it also proposes an interactive and functional emphasis on analyzing those variables assumed to determine the behaviors in question.

In phase one, stress-related situations are defined as consistent ways in which persons interact with situations which contain *unpredictable*, *ambiguous* or *uncertain* stimulus signals, as well as behavioral consequences.

There are situations linked to how people behave in social circumstances as a product of their own psychological history or personal biography, therefore it encompasses the *unique*, *idiosyncratic* and *singular* way in which a person faces situations, related not to *what* a person does, but how they do it (Ribes, 2005). An example is the situation known as risk-taking tendency, in which a person faces conditions that he/she knows are stable (in terms of the probability and quantity of stimulus consequences), or conditions that he/she knows that are variable and unpredictable but that entail major consequences. In principle, choosing the latter consequences seems to be advantageous in terms of their likelihood, quantity, or both (Ribes and Sánchez, 1992).

Through this conceptual category we emphasize a frequently overlooked phenomenon in most theories or traditional models in psychology and health, that of personality. This is a category that summarizes the psychological biography of an individual, e.g., the history of successive contacts of the person in functionally similar situations. This is therefore a category which complies with the logical function of identifying and evaluating tendencies of behavior, both along time and across situations (Ribes, 2009). Since this is a variable that refers to the individual's most distal psychological history, its plays a crucial role in predicting, with a good amount of certainty, how likely is it that a person will or will not do something in one or several interactive situations; for the case under consideration, whether a person living with a chronic condition such as HIV will actually engage in adherence behaviors in an efficient and consistent way.

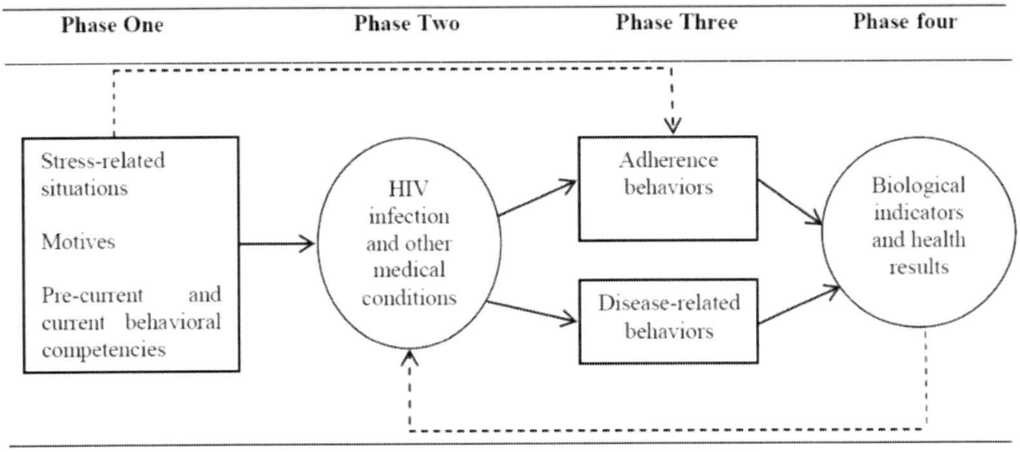

Figure 1. Psychological model for the research on adherence behaviors (Piña and Sánchez-Sosa, 2007).

The main point is, as recently suggested by Noar (2007) regarding traditional models and theories (such as health beliefs, reasoned action, planned behavior, etc.), that most of them lack a characterization of the personality phenomenon, and those which deal explicitly with the issue tend to incur in category-mistakes such as those described earlier in this section. One such example appears in the integrative change model by Fishbein et al. (Fishbein, 2000; Fishbein, Hennessy, Yzer, and Douglas, 2003) which characterizes personality as part of the distal variables without characterizing it, and placing it at the same level as *mood* and *emotions*, as if all three concepts referred to the same class of events and therefore to the same logical category. It is worth noting that the terms or words relating to emotions include other concepts, grouped with such terms as motives, moods, commotions, agitations or feelings (Ryle, 1949).

In principle, the first three would belong to the category of inclinations or propensities and the last to events or occurrences. By mixing concepts belonging to different analytical categories the model incurs in logical inconsistencies and, inadvertently, also in conceptual inconsistencies. Thus, the analysis of the behavior of one individual makes little sense in the context of another person's behavior being different.

Other individual would show a tendency to behave in a unique and idiosyncratic way both along time and between situations.[2,3,]

In the absence of the explicit recognition of the individual's psychological history these models lack *interface* or *bridging* categories which would help understand the factors that make more or less probable that, in a specific circumstance, a person will behave in a relatively stable and consistent way, again, along time and in different situations (Piña et al., 2011).

Motives (or motivation) get defined as inclinations or propensities to behave in certain way in specific socially-valued situations (Ribes, 2005). It is said that a person is motivated to practice adherence behaviors when he/she is willing to behave accordingly, after having understood the relation between such behaviors and some specific stimulus consequences. Such consequences can vary widely, ranging from interpersonal in nature (e.g., verbal praise or support from others), or intrinsic, such as perception of physical or psychological well-being. Motivational variables affect behavior by altering the effectiveness of consequences as reinforcers, in this sense the behavior-strengthening effects of reinforcement normally lead to an increase of the behavior in the future (Laraway, Snycerski, and Poling, 2004). Take, for example a person who is highly motivated to engage in adherence behaviors, not only because this is a socially expected behavior but because it has, in the past, led to a variety of positive consequences such as verbal praise by significant others or by members of the health team. If these consequences persist along the interpersonal interaction continuum, the probability of motives influencing adherence behaviors will be higher.

The behavioral competencies category summarizes what a person knows about HIV and AIDS, as well as the practice of adherence behaviors that need to occur. Such knowledge includes what is HIV, what is AIDS, which are the stimulus signaling and situations affecting the probability to practice adherence behaviors, etc. We can say that a person is behaviorally competent if he/she knows how the disease comes about, what the treatment consists of, why he/she must take medications precisely the way the health team indicates, why he/she must avoid taking substances interfering with the treatment, and above all, behave consistently with all that knowledge.

Thus, being competent involves knowing the relevant information and doing the necessary things consistently and efficiently. It should be noted that the critical underlying element to the concept of competencies in the present proposal is that it specifies criteria regarding how and what should be done by the individual in defined situations, so that a person engages in the behaviors which are expected from him/her. In contrast to traditional models, in this one, being competent involves both knowledge and sets of skills related to the practice of adherence behaviors, and not with an individual believes he/she can engage in

[2] Although some authors include one more category as part of distal variables, those described as "individual differences" are neither conceptually defined nor differentiated from the concept of personality, as if this phenomenon had little or nothing to do with individual differences.

[3] We differ from the position recently assumed by Albarracin, Rothman, DiClemente, and del Río (2010), who state that traditional models and theories overestimate the role of individual behavior, and call for analyses based on interpersonal relations and an assortment of social-structural levels as if they were an integrated whole. Although the analysis of individual behavior is indeed incomplete in the absence of a proper conceptualization of the personality phenomenon, the above proposal becomes unsustainable for two additional reasons: first, the sum of theoretical components does not necessarily equal a whole, second, the point is not to simply insure the addition of analyses stemming from diverse unrelated sources but to secure theoretical continuity. We contend that this is precisely what this proposal lacks (Piña, Fierros, García, and Ybarra, 201; Piña, Ybarra, Alcalá, and Samaniego, 2010.

such behaviors (e.g., "I believe I can take my medications") or whether the individual perceives him/herself as self-efficacious to perform it.

In last analysis, the fact that a person perceives him or herself as self-efficacious does not mean that he/she is competent of engaging in therapeutic adhering behaviors in specific places and times. In fact, a person may know that medications should be taken because he/she has been informed so, as well as "believe" that taking medication should be done because it will bring good consequences to his/her health. However once the specific conditions occur the person can either not take medication because he/she doesn't want to or because when he/she actually does it he/she does not comply with the specific efficiency criteria established by the health team (e.g., which go on an empty stomach or with food or specific fluids) that is because he/she cannot do it (as in fact sometimes occurs).

RESEARCH RESULTS AND RECENT ADVANCES

In the previous sections we have emphasized the importance of theories or models potentially applicable to the field of health psychology on the basis of two key tenets: first, such theories or models must be developed regarding the logic underlying both a general theory of behavioral processes and a theory of personality, since both logics play core roles in psychological theory construction (see Figure 2). The first describes and explains why individuals behave the way they do, on the basis of similarity criteria between psychological events that share a functional similarity with other events. The second synthesizes what one person does different to another on the basis of his/her owns biography or psychological history. This is the type of theory which plays the *interface* or *bridge* role between a general psychological processes theory and theories or models with potential application to health problems (Piña et al., 2011).

In addition, in order to avoid confusion and duplicity, we emphasize which concepts are used and how they are used (Noar and Zimmerman, 2005; Ogden, 2003). This purpose is the foundation of our proposal addressing the role of series of variables conceptually articulated within the concept of personality, e.g., motives, competencies and disease-related behaviors, as well as their relation to biological and social factors.

As part of a research project initially designed for application at an outpatient health center for prevention and treatment of persons living with HIV/AIDS in Hermosillo, the capital city of the northern of Sonora, Mexico, we started several lines of work aimed at converging in three research questions or goals: a) examining why and under which circumstances HIV-positive persons engage or not in treatment adherence behaviors; b) empirically validating the proposed theoretical model, and c) deriving a technological intervention proposal.

Regarding the first question, and within the context of the structure and needs of the health center, we started designing or adapting and validating a series of measurement instruments to collect specific data on the model's variables. The starting point involved a conceptual analysis of stress-related situations, motives and behavioral competencies (Piña, 2009, 2011). The first instrument was designed to measure psychological variables and adherence behaviors, with emphasis on motives and competential performance (past and present). Analyses yielded four factors with values higher than 1 which explained 65.5% of variance and internal consistency Cronbach's alpha coefficient of .85 (Piña, Corrales, Mungaray, and Valencia, 2006).

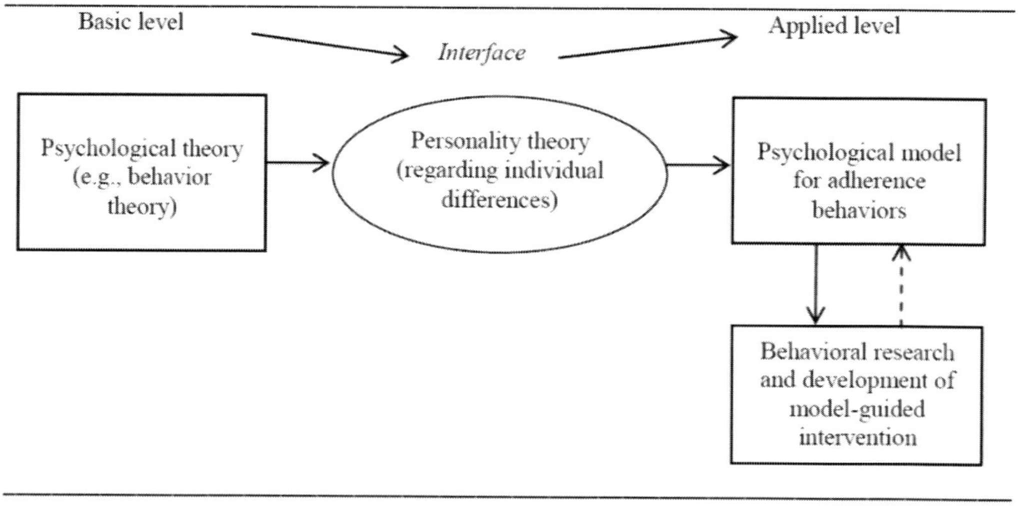

Figure 2. Relationship between theories and models in health psychology (Piña, Fierros, García, and Ybarra, 2011).

Also, a specific scale for stress-related situations including decision-making, tolerance to ambiguity, tolerance to frustration and impulsivity/non-impulsivity revealed items grouped around three factors with values higher than 1, explained variance of 70.4% and Cronbach's alpha of .90 (Piña, Valencia, Mungaray, and Corrales, 2006).

Additionally we completed the process of adaptation and validation of two more instruments. The first one, the functional social support (Duke-UNC-II), which yielded a single factor with a 6.48 value, explaining 58.6% of variance and .92 Cronbach's alpha (Piña, Corrales, and Rivera, 2007). The second was the Zung Depression Scale which yielded three factors with values higher than 1, an explained variance of 56.1% and Cronbach's alpha of .88 (Rivera, Corrales, Cázares, and Piña, 2007).

Once the psychometrical properties of the instruments were established, we explored variables presumably allowing predicting adherence behaviors. A first cross-sectional study involved 64 HIV-positive participants with or without adherence problems (Piña, Dávila, Sánchez-Sosa, Togawa, and Cázares, 2008); multiple regression analyses revealed that a combination of low levels of stress (reflected as tolerance to ambiguity) and low depression levels consistently predicted better adherence ($F = 3.298$; $p = .02$) with both variables explaining 38.2% of variance. Along similar lines (Sánchez-Sosa, Cázares, Piña, and Dávila, 2009), in a study with 68 HIV-positive participants with either high or low adherence revealed that low stress in the form of both decision-making and tolerance to ambiguity interacted with the variable motives and predicted 62.9% of variance ($F = 16.868$; $p < .001$). Finally, a cross-sectional study was carried out in a sample of 114 HIV-positive patients; overall, medication non-adherence was 29.8% ($n = 34$), meanwhile 70.2% ($n = 80$) was 100% adherent. Hierarchical regression analyses revealed three predictors of the behavior: Low stress-related to tolerance to ambiguity, high levels of current behavioral competencies and motives underlying behavior ($F = 5.5139$; $P > F = .0001$), accounting for 26.7% of variance (Piña, under review).

In light of these results, a further line of research examined the specific contribution of age, gender and time since onset of infection. Our team has so far conducted six studies, three of which are summarized as examples in the next lines. In a study including 73 HIV-positive participants the evaluation of gender allowed us to examine how the model's variables differentially affected adherence behaviors (Piña, 2012 OJO: ESTE TRABAJO ES EL DE ESTE NÚMERO QUE YA HABÍA SIDO ACEPTADO). A multivariate logistical regression analysis revealed that motives and current behavioral competencies significantly correlated with adherence. On the one hand, motives (OR = 1.75; CI 95%: 1.27-2.39; $p < .001$) revealed no reduction in statistical significance by the introduction of the gender variable (OR = 1.75; CI 95%: 1.23-2.48; $p < .005$). On the other, current competential performance (OR = 1.12; CI 95%: 1.00-1.24; $p < .05$) did lose some statistical significance upon the introduction of gender (OR= 1.11; CI 95%: 0.99-1.24; $p = .064$). Other study, with 44 HIV-positive participants used time since infection (overall mean 55 months) as criterion variable, yielded valuable information on the way this variable differentially affects psychological variables and adherence behaviors (Piña, Dávila, Sánchez-Sosa, Cázares, Togawa, and Corrales, 2009). The predictors for adherence behavior for participants with shorter time since infection included high motivational levels and low stress levels (tolerance to ambiguity) ($F = 8.130$; $p < .001$) and an explained variance of 49.7%. On the other hand, the predictors of adherence behaviors for participants who lived with virus for longer time periods were motives and low depression levels ($F = 11.057$; $p < .001$) and explained variance of 48.9%. In this same line, a more recent study with 93 HIV-positive participants examined adherence behavior as a function of time elapsed since the positivity diagnostic (overall average 42 months). Results revealed that the adherence behaviors of patients with less than 42 months since diagnostic were best predicted by high motivation, very high current competential performance and low levels of stress measured as tolerance to frustration ($F = 90.990$; $p < .001$), explaining over 80% of variance. In contrast, for patients with more than 42 months since diagnostic the best predictors were motives to behave and low stress related to decision-making, also explaining over 80% of variance ($F = 69.762$; $p < .001$) (Piña, Sánchez-Sosa, Fierros, Ybarra, and Cázares, 2011).

A third line of research focused on 100% adherent HIV-positive participants and has produced two studies. The first one involved a longitudinal study with follow up data after six months (Sánchez-Sosa, Fierros, Cázares, and Piña, 2011). Results showed that the three main predicting variables whose influence persisted over time were motives and past and present competencies. Statistical significance included $p < .001$ for motives and current behavioral competencies, and $p < .01$ for past competencies.

These results suggest that the strongest influence was exerted by immediate variables (related to more recent history) rather than mediate distal variables (e.g., stress-related situations). Additional evidence in this direction stemmed from the fact that the viral load decreased an average of 60% from the first measure to the second. The second study (Piña, García, Ybarra, Fierros, and Sánchez-Sosa, 2012), involved a path analysis on psychological variables. Results showed that motives had a relevant effect on pre-current competential performance ($F = 9.494$; $p < .005$), which in turn affected current behavioral competencies (adherence behaviors) ($F = 26.724$; $p < .001$). Meanwhile in the biological context, CD4+

lymphocytes influenced current behavioral competencies, e.g., adherence behaviors ($F = 4.411$; $p < .05$), also affected by viral load ($F = 6.260$; $p < .01$).

Finally, a fourth research line seeks to reconfirm and empirically validate the proposed theoretical model on the basis of structural equations modeling. Results from the final modeling of a study with 82 HIV-positive participants with or without adherence problems revealed that two stress-related situations: decision-making and tolerance to frustration directly influenced motives to behave, and mediated their effects on competential performance (past and present) and on adherence behaviors. Goodness of fit formulas yielded optimal effects (χ^2/df = 1/44; IAI = .93; IAIC = .93; RMSEA = .07) with a prediction power of the complete model of 68% (Piña and González, 2010). The second study sought to confirm whether social support played a relevant role with the model's predicting variables for adherence behaviors. The final model showed that motives to behave and social support were critical variables predicting adherence behaviors and these in turn affected viral load levels and CD4+ cell counts. Goodness of fit resulted in optimal values in all cases (χ^2/df = 1.29/20; GFI = .91; AGFI = .84; IFI = .97; CFI = .96; RMSEA = .07) and yielded an explained variance of 49% (González and Piña, 2011). A third study examined whether the interaction of psychological and biological variables will predict medication-adherence behaviors among one-hundred and forty one HIV-positive patients from Tamaulipas, Mexico. Eighty-two percent of the participants reported 100% adherence for antiretroviral (ARV) medication. The SEM produced a direct effect of two stress-related situations (low levels of both decision-making and tolerance to frustration) on motives to behave, this one mediating the relationship between these situations and adherence behaviors. Also, the study behavior showed a direct effect on lower levels of viral load, which in turn directly influencing higher counts of CD4+ lymphocytes. The final model fit the data very well: χ^2/df [9] = 1.480, $p = 0.149$; GFI = 0.974; AGFI = 0.940; CFI = 0.984; RMSEA = 0.053 (Ybarra, González, García, and Piña, under preparation).

Some Comments on Research Results and Perspectives

In general, the results from our program seem to allow for a series of conclusions as well as some comments and prospective considerations. On the one hand, in addition to the results yielded by the multiple lineal regression, multivariate logistical modeling and structural equations, the contribution of the predictive model's variables to adherence behaviors has been considerable. Explained variances fluctuate between 26.76% and 60% regardless of the analyses conducted, results consistently show that motives which underlie the actual practice of adherence behaviors, as well as two stress-related situations: decision-making and tolerance to frustration are key predictors of the actual occurrence of therapeutic adherence behaviors. Although the role of tolerance of ambiguity would be theoretically expected to play a relevant role, its direct influence on adherence behaviors was observed in only three of our studies, none of which employed structural modeling equations. This suggests the need to revise this variable's definition as well as the type of research questions that would help clarify these relationships in both functional and operational terms.

Also, it seems clear that, when mixed HIV-positive participants (all the way from persons with adherence problems to 100% adherent) are included in a study, the specific weight of the model's variables is different. Indeed, for 100% adherent participants the contribution of variables related to immediate history (motives and competencies) is clearly more powerful than the contribution of variables related to more mediate or distal variables (stress-related situations). This probably reflects the effect of motivational patterns that systematically and continuously reinforce competential performance a much needed outcome given the characteristics of this health condition and its treatment.

Although the present proposal involves a psychological model, we have been careful to recognize the specific role of biological and social dimensions. This has brought about a series of reflections mainly on the interaction of psychological and social variables, more specifically on what has been termed social support. Even though we are dealing with a psychological model, the explicit lack of a conceptual category covering the role of social interactions has led to a recent suggestion in the sense of adding such category to the model as an exogenous variable; such category could be designated as interpersonal interactions and would include social support (see Figure 3).

We thus propose to incorporate these types of interactions by carefully locating the various levels of behavior shown by persons living with chronic conditions starting at the individual level (where in phase one of the adherence model predominate), then to the interpersonal (which emphasize such phenomena as communication and cooperation), and then culminate with the social level proper, in which phenomena related to power and sanctions predominate.

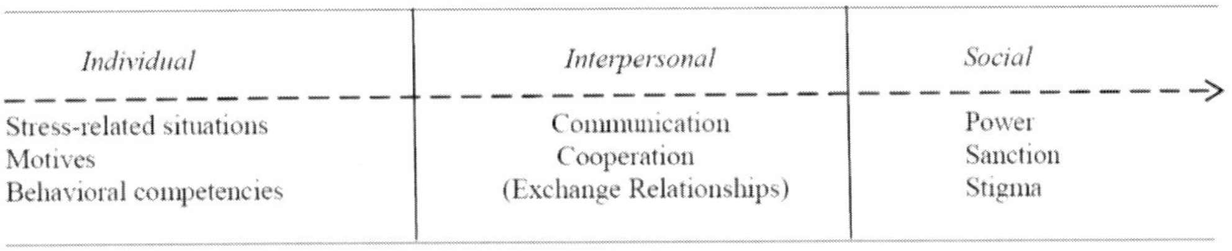

Figure 3. Interaction continuum from individual to social level (González and Piña, 2011; Piña, 2011).

This perspective seeks to provide the psychological discourse with sense, congruity and coherence along an interaction continuum, so as to stay away from the widespread tendency to incorporate variables (in health psychology models) independently of whether they keep logical and conceptual correspondence, as cautioned against by the proposed integrated model of behavioral change. As can be deduced from the previous considerations, our proposed model emphasizes its use in applied healthcare settings in a more ordered, graded and parsimonious fashion. If psychologists wish to be in a better position to design, implement and systematically evaluate intervention programs, the knowledge of the relative contribution of the variables in the model becomes crucial provided that outcomes will be different depending on what gets analyzed, how we analyze it and in relation to which other variables (Piña, 2012). Through this way of organizing health research and application we seek to obtain a sort of matrix (not to be understood as a simple set of cells encasing, for instance, HIV-positive patients). This would allow for summarizing potentially useful information allowing for functional behavioral profiles to be examined in the context of the individual, his/her interaction with the disease in question, its treatment and with other significant persons in the individual's immediate social environment (see García-Cedillo, Alfaro-Castro, Rodríguez-Delgado, and Sánchez-Armáss, 2011).

In the applied context, the present proposal attempts to avoid traditional intervention schemes that assume that, for example, an HIV-positive person does not engage in adherence behaviors because he/she "is depressed" or "stressed". The actual challenge resides in identifying those techniques or procedures most suitable for reversing as many conditions as possible so as to insure the efficient practice of such behaviors.

Within the logic of this line of reasoning, the problem is no longer that of adherence alone but all relevant behaviors related to the health condition. Traditionally many such behaviors are defined on the basis of morphological criteria (anxiety, stress, depression, social isolation, etc.); and the next assumption is that for each of those conditions there are predetermined procedures or techniques which keep some kind of univocal correspondence with such behavior morphologies. In contrast, the proposed functional profile seeks to return to the fundamental assumption that, since instrumental behavior is influenced by both the psychological history and the contextual variables of the individual, the study of applied solutions should first involve a rigorous analysis of the role they play (history and context) at a particular point in time of the interaction continuum.

This analysis will eventually reveal that, for some persons, the contribution of stress-related situations will be stronger than that of motives to behave or the availability of behavioral competencies. For others, the predominant variables may be motives, for others could be the availability of competencies, for others the influence of surrounding persons and finally, the interaction between two or more of these options of the spectrum. It should therefore become clear that procedures and techniques for behavioral change (not in the clinical sense which limits itself to eliminating "problem" behaviors) should recognize this wide array of options. Some procedures will aim at changing dispositions (stress-related situations, motives, competencies, emotional states, etc.); others at modifying specific behaviors of the patient (those linked to the disease or others seeking to establish skills and new interpersonal relation systems) and finally, procedures aimed at modifying other persons' behaviors in the interpersonal and social levels as represented in Figure 3.

In any event, the articulation of the theoretical-applied dimensions addressed in the present paper is serving as platform for a line of work seeking to link the research-intervention axes while helping HIV-positive persons at the CAPASITS community center in Hermosillo, the capital of the Mexican state of Sonora. These efforts have begun to spread to other states, such as México, Michoacán, Nuevo León, San Luis Potosí and Tamaulipas, among others. We are confident that further validation of the tenets of the present proposal that articulates theory and practice, will consolidate and advance to the extent that effective results get replicated under diverse conditions in the health sector.

REFERENCES

Ajzen, I. (1988). *Attitudes, personality and behavior.* Chicago, IL: Dorsey.

Albarracín, D., Rothman, A.J., DiClemente, R.J., and del Río, C. (2010). Wanted: A theoretical roadmap to research and practice across individual, interpersonal, and structural levels of analysis. *AIDS and Behavior, 14 (Suppl. 2),* S185-S188.

Baranowski, T. (2005). Integration of two models, or dominance of one? *Journal of Health Psychology, 10,* 19-21.

Barclay, T.R., Hinkin, C.H., Castellon, S.A., Mason, K.I., Reinhard, M., Marion, S.D., et al. (2007). Age-associated predictors of medication adherence in HIV-positive adults: Health beliefs, self-efficacy, and neurocognitive status. *Health Psychology, 26,* 40-49.

Bosworth, H.B. (2010). Medication adherence. In H.B. Bosworth (Ed.), *Improving patient treatment adherence* (pp. 69-95). New York, NY: Springer.

Enç, B. (2004). Causal theories of intentional behavior and wayward causal chaines. *Behavior and Philosophy, 32,* 149-166.

Eysenck, H.J. (1988). *Dimensions of personality.* New Brunswick, NJ: Transactions Publishers.

Fishbein, M. (2000). The role of theory in HIV prevention. *AIDS Care, 12,* 273-278.

Fishbein, M., Hennessy, M., Yzer, M., and Douglas, J. (2003). Can we explain why some people do and some people do not act on their intentions? *Psychology, Health and Medicine, 8,* 3-18.

García-Cedillo, I., Alfaro-Castro, F., Rodríguez-Delgado, M., and Sánchez-Armáss, O. (2011). Indicadores de enfermedades mentales en pacientes mexicanos con VIH/SIDA y su relación con la adherencia terapéutica. *Actualidades en Psicología, 25,* 37-55.

Garvie, P.A., Flynn, P.M., Belzer, M., Britto, P., Hu, C., Graham, B., et al. (2011). Psychological factors, beliefs about medication, and adherence of youth with human immunodeficiency virus in a multisite Directly Observed Therapy Pilot Study. *Journal of Adolescent Health, 48,* 637-640.

González, M.T. and Piña, J.A. (2011). Motivos, apoyo social y comportamientos de adhesión en personas con VIH: modelamiento con ecuaciones estructurales. *Universitas Psychologica, 10,* 597-607.

Kantor, J.R. (1959). Interbehavioral psychology. Chicago, IL: The Principia Press.

Kantor, J.R. (1978). Cognition as event and as a physic construction. *The Psychological Record, 28,* 329-342.

Kennedy, S., Goggin, K., and Nollen, N. (2004). Adherence to HIV medication: Utility of the theory of self-determination. *Cognitive Therapy and Research, 28,* 611-628.

Laraway, S., Snycerski, S., and Poling, A. (2003). Motivating operations. In J. E. Burgos and E. Ribes (Eds.), *Theory, basic and applied research, and technological applications in behavior science: Conceptual and methodological issues* (pp. 85-118). México: Universidad de Guadalajara.

Malcolm, S.E., Ng, J.J., Rosen, R.K., and Stone, V.E. (2003). An examination of HIV/AIDS patients who have excellent adherence to HAART. *AIDS Care, 15,* 251-261.

Marks, D.F. (2008). The quest for meaningful theory in health psychology. *Journal of Health Psychology, 13,* 977-981.

Moore, J. (2001). On psychological terms that appeal to the mental. *Behavior and Philosophy, 29,* 167-186.

Noar, S.M. (2007). An interventionist's guide to AIDS behavioral theories. *AIDS Care, 19,* 392-407.

Noar, S.M. and Zimmerman, R.S. (2005). Health behavior theory and cumulative knowledge regarding health behaviors: are we moving in the right direction? *Health Education Research: Theory and Practice, 20,* 275-290.

Ogden, J. (2003). Some problems with social cognition models: A pragmatic and conceptual analysis. *Health Psychology, 22,* 424-428.

Painter, J.E., Borba, C.P.C., Hynes, M., Mays, D., and Glanz, K. (2008). The use of theory in health behavior research from 2000 to 2005: A systematic review. *Annals of Behavioral Medicine, 35,* 358-362.

Piña, J.A. (2012). Psychological variables and adherence in HIV-positive patients from Mexico: A gender-based analysis. *International Journal of Hispanic Psychology, 5,* _____.

Piña, J.A. (under review). Conductas de adhesión en personas seropositivas al VIH: un análisis con base en un modelo psicológico.

Piña, J.A. (2009). Motivación en psicología y salud: motivación no es sinónimo de intención, actitud o percepción de riesgo. *Diversitas-Perspectivas en Psicología, 5,* 27-35.

Piña, J.A. (2011). *Psicología y salud: Obstáculos y posibilidades para su desarrollo en el siglo XXI.* Bogotá, Colombia: PSICOM Editores.

Piña, J.A. (2012). *El problema de la adhesión en personas con VIH: Una visión crítica desde la psicología.* Madrid: Editorial Académica Española.

Piña, J.A., Corrales, A.E., Mungaray, K., and Valencia, M.A. (2006). Instrumento para medir variables psicológicas y comportamientos de adhesión al tratamiento en personas seropositivas frente al VIH (VPAD-24). *Revista Panamericana de Salud Pública, 19,* 217-228.

Piña, J.A., Corrales, A.E., and Rivera, B.M. (2007). Validación del cuestionario de apoyo social funcional en personas seropositivas al VIH del noroeste de México. *Ciencia y Enfermería, XIII,* 53-63.

Piña, J.A., Dávila, M., Sánchez-Sosa, J.J., Cázares, O., Togawa, C., and Corrales, A.E. (2009). Efectos del tiempo de infección sobre predictores de adherencia en personas con VIH. *International Journal of Psychology and Psychological Therapy, 9,* 67-78.

Piña, J.A., Dávila, M., Sánchez-Sosa, J.J., Togawa, C., and Cázares, O. (2008). Asociación entre los niveles de estrés y depresión y la adhesión al tratamiento en personas seropositivas al VIH en Hermosillo, México. *Revista Panamericana de Salud Pública, 23,* 377-383.

Piña, J.A., Fierros, L.E., García, C.H., and Ybarra, J.L. (2011). Psicología y salud [II]. Tendiendo puentes entre la psicología básica y la aplicada: el rol del fenómeno de personalidad. *Pensamiento Psicológico, 9,* 203-212.

Piña, J.A., García, C.H., Ybarra, J.L., Fierros, L.E., and Sánchez-Sosa, J.J. (2012). Psychological and biological variables among HIV 100% adherent patients: A path-analysis. In C.H. García, R. Ballester, and J.A. Piña (Eds.), *Chronic diseases and adherence behaviors: Psychological research in Ibero-American countries* (pp. 203-220). Hauppauge, NY: Nova Science Publishers.

Piña, J.A. and González, M.T. (2010). Un modelo psicológico de adhesión en personas VIH+: modelamiento con ecuaciones estructurales. *Revista Iberoamericana de Psicología y Salud, 1,* 185-206.

Piña, J.A. and Sánchez-Sosa, J.J. (2007). Modelo psicológico para la investigación de los comportamientos de adhesión en personas con VIH. *Universitas Psychologica, 6,* 399-407.

Piña, J.A., Sánchez-Sosa, J.J., Fierros, L.E., Ybarra, J.L., and Cázares, O. (2011). Variables psicológicas y adhesión en personas con VIH: evaluación en función del tiempo de infección. *Terapia Psicológica, 29,* 149-157.

Piña, J.A., Valencia, M.A., Mungaray, K., and Corrales, A.E. (2006). Validación de una escala breve que mide situaciones vinculadas con estrés en personas VIH positivas. *Terapia Psicológica, 24,* 15-21.

Piña, J.A., Ybarra, J.L., Alcalá, I.G., and Samaniego, R.A. (2010). Psicología y salud (I): la importancia de llamarse modelo y apellidarse teórico-conceptual. *Revista Mexicana de Investigación en Psicología, 2,* 21-29.

Reynolds, N.R. (2003). The problem of antiretroviral adherence: a self-regulation model for intervention. *AIDS Care, 15,* 117-124.

Ribes, E. (2003). Concepts and theories. Relation to scientific categories. In K.A. Lattal and P.N. Chase (Eds.), *Behavior theory and philosophy* (pp. 147-163). New York, NY: Springer.

Ribes, E. (2004a). Theory, scientific research, and technical applications: how related in operant psychology? In J. E. Burgos and E. Ribes (Eds.), *Theory, basic and applied research, and technological applications in behavior science: Conceptual and methodological issues* (pp. 19-44). México: Universidad de Guadalajara.

Ribes, E. (2004b). Behavior is abstraction, not ostention: Conceptual and historical remarks on the nature of psychology. *Behavior and Philosophy, 32*, 55-68.

Ribes, E. (2005). ¿Qué es lo que se debe medir en la psicología? El problema de las diferencias individuales. *Acta Comportamentalia, 13,* 37-52.

Ribes, E. (2009). La personalidad como organización de los estilos interactivos. *Revista Mexicana de Psicología, 36,* 145-161.

Ribes, E. and López, F. (1985). *Teoría de la conducta: un análisis de campo y paramétrico.* México: Trillas.

Ribes, E. and Sánchez, S. (1990). El problema de las diferencias individuales: un análisis conceptual de la personalidad. En E. Ribes (Ed.), *Problemas conceptuales en el análisis del comportamiento* (pp. 77-97). México: Trillas.

Ribes, E. and Sánchez, S. (1992). Individual behavior consistencies as interactive styles: How related to personality? *The Psychological Record, 42,* 369-387.

Rivera, B.M., Corrales, A.E., Cázares, O., and Piña, J.A. (2007). Validación de la escala de depresión de Zung en personas con VIH. *Terapia Psicológica, 25,* 135-140.

Ryle, G. (1949). *The concept of mind.* New York, NY: Barnes and Noble.

Sánchez-Sosa, J.J. (2002). Treatment adherence: The role of behavioural mechanism and some implications for health care interventions. *Revista Mexicana de Psicología, 19,* 85-92.

Sánchez-Sosa, J.J., Cázares, O., Piña, J.A., and Dávila, M. (2009). Un modelo psicológico en los comportamientos de adhesión terapéutica en personas con VIH. *Salud Mental, 32,* 389-397.

Sánchez-Sosa, J.J., Fierros, L.E., Cázares, O., and Piña, J.A. (2011). Estudio longitudinal de variables psicológicas y conductas de adhesión en personas VIH+: efectos sobre los niveles de carga viral. In J.L. Ybarra, J.J. Sánchez-Sosa, and J.A. Piña (Eds.), *Trastornos y enfermedades crónicas: una aproximación psicológica* (pp. 137-154). México: Universidad Autónoma de Tamaulipas/El Manual Moderno.

Tarakeshar, N., Srikrishnan, A.K., Johnson, S., Vatsu, C., Solomon, S., Merson, M., et al. (2007). A social cognitive model of health for HIV-positive adults receiving care in India. *AIDS and Behavior, 11,* 491-504.

Weinstein, N.D. (2007). Misleading test of health behavior theories. *Annals of Behavioral Medicine, 33,* 1-10.

Ybarra, J.L., González, M.T., García, I., and Piña, J.A. (under preparation). *Adhesión al tratamiento antirretroviral en personas VIH-positivas: un modelo psicológico y con ecuaciones estructurales.*

(Manuscript received on 30 November 2011. Revised version accepted for publication on 29 March 2012)

In: Recent Hispanic Psychological Research ... ISBN: 978-1-62948-919-3
Editors: C. H. Garcia Cadena, A. Lopez-Espinoza et al. © 2014 Nova Science Publishers, Inc.

Chapter 13

SOCIAL SUPPORT AND MOTIVES: THEIR INFLUENCE ON TREATMENT ADHERENCE AND BIOMARKERS AMONG HIV PATIENTS FROM MICHOACAN, MEXICO

Maria Auxilio Rosas Rodriguez
and Monica Teresa González Ramirez*
Independent Researcher
Morelia, Mexico
College of Psychology
Universidad Autónoma de Nuevo León, México

ABSTRACT

Based on a psychological model, a cross-sectional study was carried out with the participation of fifty-four HIV persons under antiretroviral medication in Michoacán, Mexico, who answered three self-administered questionnaires: psychological variables and adherence behaviors, perceived social support, and depression. For data analysis a set of structural equation modeling was performed. The final model showed a direct effect of perceived social support on motives, and this one on medication-adherence behaviors, explaining both variables 61% of total variance (χ^2/df [5] = 0.368; GFI = 0.986; AGFI = 0.959; CFI = 1.000; RMSEA = 0.000); also, an effect of adherence behaviors on viral load was observed, explaining 35% of the variance; viral load in turn explains 29% of the variance of CD4+ cell count. The current study found valuable evidence of how interaction between two psychological and social variables influences positively on the consisting and efficient practice of adherence behaviors, with direct and mediated effects on both biomarkers, viral load levels and CD4+ lymphocytes cell count. We discuss the relevance of these variables in healthcare institutions context which provide specialized attention for HIV persons under antiretroviral medication in Mexico.

* Mail address: Dr. Carlos Canseco 110. Col. Mitras Centro. C. P. 64460. Tel. (52-81)- 83338233. Monterrey, Nuevo León, México. E-mail: monygzz77@yahoo.com; monica.gonzalezrz@uanl.edu.mx

Keywords: Psychological Model, HIV Patients, Social Support, Motives, Depression, Adherence Behaviors

INTRODUCTION

The introduction of antiretroviral therapy (ARVT) in the middle of the last decade led to a radical change in the care provided to people living with HIV or AIDS (PCVS), from a determined point in typical palliative cares of terminal phase to another in which clinical progression control of the disease is particularly emphasized (Pasche-Orlwo, Chen, Palepu, Melli, Faber, and Samet, 2006). Certainly, in order that such therapy is one hundred percent effective it is essential PCVS practice the adherence behaviors in strict correspondence with instructions provided by health personnel; meaning, it is necessary those people consume antiretroviral drugs in the doses and frequency expected, so as to prevent resistance medications or viral mutations that accelerate the transit from an asymptomatic state to one as AIDS as such (Anema, Wood, and Montaner, 2008).

From the above, we can state consistent and efficient practice of adherence behaviors constitutes an instrument that facilitates PCVS to maintain stable immune system functionality as much as possible (Villa and S.a., 2006), thereby contributing to both reduce the amount of circulating virus in the organism and an increase of CD4+ cell count (Hirsch Gunthard, Schapiro, and Brun-Vezinet, 2008; Ironson, O' Cléirigh, Fletcher, Laurenceau, Balbin and Klimas, 2005). As it is well known, both are two of the main biological markers used today to evaluate health conditions, potential risk of developing opportunistic infections and die from HIV/AIDS, especially among PCVS with adherence problems (Giordano, Gifford, White, Suarez-Almazor, Rabenek, Hartman et al., 2007;) Wood, Hogg, Yip, Harrigan, O´Shaughenessy, and Montaner, 2003).

Indeed, in several studies in its longitudinal section or in others in which intervention programs have been used (i.e., behavioral or cognitive-behavioral), has been revealed how psychological or social nature variables influence on the practice of the aforementioned behaviors, but both biological markers as well.

In one of them, carried out in South Africa during five years, Ford, Darder, Spelman, Maclean, Mills, and Boulle (2010), who worked with a sample of 207 PCVS, indicate that 87% of the first measurement reported to be 100% ARVT adherence, while remaining 13% had adherence problems; it was precisely this group which after five years presented virological failure on a ratio of 2.7 times more than its counterpart, the group of adherents. Likewise, Sanchez-Sosa, Irons, Cazares, and Pina (2011), who worked with a sample of 70 PCVS, 100% adherents to ARVT adherents in the State of Sonora, in the Northwest of Mexico, found that in two measurements, with a difference of six months, a high motivation and optimum competence performance (in past and present) were decisive factors in the reduction of viral load levels in almost 60%, among measurements.

With regard to the studies that have been used intervention programs, Molassiotis, Lopez-Nahas, Chung, and Lam (2003), who worked with a PCVS sample in China, based on a program that considered individualized education and positive reinforcement, conclude that measurements on the monthly, quarterly and semestral baseline, adhesion percentages improved from 80.2% to the beginning of the program to 97.5% six months of the persons exposed to the program, being observed as well a substantial increase in CD4+ cell count, going from an average of 275 cells/ml on base line to 325 cells/ml six months later. In a similar direction, Wagner, Kanouse, Golinelli, Miller, Daar, Witt et al (2006), worked on comparing the effectiveness of cognitive-behavioral vs. improved treatment and conventional therapy group, in a group of 230 PCVS in the United States of America; After base line, four measurements were conducted in weeks four, 12, 24, 48, being found that proportion of doses taken in percentages equal or higher than 90% were always greater in the intervention group; when comparing effects of program about amount of virus circulating in the body and other health results, notwithstanding that in the intervention and improved treatment groups, percentages of reduction higher viral load levels were observed, which in relation to the control group, differences between groups were not statistically significant.

This series of studies are important because they allow a more complete understanding of what and how some psychological or social variables are keys not only to predict practice of adherence behaviors, but also about how those same variables can positively influence biological functionality into PCVS exposed to ARVT regimes. However, the question we ask at this moment is if other types of studies, in particular, of cross-cutting, could also bring light on such matters.

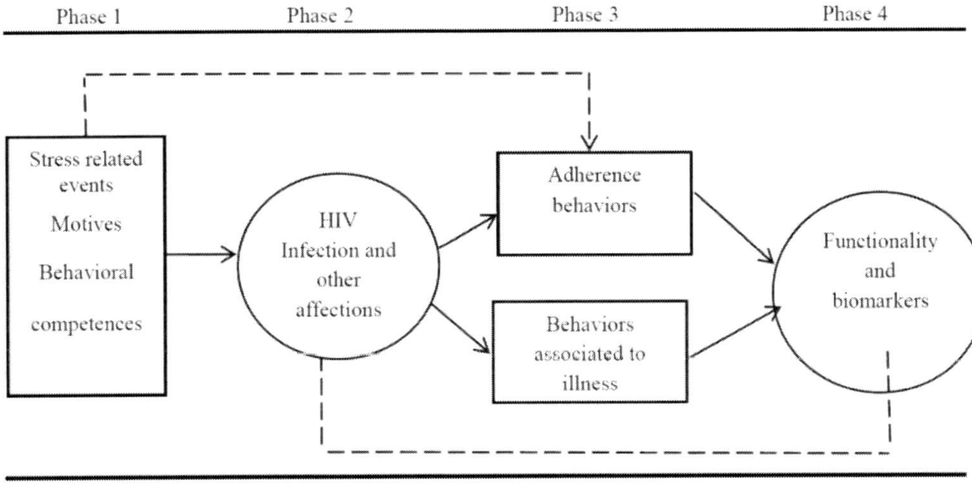

Figure 1. Simplified version of adherence psychological model of Piña and Sanchez-Sosa (2007).

Recently, based on a psychological adherence model (Pina and Sanchez-Sosa, 2007) some research works have been developed in which these matters have been addressed. For example, in one of them (Gonzalez and Pina, 2011), where 69 PCVS participated from the State of Sonora, in Northwest of Mexico, the objective considered was to test which variables about referred model, as well as an exogenous variable, social support would predict adherence behaviors and what sense both viral load levels and CD4+ cell count are related; with structural equations modeling, it was showed that motive to behave and social support were two critical variables influenced those behaviors ($\chi 2$/gl 1.29/20; $p < 0.001$; IBA = 0.91; IBAC = 0.84; IAI = 0.97; IAC = 0.96; RCMEA = 0.07), by explaining both variables 49% of total variance; on the other hand, a good adherence allowed to explain 9% of variance in the low/intermediate levels of viral load, while these ones explained 11% of the variance in CD4+ cell counts.

This work was prepared from previous summarized outcomes and in order to continue this research line. Its theoretical justification is found in adherence psychological model proposed by Pina and Sanchez-Sosa (2007). From this, we can assume consistent and efficient practice of adherence behaviors to treatments can be affected when performing by variables including stress related events , past competences a person has used and their translation into efficient performance in the present, motives (all variables covered in phase one), as well as by other behaviors, associated with the disease (as part of phase three,) which include anxiety, social isolation, depression, anger, and impulsiveness, among others (Figure 1).

Stress related events refers to all interactive or social situations a person experiences when suffering a chronic disease that can generate stress, which in this context is defined as a *biological reaction* produced by situations characterized by: a) difficulty or impossibility of predicting the stimulus consequences before which the individual responds (unpredictability); (b) because events or stimulus signals may occur or be interpreted in ambiguous way (*ambiguity*), or, c) because the consequences are perceived as independent from person's behavior (*uncertainty*) (Ribes, 1990).

In another area, motives refer to a variable which involves choice or preference for objects, events or people in an interactive situation with socially valued consequences. It is concepts applied to circumstances in which making or behave in certain way, it is considered timely and relevant, provided that a person *wants* to do things (Ribes, 2005). Therefore, motives refers to a *tendency* or a *propensity* to behave in a certain way, in so far as this way of behave has been associated in the past with obtaining positive reinforcement consequences (Pina, 2009).

Finally, within the same phase one, there are behavioral competences defined as the set of resources available for a person to respond efficiently to demands or requirements within a specific circumstance.

With respect to HIV infection, be competent would imply to know: a) what is HIV; (b) what are the clinical stages of infection; (c) what is the role of biological markers, that is, viral load levels and CD4+ cell counts, and d) what are the medications existing in the market, how they have to be administered and why; then, be competent means that a person *can* do things in a consistent and efficient manner. Competencies, as well as motives, is a concept giving account immediately and continually modifiable psychological history, since meanwhile encompasses knowledge, abilities and skills enabling to produce results or specific achievements, all of these are cumulative and susceptible to be seen modified by demands or explicit requirements within an interactive situation.

One of the assumptions of psychological model referred, is that depending on the interaction between these variables, adherence behaviors (phase 3) will be facilitated or not. Once translated into instrumental behaviors, a higher probability to keep a stable biological functionality (modulation), and low levels of vulnerability of the body will be generated, which in the future will bring optimum health results (within phase four). Secondly, occurrence of other resulting pathologies that are associated with HIV would be less probable, cases like pulmonary tuberculosis infection, pneumonia due to *Pneumocystis jirovecii* and Kaposi's sarcoma among others (as part of phase two).

On the other hand, adherence behaviors may be affected performing other behaviors associated to the disease (Ribes, 1990). They are behaviors, as author indicates, which can be correlated with a disease drawn from treatments or others that may eventually arise without necessarily having a biological pathology. In HIV infection, it has been fully demonstrated antiretroviral medications consumption often produce many side-effects (e.g., nausea, vomiting, stomach irritability, etc.) and encourage the presence of a diversity of unspecified arising behaviors as a reaction to the disease as such, which would labeled in general context of emotional/affective states, among which we find depression, anger, impulsiveness, tension, negative mood, etc. In essence, there are behaviors characterized because they interfere both with psychological and social adjustment of people suffering a chronic disease, as well as the treatment itself and their potential effectiveness (Edo and Ballester, 2006, Gordillo, Fekete, Platteau, Antoni, Schneiderman, and Nöstlinger, 2009).

Based on this psychological adherence model, in the present study the following hypotheses were divided: a) social support, as exogenous variable, should positively influence on the underlying motives to practice adherence behaviors, as well as low levels of depression; (b) these three variables should influence positively and directly on the aforementioned behaviors, and c) competence practice of adherence behaviors should influence on low levels of viral load, which in turn, will influence increase in CD4+ cell count.

Table 1. Clinical and socio-demographic characteristics of participants (n = 54)

	N	%
Gender		
Male	43	79.6
Female	11	20.3
Sexual orientation		
Homosexual	21	38.8
Bisexual	11	20.3
Heterosexual	22	40.7
Marital status		
Single	29	53.7
Married	7	12.9
Divorced	3	5.5
Free union	6	11.11
Separated	6	11.11
Widow	3	5.5
Belonging to a support group	11	20.3
Does exercise	33	61.11
	X	
Age	36.07	
Schooling	10.4	
Years of diagnosis	6.5	
Viral load	2332.63	
CD4+ cell	523.52	

METHOD

Participants

A convenient sample was selected from total of PCVS, who were receiving attention in different health institutions based in the city of Morelia, capital of Michoacán State (in central Mexico). The following were considered as inclusion criteria: a) an age equal or older than 18 years; (b) diagnosed as HIV-positive at least six months prior to the study; (c) they were under an ART treatments; d) that they could read and write, and e) that they have recent results of viral load and CD4+ cell count. It was initially considered a universe of 97 PCVS, 43 out of them failed to meet some of these criteria, particularly not having updated results of CD4+ cell count and viral load levels. Therefore, final sample was composed of 54 PCVS, with an average age of 36.07 years; also, 28 participants (53.7%) were singles at the time of the study, while educational level average was 10.4 years (equivalent to secondary school level); remaining social-demographic characteristics and clinics are summarized in table 1.

Instruments and Measures

Questionnaire of psychological variables and adherence behaviors (VPAD-24) designed and validated in Mexico (Pina, Corrales, Mungaray, and Valencia). It consists of 24 questions grouped into four factors: first factor includes measurement of adherence behaviors (medicine consumption, punctual appointments attendance and avoid the consumption of substances such as alcohol, mainly) and variables related to treatment. Second factor consists of motives underlying these behaviors; three and four factors, both, consist in performing respectively past and present competences.

For purposes of this study, only the measurement of adherence behaviors related to consumption of medicines and underlying motives, was considered, being part of factor two. Adherence behaviors were defined in a Likert-type scale, with five –level answer items, ranging from one (I did not consume them any day of the week) to five (I consumed them seven days a week); on the other hand, motives factor included four questions in a Likert-type scale with four-level answer items, ranging from one (it was not a decisive motive) to four (it was a decisive motive); the following is an example of the question: "From motives listed above, could you tell us what was the decisive motive to make you consume medicine every day of the week?" (i.e. I did it because I want to keep myself healthy, as much possible time); the lower score, the lower motivation to practice adherence behaviors and vice versa.

Questionnaire of social support (Duke-UNC-11) adapted and validated in Mexico by Piña, Corrales, and Rivera (2007). It contains 11 questions about affective support and confidence evaluation from significant or not significant people from immediate social environment.

The questions were in a Likert- type scale with four-level answer items, ranging from one (much less than what I want/hope) to four (more than what I want/hope); the following is an example of a question: I get visits from my family or friends. The lower score, the lower evaluation of social support received, and vice versa.

Zung's depression scale used (EZD-20), adapted and validated in Mexico by Rivera, Corrales, Cazarez, and Pina (2007). It includes 20 questions about depressive mood, as well as symptoms in their physical and psychological modalities. All the questions were in a

Likert-type scale with four-level answer items, ranging from one (very few times) to four (most of the time); the following is an example of a question: I feel bored, discouraged and sad. The lower score, the lower depression evaluation in each condition, and vice versa.

Biological markers: data about infection time in months (from seropositive HIV diagnosis), viral load levels and CD4+ cell count.

Procedure

Study managers attended different institutions and requested authorization from relevant authorities to apply it. Once it was granted, PCVS from each institution were invited to voluntarily participate. Prior to its beginning, objectives pursued were explained to all participants and they were reiterated their participation would be voluntary, as well as anonymous and confidential, adding that if they agree it would be necessary to review clinical records in order to obtain data about HIV-positive diagnosis date, viral load levels, CD4+ cell count and treatment regime to which they were exposed. Those who agreed to participate read and signed informed consent. Original version project was approved by committees of research and/or ethics of each institution in which study was conducted.

Statistical Analysis

Statistical SPSS packages (version 13.0) and AMOS (version 7.0) were used for analyzing data. An initial analysis showed averages, standard deviations and range of values for different variables; Cronbach's alpha coefficient (α) was used to estimate internal consistency of each subscale.

Pearson r coefficient was used in order to analyze correlation between adherence behaviors, variables contained in instruments and two biological markers. In addition, and in order to prove capacity of prediction of theoretical model, it was adopted a two-step strategy: the first one consisted in analyzing influence of social support perceived on motives, and from both, on adherence behaviors; the second one consisted of both incorporate depression variable and its relationship with both social support and motives, as well as their possible influence on those behaviors; both were proved as well regarding eventual effect of adherence behaviors on viral load levels and of the latter, CD4+ cell count. Goodness of fit was estimated from verifying coefficients were significant and there would have optimal correspondence between variances/co-variances original matrix, as well as the one produced based on estimated parameters by several absolute statistical goodness-of-fit: chi-square (χ^2), ratio between Chi-square and degrees of freedom (χ^2g. l.), goodness of fit (GFI) and of adjusted goodness of fit (AGFI); similarly, other fit indices increase: normed fit index (NFI)), non-normed fit index (NNFI), comparative fit index (CFI), incremental fit index (IFI) and root of mean square of error of approximation (RMSEA). A non significant Chi-square was expected, values equal or higher than .90 in GFI, AGFI, AGFI, NFI, NNFI, CFI and IFI, as well as those lower than .08 in RMSEA, would suggest relevance of model data (Bentler, 1990;) Bentler and Bonnet, 1980; Bollen, 1989; Browne and Cudeck, 1993).

RESULTS

As we can see in table 2, scores obtained in different measures were low in case of motives ($\overline{X}$ = 10.1 from a possible range of 4 to 20), high in perceived social support ($\overline{X}$ = 43.7 from possible range of 11 and 55 points) and intermediate in depression ($\overline{X}$ = 37.8 from possible range of 20-60 points). Cronbach's alpha coefficient (α) values were optimal.

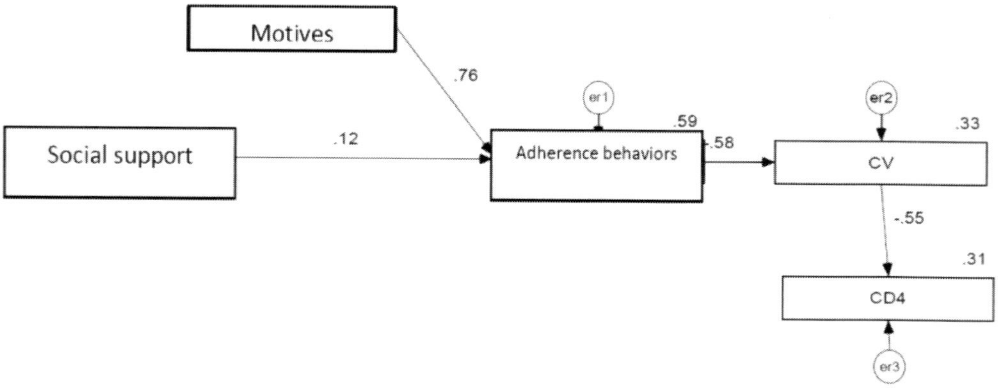

Figure 2. Model 1, copies Gonzalez and Piña model (2011).

On the other hand, table 3 summarizes correlations between dependent and independent variables (psychological, social and biological). In general terms, high and significant correlations between variables were found.

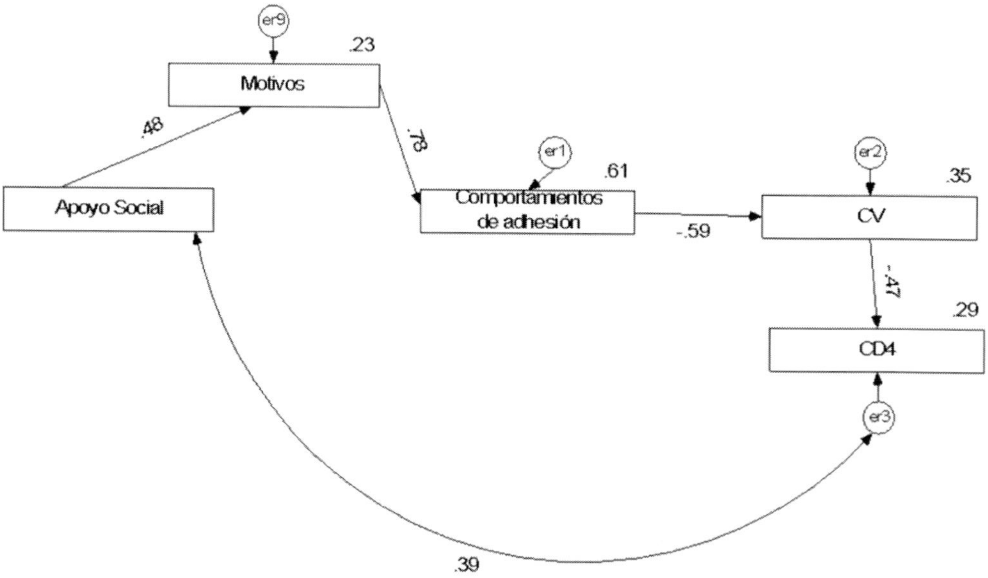

Figure 3. Model 2 with better adjustment.

Concerning modeling with structural equations, first model estimated (Figure 2) is a replica of the one reported by González and Pina (2011). In such model, social support did not directly influence adhesion behaviors (β. 118; p. 178); while motives did show a significant effect on them (β. 760; p. 001). Likewise, effect of adherence behaviors on viral load was significant (β. 577; p. 001) and of the latter on CD4+ (β-. 554; p. 001). Finally, fit of model was not optimal, as seen in table 4.

From the foregoing, it was evaluated social support indirect effect on adherence behaviors, by estimating a social support direct effect on motives to practice them (Figure 3). In this second model, all parameters were significant and adjustment improved significantly (table 4): social support effect on motives variable was significant (β. 485; p. 001), meanwhile social support over adherence behaviors was indirect (β. 380; p. 05) mediated by motivation, explaining 60% of variance of aforementioned behaviors. Finally, they explained 35% of viral load variance, while the latter explains 29% of CD4+ cell count variance.

Table 2. Univariate statistics and reliability of measures

Variable	Scoring	X	Standard bias	α
Adherence Behaviors	1-5	4.61	0.7	---
Motives	4-20	10.1	6.3	.94
Social support	11-55	43.5	10.0	.93
Depression	20-80	37.8	8.8	.89

Table 3. Correlation between dependent and independent variables, including biomarkers

	1	2	3	4	5
1. Adherence behavior					
2. Social support	.467				
3. Motives	.784	.485			
4. Depression	-.464	-.640	-.418		
5. Viral load	-.593	-.280	-.446	.310	
6. CD4+	.476	.454	.408	-.372	-.559

* p < .01 in all the cases.

Table 4. Indicators of structural models' goodness of fit

				Absolute fit indexes			Incremental fit indexes			
Models	X^2	gl	X^2/gl	GFI	AGFI	RMSEA	NFI	TLI	CFI	IFI
1	2.604	6	3.767	.857	.642	.229	.807	.742	.845	.851
2	1.841	5	0.368	.986	.959	.000	.984	1.059	1.000	1.028
3	10.010	9	1.112	.945	.871	.046	.933	.987	.992	.993

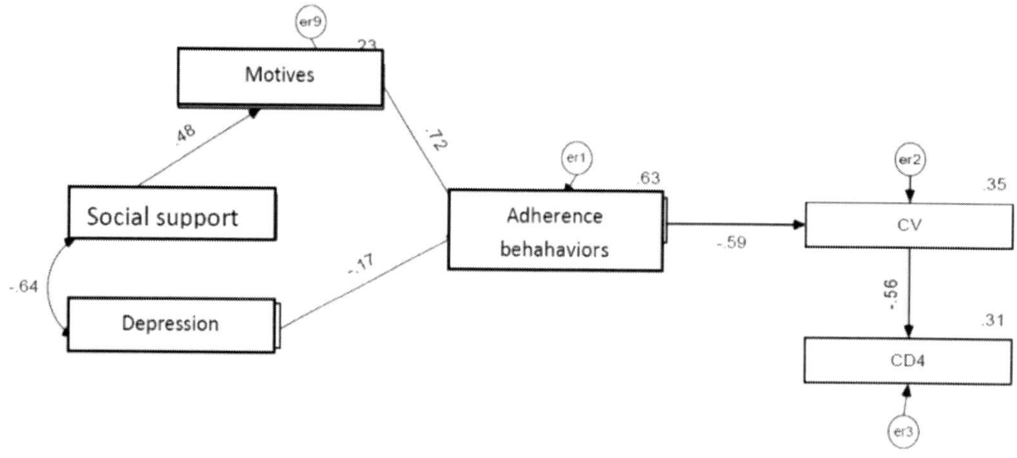

Figure 4. Model 3, including depression variable.

Finally, interaction between social support, motives and depression variables with respect to adherence behaviors was evaluated (Figure 4). As in previous model, in this new account was found a social support direct influence on motives (β. 485; p. 001), as well as on adherence behaviors (β. 724; p. 001). An outstanding fact in this new model was covariance of social support on depression, in the sense that a lesser social support is related to a higher depression, and vice versa (r-. 640; p. 001). Also, it is important to stand out that effect of depression variable on adherence behaviors was not significant (β-. 168; p. 057), while an adherence behaviors direct effect on viral load levels was observed (β. 588; p. 001), which also influenced directly on CD4+ cell count (β-. 557; p. 001). As summarized in table 4, values of remaining indicators were optimal, excepting AGFI.

DISCUSSION

Results of this study corroborate beneficial role of social support on motives underlying consistent and efficient practice of adherence behaviors in PCVS. It also was revealed effect of these behaviors viral load levels, and these on CD4+ cell count. As it is well known, social support is a critical variable in prediction of optimal adherence to treatments, but above all, in obtaining better health outcomes for people living with chronic diseases in general, and with VIH/AIDS in particular (Martos and Pozo, 2011;) Stanton, Revenson, and Tennen, 2007). Thus, agreeing with findings reported by other authors (e.g., Dilorio, McCarty, DePadilla, Resnicow, McDonnell, Yeager et al., 2009) Littlewood, Vanable, Carey, and Blair, 2008), here we found a social support direct effect on motivation, variable which mediated influence of the first one on adherence behaviors.

In light of the psychological model that served as support to this study, which defined social support as a variable where interpersonal relations were involved as interchanging relations - including mainly communication and cooperation (Gonzalez and Pina, 2011), it is understandable why a high score in variable influenced directly and decisively on motives underlying practice of adherence behaviors. In fact, it has been recently demonstrated that a good social support provision from immediate social environment significant people (e.g., relatives or close friends) tends to positively affect PCVS psychological conditions, facilitating a better psychological health and development of behavior patterns allowing them to adjustment to disease and every entailing item, as it would be the case of a competitive respond to requirements imposed by treatment, interchanges of work social type in general, and so on (Reich, Lounsbury, Zaid-Muhammad, and Rapkin, 2010;) Sikkema, Watt, Drabkin, Meade, Hansen, and Pence, 2010).

From the above, we can state it comes once PCVS get in contact with other significant persons from their immediate social environment, provoking communication and cooperation relations are translated into socially valued and reinforced practices, which, throughout the intervention process will facilitate a better fit in social life both to disease itself and treatment of those ones (GengNash, Kambagu, Zhang, Braistein, Christopoulos et al., 2010; Turner-Cobb, Gore-felton, Marouf, Koopman, Kim, Israelski et al., 2002).

However, the foregoing would allow understanding why an optimal social support influenced directly and positively on the motives variable. This one, which implies choice or preference for objects, events, or people contacted in socially valued situations, has as a purpose to give sense to behavior, whose central component is reinforced practices; it is precisely in these practices where positive reinforcement acquires functional properties relevant to subsequent practice of adherence behaviors in its different forms (e.g., to consume antiretroviral drugs, to attend doctor's appointments on time, to do laboratory tests, and so on). In other words, what it would be causing is a functional change in PCVS behavior's system that would affect their individual and interpersonal sphere that eventually will be maintained over time because of the outcomes obtained from such positive consequences (Pina and Gonzalez, 2010).

Therefore, even though social support and motives are two variables with different generalization range (which, we insist, the first one has been redefined as interpersonal relationships, meanwhile the second one as a typically psychological variable), both have and underlying common component: they are linked with what people do in different social circumstances and with positive consequences obtained by practicing different behaviors, exchange and adherence, respectively (Gonzalez and Pina, 2011;) Knowlton, Yang, Bohnert, Wissow, Chander, and Arnsten, 2010). Certainly, in other studies – subject to later empirical confirmation -it must be analyzed which types of consequences operate in each of these levels and, most important, if those who would do so at a relations interchange level are general to individual level or not. This, which evidently is an origin theoretical problem, looks interesting because we assume it could give us a light on how through continuous interaction, ranging from psychological to social (passing by interchange relations), they are going structuring relations between behaviors-consequences that eventually might be functionally relevant sometime and in certain social circumstances but not in another one.

With respect to influence of both variables on intermediate depression levels, here it is convenient to consider the matter carefully. As a starting point, it is necessary to recognize there is an interaction and effects between variables justly operating with different generalization range. Social support operates at social level, while motives and depression at the psychological level. However, as it has been suggested recently, the fact PCVS are part of networks or groups which provides informative, emotional or instrumental social support, seems to favor a better psychological level performance, particularly with the so-called be psychological "welfare", by reducing substantially problems associated, for example, with emotional and affective states which mainly include stress, anxiety and depression (Gordillo et al., 2009;) Munoz, Bayonne, Sanchez, Arevalo, Sebastian, Arteaga et al., 2010).

However. the issue, regardless this sample's PCVS reported intermediate levels in the last one of variables- depression- and that a good perception of social support influenced on it, their influence on adherence behaviors was null, meaning, it was not statistically significant. With regard to this, we can mention that if a good social support is perceived and at the same time those are highly motivated to practice these behaviors, probability both promote a better psychological and social adjustment will be higher, and, in consequent, they will limit possible negative effect of intermediate levels of depression. In other words, if we start from understanding that depression, behaviors associated with the disease, constitutes a relevant epidemiological co-morbid condition between PCVS (Kacanek, Jacobson, Spiegelman, Wanké, Isaac, and Wilson, 2010;) Pina, Davila, Sanchez-Sosa, Togawa, and Cazares, 2008; Simoni, Safren, Manhart, Lyda, Grossman, Rao et al., 2011; Sueoka, Goulet, Fiellin, Rimland, Butt, Gilbert et al., 2010). The fact that in this study intermediate levels ($\overline{X}$ =37.8 of a possible range of 20 to 80 points) in the variable were reported, it would lead us that in some sense, there is a psychological and social adjustment both towards disease itself and therapy which, we insist, limits its negative influence.

On the other hand, if we consider overall effects produced by social support and motives variables on adherence behaviors, we would understand why we finally found their influence over them became, in other times, in a positive influence on both biological markers. Certainly, we must remember first one influenced the second one, who mediated its influence on above behaviors.

Since we generally worked with a PCVS sample, which reported intermediate to high levels of adherence, it is therefore understandable that a good perception of social support and a high motivation explain a high variance of the adherence behaviors, and in turn, they do the same on viral load levels and CD4+ cell count. Then, a consistent practice and efficient behaviors we are dealing with (in terms of competence), will gradually favor to reduce the first ones and increase the second ones, as it was fully demonstrated in this study.

Nonetheless all what has been said so far, this time is needed to recognize both limitations. First, to work with a small sample surely limited the different models analyzed role of depression variable. Second, to include only two variables of model and an exogenous one (social support), cannot allow us to get any definite conclusions about the joint role of theoretical model that served as a support to this study.

Then, it is necessary to drive many others ensuring not only a PCVS broader and more representative sample inclusion, from the same region of Michoacán, but model remaining variables as well, in particular stress related events and both types of behavioral competencies, past and present ones.

For this purpose, a study with a highly representative sample in at least seven federal entities in our country, including Michoacán, is being prepared, in which, together with model's variables (stress related events with stress, motives, competencies and depression), measurement of social support will be promoted as interchange relations under their communication and cooperation modalities, as well as other behaviors associated with the disease, classified as anxiety, anger, and impulsiveness, all defined in strictly behavioral terms and according to theoretical logic of adherence psychological model used herein.

Finally, we hope the information obtained from this study will enable us to contribute with Mexican health authorities to design, implement and evaluate behavioral intervention programs aimed to two objectives: promoting a better fit at psychological and social levels that, as a natural consequence, facilitate a consistent and efficient practice of adherence behaviors in PCVS with direct effects on two clinical markers par excellence, viral load levels and CD4+ cell count, as well as clinical course of disease.

REFERENCES

Anema, A., Wood, E., and Montaner, J. (2008). The use of highly active antiretroviral therapy to reduce HIV incidence at the population level. *Canadian Medical Association Journal, 179*, 13-14.

Bentler, P.M. (1990). Comparative fit indexes in structural models. *Psychological Bulletin, 107*, 238-246.

Bentler, P.M. and Bonett, D.G. (1980). Significance tests and goodness of fit in the analysis of covariance structures. *Psychological Bulletin, 88*, 588-606.

Bollen, K.A. (1989). A new incremental fit index for general structural equation models. *Sociological Methods and Research, 17*, 303-316.

Browne, M.W. and Cudeck, R. (1993). Alternative ways of assessing model fit. In K.A. Bollen and J.S. Long (Eds.), *Testing structural equation models* (pp. 136-162). Newbury Park, CA: Sage.

Edo, M.T. and Ballester, R. (2006). Estado emocional y conducta de enfermedad en personas con VIH/SIDA y enfermos oncológicos. *Revista de Psicopatología y Psicología Clínica, 11*, 79-90.

Ford, N., Darder, M., Spelman, T., Maclean, E., Mills, E., and Boulle, A. (2010). Early adherence to antiretroviral medication as a predictor of long-term HIV virologic suppression: Five-year follow up of an observational cohort. *PLos One, 5*: e10460.

Geng, E., Nash, D., Kambugu, A., Zhang, Y., Braitstein, P., Christopoulos, K., et al. (2010). Retention in care among HIV-infected patients in resource-limited settings. *Current HIV/AIDS Reports, 7*, 234-244.

Giordano, T.P., Gifford, A.L., White, A.C., Suarez-Almazor, M.E., Rabenek, L., Hartman, C., et al. (2007). Retention in care: A challenge to survival with HIV infection. *Clinical Infectious Diseases, 44*, 1493-1499.

González, M.T. and Piña, J. (2011). Motivos, apoyo social y comportamientos de adhesión en personas con VIH: modelamiento con ecuaciones estructurales. *Universitas Psychologica, 10*, 597-607.

Gordillo, M.V., Fekete, E.M., Platteau, T., Antoni, M.H., Schneiderman, N., and Nöstlinger, C. (2009). Emotional support and gender in people living with HIV: effects on psychological well-being. *Journal of Behavioral Medicine, 32*, 523-531.

Hirsch, M., Günthard, H., Schapiro, J., and Brun-Vézinet, F. (2008). Antiretroviral drug resistance testing in adult HIV-1 infection: 2008. Recommendations of an International AIDS Society-USA Panel. *Clinical Infectious Diseases, 47*, 266-271.

Ironson, G., O'Cleirigh, C., Gletcher, M., Laurenceau, J., Balbin, E., and Klimas, N. (2005). Psychosocial factors predict CD4 cell count decline, and viral load change in men and women with human immunodeficiency virus in the era of highly active antiretroviral treatment. *Psychosomatic Medicine,* 67, 1013-1021.

Kacanec, D., Jacongosn, D.L., Spiegelman, D., Wanke, C., Isaac, R., and Wilson, I.B. (2010). Incident depression symptoms are associated with poorer HAART adherence: A longitudinal analysis from the Nutrition for Healthy Living Study. *Journal of Acquired Immune Deficiency Syndromes, 53,* 266-272.

Knowlton, A.R., Yang, C., Bohnert, A., Wissow, L., Chander, G., and Arnsten, J.A. (2010). Informal care and reciprocity of support are associated with HAART adherence among men in Baltimore, MD, USA. *AIDS and Behavior* (Published online 15 July 2010).

Littlewood, R.A., Vanable, P.A., Carey, M.P., and Blair, D.C. (2008). The association of benefit finding to psychosocial and health behavior adaptation among HIV+ men and women. *Journal of Behavioral Medicine, 31,* 145-155.

Martos, M.J. and Pozo, C. (2011). Apoyo funcional *vs.* disfuncional en una muestra de pacientes crónicos: su incidencia sobre la salud y el cumplimiento terapéutico. *Anales de Psicología, 27,* 47-57.

Molassiotis, A., Lopez-Nahas, V., Chung, W.Y., and Lam, S.W. (2003). A Pilot study of the effects of a behavioral intervention on treatment adherence in HIV-infected patients. *AIDS Care, 15,* 125-135.

Muñoz, M., Bayona, J., Sánchez, E., Arévalo, J., Sebastián, J.L., Arteaga, F., et al. (2010). Matching social support to individual needs: A community-based intervention to improve treatment adherence in a resource-poor setting. *AIDS and Behavior* (Published online 10 April 2010).

Pasche-Orlwo M.K., Cheng, D., Palepu, A., Melli, S., Faber, V., and Samet J. (2006). Health literacy antiretroviral adherence and HIV-RNA suppression: a longitudinal perspective. *Journal of General Internal Medicine, 21,* 835-840.

Piña, J.A. (2009). Motivación en psicología y salud: motivación no es sinónimo de intención, actitud o percepción de riesgo. *Diversitas-Perspectivas en Psicología, 5,* 27-35.

Piña, J.A., Corrales, A.E., Mungaray, K., and Valencia, M.A. (2006). Instrumento para medir variables psicológicas y comportamientos de adhesión al tratamiento en personas seropositivas frente al VIH(VPAD-24). *Revista Panamericana de Salud Pública, 19,* 217-228.

Piña, J.A., Corrales, A.E., and Rivera, B. (2007). Validación del cuestionario de apoyo social funcional en personas con VIH del noroeste de México. *Ciencia y Enfermería, 13,* 53-63.

Piña, J. A. and Sánchez-Sosa, J. J. (2007). Modelo psicológico para la investigación de los comportamientos de adhesión en personas con VIH. *Universitas Psychologica, 6,* 399-407.

Piña, J. A., Dávila M., Sánchez-Sosa, J.J., Togawa, C., and Cázares, O. (2008) Asociación entre los niveles de estrés y depresión y la adhesión al tratamiento en personas seropositivas al VIH en Hermosillo, México. *Revista Panamericana de Salud Pública, 23,* 377-383.

Piña, J.A. and González, M.T. (2010). Un modelo psicológico de adhesión en personas VIH+: Modelamiento con ecuaciones estructurales. *Revista Iberoamericana de Psicología y Salud, 1,* 185-206.

Reich, W.A., Lounsbury, D.W., Zaid-Muhammad, S., and Rapkin, B.D. (2010). Forms of social support and their relationship to mental health in HIV-positive persons. *Psychology, Health and Medicine, 15,* 135-145.

Ribes, E. (1990). *Psicología y salud. Un análisis conceptual.* Barcelona: Martínez Roca.

Ribes, E. (2005). ¿Qué es lo que se debe medir en psicología? La cuestión de las diferencias individuales. *Acta Comportamentalia, 13,* 37-52.

Rivera, B.M., Corrales, A.E., Cázares, O., and Piña, J.A. (2007). Validación de la escala de depresión de Zung en personas con VIH. *Terapia Psicológica, 25,* 135-140.

Ruiz, M. (2000). *Introducción a los modelos de ecuaciones estructurales.* Madrid: Ediciones UNED.

Sánchez-Sosa, J.J., Fierros, L.E., Cázares, O., and Piña, J.A. (2011). Estudio longitudinal de variables psicológicas y conductas de adhesión en personas VIH+: efectos sobre los niveles de carga viral. En J.L. Ybarra, J.J. Sánchez-Sosa, and J.A. Piña (Eds.), *Trastornos y enfermedades crónicas: una aproximación psicológica* (pp. 137-154). México: Universidad Autónoma de Tamaulipas/El Manual Moderno.

Sikkema, K.J., Watt, M.H., Drabkin, A.S., Meade, C.S., Hansen, N.B., and Pence, B.W. (2010). Mental health treatment to reduce HIV transmission risk behavior: A positive prevention model. *AIDS and Behavior, 14,* 252-262.

Simoni, J.M., Safren, S.A., Manhart, L.E., Lyda, K., Grossman, C.I., Rao, D., et al. (2011). Challenges in addressing depression in HIV research: Assessment, cultural context, and methods. *AIDS and Behavior, 15,* 376-388.

Stanton, A.L., Revenson, T.A., and Tennen, H. (2007). Health psychology: Psychological adjustment to chronic disease. *Annual Review of Psychology, 58,* 565-592.

Sueoka, K., Goulet, J.L., Fiellin, D.A., Rimland, D., Butt, A.A., Gilbert, C., et al. (2010). Depression symptoms and treatment among HIV infected and uninfected veterans. *AIDS and Behavior, 14,* 272-279.

Turber-Cobb, J.M., Gore-Felton, C., Marouf, F., Koopman, C., Kim, P., Israelski, D., et al. (2002). Coping, social support and attachment style as psychosocial correlates of adjustment in men and women with HIV/AIDS. *Journal of Behavioral Medicine, 25,* 337-353.

Villa, C. and Vinaccia, S. (2006). Adhesión terapéutica y variables psicológicas asociadas en personas con diagnóstico de VIH/SIDA. *Psicología y Salud, 16,* 51-62.

Wagner, G.J., Kanouse, D.E., Golinelli, D., Miller, L.G., Daar, E.S., Witt, M.D., et al. (2006). Cognitive-behavioral intervention to enhance adherence to antiretroviral therapy: a randomized controlled trial (CCTG 578). *AIDS, 20,* 1295-1302.

Wood, E., Hogg, R.S., Yip, B., Harrigan, R., O´Shaughnessy, M.V., and Montaner, J.S.G. (2003). Effect of medication adherence on survival of HIV-infected adults who start highly active antiretroviral therapy when $CD4^+$ cell count is 0.200 to 0.350 x 10^9 cell/l. *Annals of Internal Medicine, 139,* 810-816.

(Manuscript received on October 20, 2011. Revised version accepted for publication on November 17, 2011)

In: Recent Hispanic Psychological Research ... ISBN: 978-1-62948-919-3
Editors: C. H. Garcia Cadena, A. Lopez-Espinoza et al.

Chapter 14

Psychological Variables and Adherence Behaviors among HIV+ Patients: A Gender-Based Analysis

Julio Alfonso Piña López* and Ramón Alberto Rascón Pacheco
Independent Researcher, Hermosillo, México
Unit of Epidemiological Research and Health Services
Instituto Mexicano del Seguro Social, México

Abstract

A retrospective and cross-sectional study was performed in order to identify gender differences in psychological variables associated with adherence behaviors among 74 HIV+ patients from Sonora, Mexico, who answered two self-administered questionnaires: 1) Psychological variables underlying adherence behaviors, and 2) Stress-related situations. Statistically significant differences were observed among non-adherent and 100% adherent patients (χ^2 [1] = 26.162; $p < .001$), as well as among men (83.7%) and women (72%) practicing adherence behaviors all days of the week ($Z = -4.907$; $p < .001$); finally, a multivariate logistic regression analysis showed that motivation variables (corrected OR = 1.75; 95% CI: 1.27-2.39), as well as current behavioral competencies (corrected OR = 1.12; 95% CI: 1.00-1.24) were psychological variables associated with adherence behaviors. Results show that motivation and optimal current competent performance are psychological variables operating in different way in both VIH+ men and women; this issue must be taken into account in order to improve the effectiveness of interdisciplinary intervention programs regarding Mexican health care institutions.

Keywords: Gender, Psychological Model, Adherence, Motivation, Behavioral Competences

* Mail address: Guillermo Prieto No. 18. Col. Constitución. Hermosillo, Sonora, C.P. 83150 (México). E-mail: ja.pina@yahoo.com.mx.

INTRODUCTION

Multiple studies have been conducted around the world, whose main objective is to identify possible differences between men and women regarding adherence behavior practice to antiretroviral treatment (ART). Up to date, results have been conflicting, since meanwhile those differences, in some results, have not been evident with respect to statistics meaning terms (Applebaum, Richardson, Brady, Brief, and Keane, 2009; Ballester, Garcia, Reinoso, and Campos, 2002; Silva, Ximenes, Miranda Filho, Arraes, Mendes et al., 2009), in others it is claimed men are more adherent than women (Berg, Demas, Howard, Schoembaum, Gourevitch, and Arnsten, 2004; Waldrop-Valverde, Jones, Jayaweera, Gonzalez, Romero, and Ownby, 2009).

However, beyond if those differences eventually exist, what finally must be our interest is how to get a better and more thorough understanding of their "why", meaning, what it would be required is to identify which psychological variables affect, and in what sense, HIV+ patients of both genders in a certain moment, or through a continuous interaction. As example, we can mention that in a work carried out in Mexico based on psychological model to research adherence behaviors of people living with chronic illnesses (Piña and Sanchez-Sosa, 2007); although it is true that a statistically significant difference was found between men and women in ART adherence behaviors, the most interesting from results were psychological variables that predicted a high motivation and low levels of stress linked to both ambiguity tolerance and frustration tolerance, with variances explained in percentages come to 51.6 and 30.6%, respectively (Davila, Piña, and Sanchez-Sosa, 2008).

In the frame of health psychology, the aforementioned is a key issue, especially if there is a genuine interest to fully comply with such understanding of the recent mentioned case, in its purest theoretical sense.

We refer to the fact that today, more than ever, to justify theoretically the design and guidance of applied cross-sectional studies has become essential, and to be remarkable as well for providing elements that make possible to translate findings into intervention proposals, susceptible to be evaluated and systematically replied (Piña, Ybarra, Alcala, and Samaniego, 2010); that is exactly the double premise that provoked the psychological model development served to sustain this study.

It is an interactive and functional model in which interaction between a group of psychological and biological variables through four phases is proposed (Figure 1). In phase one, three process psychological variables are included: stress related events (SRE), motives and skill-based performance; phase two is dedicated to HIV seropositive diagnosis and other affections; third one deals with two type of behaviors, adherence and those types associated to diseases; finally, fourth one discusses phenomena implied in biological reactivity (modulation and vulnerability) and health results (mainly, T-CD4+ account cells and viral load levels).

Stress related events are understood as those situations (from daily life or those derived from disease and treatment itself) facilitating the presence of states of stress permanently related, which in our model 3 has been mainly considered: decision making, ambiguity tolerance and frustration tolerance; they are situations related to experimental phenomena known in literature as uncertainty, ambiguity and unpredictability, in which stimulus signals or response consequences acquire special relevance (Ribes, 1990). Since each situation is identified as a functional "profile" describing a particular type of interaction in a certain circumstance, theoretically talking, based on such conceptual category, it would be possible to measure behavioral tendencies, meaning, behavior consistencies in and through time (Ribes, 2009).

Motives mean inclinations or tendencies to behave in a way or other in social circumstances where there is a good probability to obtain positive stimulus consequences (flatteries, verbal or affective expressions of support, etc.); regarding our subject, to say a HIV+ patient is motivated, it would imply he wants to do the things (to consume medicaments) because he has learned to relate practice of those behaviors with determined consequences of stimulus; such consequences could be eventually granted by the own health personnel or other significant persons from his social immediate environment (understanding couple, relatives or close friends, mainly), or could be drawn from the own knowledge about health condition from the same patients. (Piña, 2009).

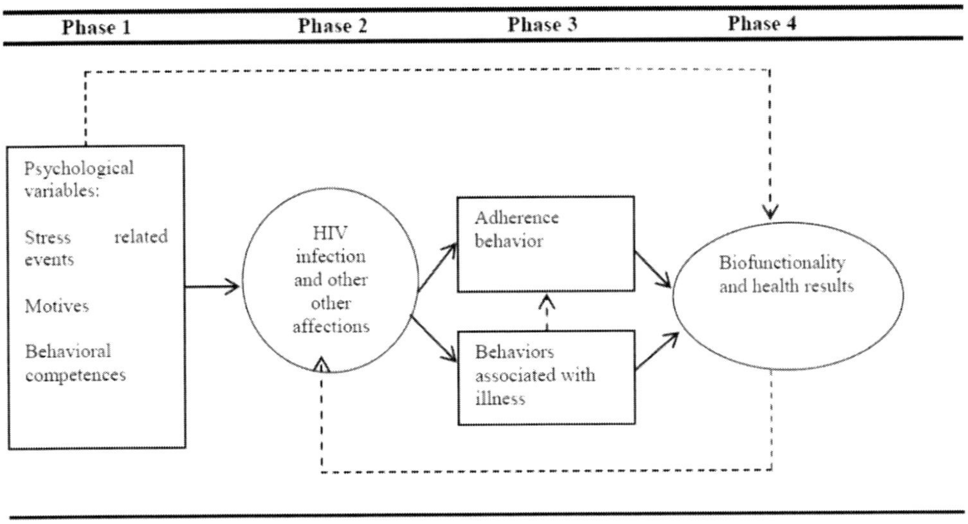

Figure 1. Graphic display of adherence psychological model of Piña and Sanchez-Sosa (2007).

Regarding skill-based performance (including knowledge, skills and abilities), we refer it to different behaviors allowing HIV+ patient to carry out efficiently in situations demanding a particular type of behavior, since he knows what he has and additionally because he can do what is expected; here, a wide rank of behaviors acquires importance, some of them are related to prescribed medicaments consumption, others to attending devotedly doctor's appointment and to make periodical clinic and laboratory tests, etc.

Once a person is diagnosed with HIV infection (phase two) and treatment regime has been agreed with medical personnel, it is expected patient practices adherence behaviors assigned in phase three, especially those concerning antiretroviral medicaments consumption; or, those behaviors may be affected by process psychological variables of phase one, in addition to other behaviors; those associated to illness (CAE) of the same phase three, which are grouped in general categories including depressive states and phenomena like anger, impulsiveness and social isolation, among others. If adherence behaviors are practiced efficiently (meaning, in skill-based terms), it is highly probable to keep an optimum functioning of biological reactivity, and to observe as well optimum health results (low levels of viral load and high T-CD4+ cell count, as part of phase four; this last one would be translated in a minor risk to develop other affections typical of phase two, those known as opportunistic infections, or those that are part of HIV diagnosis as such.

This study, having a psychological model as theoretical support to research adherence behaviors, whose objective was to identify differences per gender when associating a group of psychological variables (stress related events, motivation and behavioral competences), and the behaviors mentioned in a HIV+ patients representative sample in the State of Sonora (in the Northwest of Mexico) exposed to regimes of treatment with antiretroviral medicaments.

METHOD

Participants

Previously to its instrumentation, this retrospective and cross-sectional study was approved by the Committee of Research and Quality of the Ministry of Public Health in the State of Sonora, in the Northwest of Mexico. Initially, an interdisciplinary team (composed of physicians, psychologists and social workers) invited to participate in this study a group of little less HIV+ 200 patients, who were receiving treatment in a health institution in the city of Hermosillo, Capital of the State of Sonora; from that amount, 94 patients accepted to participate. The following were considered eligibility criteria: 1) to have a confirmed seropositive HIV diagnosis of at least six months previous to study beginning; 2) to have 18 years old or older; 3) to be under an ART treatment, and 4) to have at least the last laboratory results in which viral load and T-CD4+ cells count are specified. Since 20 of the patients did not comply with all of those criteria, definitive sample was composed of 74 patients, 49 out of them (66.2%) were men and 25 (33.8%) were women, with an age median of 37.5 years old (DE = 10.3); other sociodemographic and clinical characteristics were summarized in Table 1.

Instruments and Biological Measures

Psychological variables and adherence behaviors (VPAD-24), designed and validated in Mexico (Piña, Corrales, Mungaray, and Valencia, 2006) is composed of 24 questions grouped in four factors (Global Cronbach $\alpha = .87$ to this sample): the first includes specific questions about behaviors related to medicaments consumption, alcohol or drugs substances, as well as contraindicated food. For this work purposes, behaviors measures related to medicaments consumption were the only included, defined by a Likert type scale with response options going from one (I did not eat them during the week) to five (I ate them the seven days of the week), for analysis purposes, variable were dichotomized later so as to differentiate between non adherent patients (who responded to options one, two, three and four), and 100% of adherent ones (who responded to option five).

The second factor includes four questions about motives lying in the practice of behaviors in question, defined by a Likert Type format with answer's options going from one (it was not a determinant motive) to four (it was a sufficient determinant motive); for example, if a patient responded he had consumed medicaments the seven days of the week, immediately after he was questioned about motives influencing to practice such behaviors, he answered: "because I have experienced their benefits", "because physician asked me to", "I did it because of close people", and "because I want to keep myself healthy as much as I can". Reliability of measure was high among questions composing subscale (Table 1).

Third and fourth factors measure respective present and past skill-based performance. Four questions of current competence subscale were in a Likert type format with five level-answer going from one (it is very difficult) to five (it is not hard), which were related to patients efficient performance concerning personal and social situations that eventually could interfere with adherence behaviors practice; a question example with respect to personal competence was the following: How hard is for you to prevent situations provoking you depression or sadness? One question regarding environment implied in social interaction was: How hard is for you to start or to keep social bonds with people from your immediate environment?

Table 1. Socio-demographic and clinical characteristics of participants (n = 74)

		N	%	Median	Interquartile rank	α
Sex:						
Man		49	66.2			
Woman		25	33.8			
Age:				37.5.	29-64	
Marital status:						
Single	41	55.4				
Married	10	13.5				
Free union		16	21.6			
Separated		5	6.8			
Widow		2	2.7			
Time of infection (months):				52.6	21-84	
Viral load:						
< 400 copies/mL. 401-		24	32.4			
30 mil copies/mL		30	40.5			
.> 30 mil copies/mL.		20	27.1			
T CD4+ cells:						
> 200 cells/mL.	48	64.9				
201-400 cells/mL.	4	22	29.7			
> 400 cells/mL.		5.4				
Motives						.90
Current competences						.86
Past competences						.76
Frustration tolerance						.80
Decisions making						.90
Ambiguity tolerance						.92

Finally, past competences were defined in a Likert type format with five level- answers going from one (never) to five (always). These subscale's five level-answers were related with the efficient performance previous to HIV seropositivity diagnosis and other illnesses, in this way, if, for example, patients get a cold, get sick of stomach, get a sore throat, etc., then, they were asked how frequency they had practiced adherence behaviors and those linked to illness care: "to prevent consuming substances like alcohol", "consuming medicines as they were prescribed" and "to make lab exams or other necessary indicated by the physician".

Stress related events (SVE-12), which is a scale designed and validated in Mexico (Piña, Valencia, Mungaray, and Corrales, 2006). It includes 12 answers about three situations, meaning, frustration tolerance, decision making and ambiguity tolerance; all the questions were in a 10 points scale going from one ("it is not a disturbing situation") to 10 ("it is a very disturbing situation"). Frustration tolerance (which corresponds to unpredictability phenomenon) was composed of six questions, being an example the following: "You are receiving a treatment and accomplish with your doctor's indications, but you do not receive positive feedback from anyone"; consequently, the result for you is...On the other hand, in decision making (which corresponds to uncertainty phenomenon) there were three questions, one of them stated the following: "In this moment, you are receiving a treatment for the illness, but from other people's pressure, you decide to take a different treatment"; consequently, the result for you is...Likewise, in tolerance to ambiguity situation (which corresponds to the phenomenon of the same name) three questions were included, being an example the following: "In this moment, you are receiving treatment for the illness, but you do not know if medicaments will provoke secondary effect"; consequently, the result for you is...

Finally, three biological measures were extracted from clinical history: infection time (in months), T-CD4+ cells count and viral load levels.

Procedure

Previously to instruments administration, HIV+ patients were individually invited so they can cooperate voluntarily in this study. Those who accepted were provided with an informed consent (in which purposes of the study as well as commitment from parties, meaning, responsible persons and participants), which was read and signed. Next, they received the instruments and indications about how to answer were given; it was clarified that in case of any doubt, they could ask research team members (previously trained by this work's author) so they can be cleared; instruments administration varies from 35 to 45 minutes. None of the patients received any economical remuneration.

Data Analysis

For statistical treatment of data, STATA program (MAC OS-X 9.0 version) was used. According to objective proposed and from reclassification dependent variable (in a dichotomous format) and independent ones (considering median values), non parametrical tests including Pearson χ^2, Wilcoxon and Mann-Whitney U were used. In a first moment, unvaried statistics of variables of interest were obtained; Pearson χ^2 was used to estimate possible differences between non HIV+ patients and HIV+ patients and 100% adherent ones; next, Wilcoxon test ranks were used to evaluate possible differences between non patients and patients and 100% adherent ones according to gender variable; likewise, Mann-Whitney U test was used in order to estimate possible differences (both adherence percentages and gender) with respect to scores obtained per each one of independent variables (model psychological variables).

Finally, a series of multivariate logistic regression analysis were conducted, adjusted to gender variable. It deals with an advantaging procedure which only needs to know if event happened or not (i.e., to practice or not adherence behaviors) so as to be in conditions for using a dichotomous value of dependent variable. From such value, by applying logistic regression, it can be predicted estimate regarding probability the event occurs or not, value pertaining to odds ratio (RM and its confidence interval, or CI), which essentially constitute the measure of changes according to probabilities (Hair, Anderson, Tatham, and Black, 2000).

Table 2. Univariate statistics and median values of adherence model psychological variables (analysis per adherence percentage)

Variable	Group	N	Rank of X	U	Z	P
Motives	Non -adherent	15	18.5	157.5	-3.969	.001
	100% adherent	59	41.7			
Current competences	Non- adherent	15	27.7	296	-1.923	.05
	100% adherent	59	39.4			
Past competences	Non- adherent	15	29.2	319	-1.588	nsa
	100% adherent	59	39			
Frustration tolerance	Non adherent	15	36.8	432.5	- .036	ns
	100% adherent	59	37			
Decisions making	Non- adherent	15	35.2	408.5	- .365	ns
	100% adherent	59	37.4			
Ambiguity tolerance	Non- adherent	15	39.1 3	402.5	- .449	ns
	100% adherent	59	6.4			

[a]ns (non significant).

RESULTS

Based on medicaments consumption through all the week, 15 (20.3%) patients reported to be non-adherent, meanwhile 59 (79.7%) were 100% adherent, a significant difference (χ^2 [1] = 26.162; $p < .001$). When comparing practice of adherence behaviors regarding gender, Wilcoxon ranks test showed a significant difference ($Z = -4.907$; $p < .001$), being the group of men which practiced more frequently adherence behavior, meaning, seven days a week (83.7% vs. 72% of women).

So as to calculate possible difference in psychological differences according to adherence percentages, Mann-Whitney U test was used. Such as it can be observed in Table 2, only two statistically significant differences were found: in motives' variables (Z = -3.969; p < .001) and in current competence performance (Z = -1.924; p < .005), in both cases with HIV+ 100% patients, having a higher score in Median ranks.

Using the same procedure, but now with the purpose of calculating possible differences according to gender variables, results are summarized in Table 3.

Similarly to previous analysis, in this one there were found statistically significant differences in the same variables: motives (Z = -2.565; p < .01) and current behavioral competences (Z = -2.619; p < .005), with median ranks, showing a higher motivation to practice adherence behaviors in women and a better competence performance in men.

Table 3. Univariate statistics and median values of adherence model psychological variables (analysis per gender)

Variable	Group	N	Rank of X	U	Z	P
Motives	Men	49	32.7	379.5	-2.565	.001
	Women	24	45.6			
Current competences		49	41.4	368	-2.619	.005
	Men Women	24	27.8			
Past competences		49	35.8	533	- .647	ns[a]
	Men Women	24	39.9			
Frustration tolerance	Men	49	37.7	553	- .463	ns
	Women	24	35.5			
Decisions making		49	34.2	455	-1.577	ns
	Men Women	24	42.5			
Ambiguity tolerance		49	34.7	476.5	-1.326	ns
	Men Women	24	41.6			

[a]ns (non significant).

In order to visualize results from both analyses, "Box" graphics was used (Figure 2). As it can be seen there, each one of six psychological variables was divided in pairs: the first one corresponds to non-adherent and the second one to 100% adherent; likewise, in each pair male patients are located (left side) and women (right side). Lines inside each graphics represent median scores obtained from a group of patients in each process psychological variable.

Finally, in Table 4, multivariate logistic regression analysis results are described. It was found process psychological variables were associated significantly with adherence behaviors: on one side, motives (RM = 1.75; IC 95%: 1.27-2.39; p < .001), by observing statistical effect significance was no lost when introducing gender variable (RM = 1.75; IC 95%: 1.23-2.48; p < .005); on the other side, current competent performance (RM = 1.12; IC 95%: 1.00-1.24; p < .05), with a statistical effect significance once gender variable was introduced (RM = 1.11; IC 95%: 0.99-1.24; p = .064).

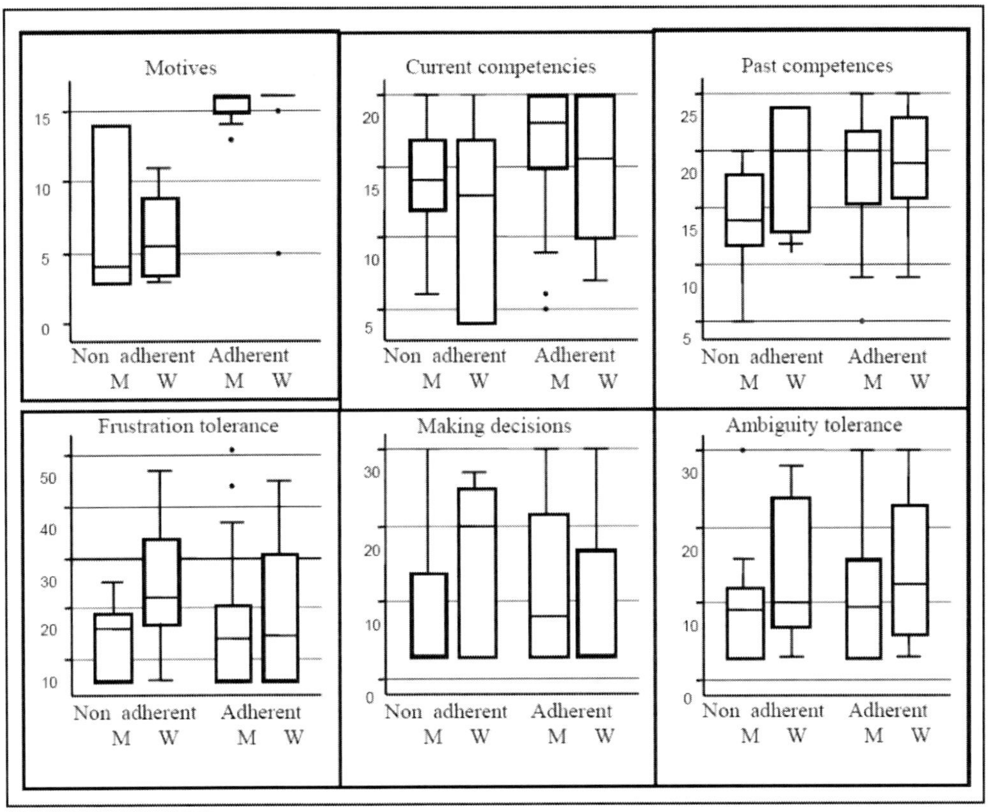

Figure 2. Frequencies distribution (Median values) of psychological variables between non adherent and 100% adherent, as well as between men (M) and women (W).

Table 4. Logistic regression analysis and adherence behaviours

Variables	Analysis	RM	IC 95%	Ji^2	P
Motives	Raw	1.75	1.27-2.39	3.47	.001
	Corrected	1.75	1.23-2.48	3.14	.002
Current behavioral competences	Raw	1.12	1.00-1.24	2.00	.046
	Corrected	1.11	.99-1.24	1.85	.064
Past behavioral competences	Raw	1.08	.97-1.20	1.43	.151
	Corrected	1.08	.98-1.20	1.56	.118
Frustration tolerance	Raw	.99	.94-1.04	- .31	.760
	Corrected	1.00	.95-1.04	- .13	.724
Decisions making	Raw	.99	.93-1.04	- .46	.649
	Corrected	.99	.93-1.04	- .47	.641
Ambiguity tolerance	Raw	1.00	.93-1.06	-.12	.901
	Corrected	1.00	.94-1.07	.08	.935

Discussion

A first group of data of interest showed in this work, has to do with high percentages of adherence obtained from the sample, as a whole, (79.7%), as well as those found both in men (83.7%) and in women (72%). In general terms, it is about higher percentages than those reported in studies carried out in different countries of the world (Breton, Lewden, Spire, Salmon, Brun-Vézinet, Duong et al., 2007; Hermann, McKinnon, John, Hylands, Matínez, Cain et al., 2008), although they are pretty similar to those obtained by other authors (Kuoanfack, Laurent, Peytavin, Ciaffi, Ngolle, Mawamba et al., 2008; Peltzer, Friend-du Preez, Ramlagan, and Anderson, 2010).

A second group of data regarding variation observed in process psychological variables, once they were analyzed according to both adherence and gender percentages. It comes to our attention, on one side, the behavior of motives' variables and the two types of competences, whose scores were high among HIV+ 100% adherent patients, information consisting in other studies' reports from our research team (Piña and González, 2010; Sanchez-Sosa, Cázares, Piña, and Davila, 2009). On the other hand, and concerning analysis according to gender variable, it is important to emphasize that even it is true there were found statistically significant differences in motives' variables and current competences, following the logic of results obtained in a previous study (Davila et al., 2008), we expected were women and not men, who obtained higher scores in competence performance.

This last condition is a key point , since according to proposal exposed at the beginning of this work, the matter has partially to do with if eventually differences exist or not in adherence behaviors between men and women; in effect, the essential of the discussion, from our point of view, is to understand why these differences appear. Today, there is already a strong group of knowledge in which it is stated how HIV+ patients of both gender used to react differently both to illness and antiretroviral treatment; that can be caused by variables influence including biological reactivity itself, meaning, to conditions of the body in a particular moment, or through all the interaction (Ford, Darder, Spelman, Maclean, Mills, and Boulle, 2010; Nachega, Trotta, Nelson, and Ammassari, 2009); to neurocognitive functioning (Lovejoy and Suhr, 2009); to the presence of more or less permanent depression or stress states, as well as lack of emotional and social support networks, mainly (Bottonari, Safren, McQuaid, Hsiao, and Roberts, 2010; Gordillo, Fekete, Platteau, Antoni, Schneiderman, and Nöstlonger, 2009).

With respect to our study, these differences were evident in two of the six psychological variables analyzed, meaning, motives and current competent performance, whose influence has been fully confirmed in HIV+ patients requiring to practice adherence behaviors, as well as other related to health care (Piña, Davila, Sanchez-Sosa, Cázares, Togawa, and Corrales, 2009). It deals essentially with two variables sharing the characteristic of being potentially modifiable, either because of the influence of the own situations linked to stress, or the influence of context variables (including people coming into contact with, what kinds of social circumstances, etc.) in which patients are interacting.

Returning to theoretical model used in this work, the motives one is a critical variable allowing us to understand why those patients practice adherence behaviors as it is expected they do. Motives always happen as a psychological phenomenon once a patient interacts with other significant persons from their environment in social circumstances where a reasonable probability of obtaining positive stimulus consequences exists. In our sample, women were the ones more motivated than men (rank of X = 45.6 y de 32.7, respectively), which would be reflecting a tendency to do the things due to stimulus consequences that come with instrumental execution of adherence behaviors. At this point, it is convenient to remind specific questions about lying motives to practice such behaviors involved in two of the four cases to other significant persons of immediate social environment (i.e., health personnel, relatives or family), which would suggest it is possible that women of this sample were exactly more "sensitive" to use a colloquial expression to positive influence of those other persons.

In the opposite sense, it was more evident in men (rank of X = 41.4 vs. 27.8 of women) the important role of current competent performance variable. It constitutes a variable concerning "to be able2 to do the things concerning concrete demands faced by HIV+ patients which would imply to know what and how many medicaments exist, which are accompanied with liquids or food, at what time they have to be taken, etc., but take them efficiently, that is, by practicing adherence instrumental behaviors.

In regard to this point, it is convenient to stand out that when we talk about behavioral competences, we are referring to knowledge, skills and particular abilities, and not to a diversity of "beliefs", "ideas" or "thoughts" about if a HIV+patient knows if he can or not to do the things (i.e., DiLorio, McCarthy, DePadilla, Resnicow, McDonnell, Yeager et al., 2009; Johnson, Neilands, Dilworth, Morin, Remien, and Chesney, 2007); to be competent implies, then, that something can be done because there are knowledge, skills and abilities to do it to greater extent since it has been done before.

In this general framework, it has to be cleared that both motivation and current behavioral competences are part of the person history, even if it deals with a history of changes, in the sense that it is not a determined beginning and ending history; by such virtue, it is not about a history concluded in a moment a measurement is carried out, but it is one which differential role of stimulus consequences is a key point to identify a greater or lesser motivation, as well as translation of those competences into adherence behaviors way.

For all of the above, we have emphasized on the value of knowing the role of different psychological variables and the way in which they are related to determined stimulus consequences where their influence is analyzed about adherence behaviors. We cannot ignore we are working with HIV+ patients, whose psychological stories (and the way such stories determined the way of interacting with objects, events and other persons today) are undeniably different. This last condition could help us to understand the results showed in intervention studies, in which differential effects in psychological and biological levels produced by cognitive-behavioral strategies application have been found (Wagner, Kanouse, Golinelli, Miller, Daar, Witt et al., 2006), facilitating both adherence behaviors practice (Javanbakht, Prosser, Grimes, Weinstein, and Farthing, 2006).

Nonetheless findings reported this time that it is convenient to recognize three limitations. Maybe the most important was sample size, limited only to a little more than one third of HIV+ patients of the country's region where they are under treatment regimes with antiretroviral medicaments. Second limitation was not to state the influence of events variable related to stress, which has demonstrated to play a first role in some studies carried out based on adherence psychological model (Piña et al., 2009; Piña, Davila, Sanchez-Sosa, Togawa, and Cázares, 2008; Sanchez-Sosa et al., 2009). Finally, in this occasion was not possible to include other variables analysis, which even they are inscribed in what we have called interpersonal and social levels of interaction, they are essential as well so as to be able to evaluate their relative weight, once they interact with our model psychological variables; we refer to those of support and social position (i.e., Arrivillaga, Ross, Useche, Alzate, and Correa, 2009).

By all means, and recognizing such limitations, we consider that our study initially contributes to a more complete understanding of what and how a group of psychological variables affects differentially HIV+ men and women under treatment. It is fair to say that from such understanding, we will be in better conditions to design, instrument and evaluate interdisciplinary intervention programs adjusting their needs, since we cannot ignore there are no two HIV+ patients with the same psychological background and behaving currently in the same way. That is why it was so important to justify research works in articulated theoretical models grouping in its structure, concepts related to psychological history (distal and immediate) with those of current social context.

References

Applebaum, A.J., Richardson, M.A., Brady, S.M., Brief, D.J., and Keane, T.M. (2009). Gender and other psychosocial factors as predictors of adherence to highly active antiretroviral therapy (HAART) in adults with comorbid HIV/AIDS, psychiatric and substance-related disorders. *AIDS and Behavior, 13,* 60-65.

Arrivillaga, M., Ross, M., Useche, B., Alzate, M.L., and Correa, D. (2009). Social position, gender role, and treatment adherence among Colombian women living with HIV/AIDS: Social determinants of health approach. *Revista Panamericana de Salud Pública, 26,* 502-510.

Ballester, R., García, S., Reinoso, I., and Campos, A. (2002). Gender differences in adherence to treatment and illness behavior in HIV/AIDS patients: an exploratory study in Spain. *International Journal of Psychology and Psychological Therapy, 2,* 219-236.

Berg, K.M., Demas, P.A., Howard, A.A., Schoembaum, E.E., Gourevitch, M.N., and Arnsten, J.H. (2004). Gender differences in factors associated with antiretroviral adherence. *Journal of General Internal Medicine, 19,* 1111-1117.

Bottonari, K.A., Safren, S.A., McQuaid, J.R., Hsiao, C-B., and Roberts, J.E. (2010). A longitudinal investigation of the impact of life stress on HIV treatment adherence. *Journal of Behavioral Medicine, 33,* 486-495.

Breton, G., Lewden, C., Spire, B., Salmon, D., Brun-Vézinet, F., Duong, M., et al. (2007). Characteristics and response to antiretroviral therapy of HIV-1-infected patients born in Africa and living in France. *HIV Medicine, 8,* 164-170.

Davila, M., Piña, J.A., and Sánchez-Sosa, J.J. (2008). Psychological variables and treatment adherence behaviors among persons living with HIV: a gender-based analysis [In Spanish]. En S. Rivera, R. Díaz-Loving, R. Sánchez, and I. Reyes-Lagunes (Coords.), *La psicología social en México. Vol. XII* (pp. 61-66). México: Asociación Mexicana de Psicología Social.

DiLorio, C., McCarthy, F., DePadilla, L., Resnicow, K., McDonnell, M., Yeager, K., et al. (2009). Adherence to antiretroviral medication regimens: A test of a psychosocial model. *AIDS and Behavior, 13,* 10-22.

Ford, N., Darder, M., Spelman, T., Maclean, E., Mills, E., and Boulle, A. (2010). Early adherence to antiretroviral medication as a predictor of long-term HIV virologic suppression: Five-year followup of an observational cohort. *PloS One, 5:* e10460.

Gordillo, V., Fekete, E.M., Platteau, T., Antoni, M.H., Schneiderman, N., Nöstlinger, C., et al. (2009). Emotional support and gender in people living with HIV: effects on psychological well-being. *Journal of Behavioral Medicine, 32,* 523-531.

Hair, J.F., Anderson, R.E., Tatham, R.L., and Black, W.C. (2000). *Análisis multivariante.* Madrid: Prentice Hall.

Herrmann, S., McKinnon, E., John, M., Hylands, N., Martínez, O.P., Cain, A., et al. (2008). Evidence-based, multifactorial approach to addressing non-adherence to antiretroviral therapy and improving standars of care. *Internal Medicine Journal, 38,* 8-15.

Javanbakht, M., Prosser, P., Grimes, T., Weinstein, M., and Farthing, C. (2006). Efficacy of an individualized adherence support program with contingent reinforcement among nonadherent HIV-positive patients. *Journal of the International Association of Physicians in AIDS Care, 5,* 143-150.

Johnson, M.O., Neilands, T.B., Dilworth, S., Morin, S.F., Remien, R.H., and Chesney, M.A. (2007). The role of self-efficacy in HIV treatment adherence: Validation of the HIV treatment adherence self-efficacy scale (HIV-ASES). *Journal of Behavioral Medicine, 30,* 359-370.

Kuoanfack, C., Laurent, C., Peytavin, G., Ciaffi, L., Ngolle, M., Mawamba, Y., et al. (2008). Adherence to antiretroviral therapy assessed by drug level monitoring and self-report in Cameroon. *Journal of Acquired Immune Deficiciency Syndromes, 48,* 216-219.

Lovejoy, T.I. and Suhr, J.A. (2009). The relationship between neuropsychological functioning and HAART adherence in HIV-positive adults: a systematic review. *Journal of Behavioral Medicine, 32,* 389-405.

Nachega, J.B., Trotta, M.P., Nelson, M., and Ammassari, A. (2009). Impact of metabolic complications on antiretroviral treatment adherence: Clinical and public health implications. *Current HIV/AIDS Report, 6,* 121-129.

Peltzer, K., Friend-du Preez, N., Ramagian, S., and Anderson, J. (2010). Antiretroviral treatment adherence among HIV patients in KwaZulu-Natal, South Africa. *BMC Public Health, 10.*111

Piña, J.A. (2009). Motivation in health psychology: motivation is not synonymous of intention, attitude or risk perception [In Spanish]. *Diversitas-Perspectivas en Psicología, 5,* 27-35.

Piña, J.A., Corrales, A.E., Mungaray, K., and Valencia, M.A. (2006). Instrument for measuring psychological variables and adherence to treatment behaviors in persons who are seropositive for HIV (VPAD-24) [In Spanish]. *Revista Panamericana de Salud Pública, 19,* 217-228.

Piña, J.A., Dávila, M., Sánchez-Sosa, J.J., Cázares, O., Togawa, C., and Corrales, A.E. (2009). Effects of length of infection on predictors of adherence in persons with HIV [In Spanish]. *International Journal of Psychology and Psychological Therapy, 9*, 67-78.

Piña, J.A., Dávila, M., Sánchez-Sosa, J.J., Togawa, C., and Cázares, O. (2008). Association between stress and depression levels and treatment adherence among HIV-seropositive individuals in Hermosillo, Mexico [In Spanish]. *Revista Panamericana de Salud Pública, 23,* 377-383.

Piña, J.A. and González, M.T. (2010). A psychological model of adherence in HIV+ people: Structural equation modeling [In Spanish]. *Revista Iberoamericana de Psicología y Salud, 1,* 185-206.

Piña, J.A. and Sánchez-Sosa, J.J. (2007). Psychological model for investigation of therapeutic compliance behaviors in people with HIV/AIDS [In Spanish]. *Universitas Psychologica, 6,* 399-407.

Piña, J.A., Valencia, M.A., Mungaray, K., and Corrales, A.E. (2006). Validation of a short scale that measures stress related events in HIV positive patients [In Spanish]. *Terapia Psicológica, 24,* 15-21.

Piña, J.A., Ybarra, J.L., Alcalá, I.G., and Samaniego, R.A. (2010). Psychology and health: the importance to be named model and to be surnamed theoretical-conceptual [In Spanish]. *Revista Mexicana de Investigación en Psicología, 2,* 21-29.

Ribes, E. (1990). *Psychology and health. A conceptual analysis* [In Spanish]. Barcelona: Martínez Roca.

Ribes, E. (2009). Personality as the organization of interactive styles [In Spanish]. *Revista Mexicana de Psicología, 26,* 145-161.

Sánchez-Sosa, J.J., Cázares, O., Piña, J.A., and Dávila, M. (2009). A psychological model for therapeutic adherence behaviors in persons with HIV [In Spanish]. *Salud Mental, 32,* 389-397.

Silva, M.C., Ximenes, R.A., Miranda Filho, D.B., Arraes, L.W., Mendes, M., Melo, A.C., et al. (2009). Risk-factors for non-adherence to antiretroviral therapy. *Revista del Instituto de Medicina Tropical de São Paulo, 51,* 135-139.

Wagner, G.J., Kanouse, D.E., Golinelli, D., Miller, L.G., Daar, E.S., Witt, M.D., et al. (2006). Cognitive-behavioral intervention to enhance adherence to antiretroviral therapy: a randomized controlled trial (CCTG 578). *AIDS, 20,* 1295-302.

Waldrop-Valverde, D., Jones, D.L., Jayaweera, D., Gonzalez, P., Romero, J., and Ownby, R.L. (2009). Gender differences in medication management capacity in HIV infection: The role of health literacy and numeraly. *AIDS and Behavior, 13,* 46-52.

(Manuscript received on October 15, 2010. Revised version accepted for publication on March 20, 2011)

In: Recent Hispanic Psychological Research ... ISBN: 978-1-62948-919-3
Editors: C. H. Garcia Cadena, A. Lopez-Espinoza et al. © 2014 Nova Science Publishers, Inc.

Chapter 15

A Correlation Study of Abilities-Coping and Adherence to Antiretroviral Therapy in HIV/Aids Persons*

***Maria Morna González Vera*#**
Universidad Nacional de San Luis
San Luis, Argentina

Abstract

Antiretroviral treatments (ARTs) stop the replication of HIV, but it is a major requirement for people with HIV/AIDS (PWHA) to display adherence behaviors equal to or higher than 90%. Since the disease and its treatment are considered highly stressful, PWHA are required for implementing a variety of coping skills (CSs) that enable to cope with them efficiently.

This study explores the relationship between adherence to the ART and CSs in a group of 158 PWHA receiving attention at Hospital Muñiz, in the Autonomous City of Buenos Aires, Argentina.

Two assessment methods were applied: an *ad hoc* questionnaire to measure adherence, and the Moos Coping Scale (form B). The main correlations were found between stress management strategies with problem-solving behaviors ($p = .00$), cognitions oriented towards problem-solving ($p = .00$), cognitive avoidance-resignation ($p = .04$), emotions oriented towards problem-solving ($p = .00$), and social support ($p = .00$). Meanwhile, social support turned out to be positively related to problem-solving behaviors ($p = .00$), negatively to strategies of problem-avoidance ($p = .00$), avoidance/emotional release ($p = .00$), as well as with an avoidance index ($p = .00$). This study revealed the relationship between adherence to the ART and different coping strategies, which lead to the conclusion that acquaintance with these strategies, could help to predict, with a reasonable degree of certainty, the probability of adherence to the ART by patients with HIV.

---

* The author thanks Lilia Mabel Labiano and Marcos Jofré Neila (Universidad Nacional de San Luis, Argentina) for their helpful comments on earlier draft.

Mail Address: Jean Jaures 367, 12, "G" (C1215ACE). Ciudad Autónoma de Buenos Aires, Argentina. E-mail: mornagonzalezvera@gmail.com

Keywords: Adherence, Coping Strategies, Antiretroviral Therapies

Introduction

Nonetheless today we can count on more and more powerful medicaments preventing clinical progression of HIV infection (that are part of the known antiretroviral treatment or ART), which must be consumed to life and according to some criteria that must be followed up; meaning, in order that treatment is effective, it is required to practice consistently and efficiently adherence behaviors (Krueger, Berger, and Felkey, 2005; Simpson, Eurich, Majumdar, Padwal, Tsuyuki, Varney et al., 2006), which, in percentage terms, must be equal or higher than 90% (Bangsberg, 2006).

As it is well known, due to illness characteristics and complexity of ART, persons living with HIV/aids (PCVS) are found regularly under an excessive pressure, and we have to add as well the fact illness bears, in countries like ours, the burden of social stigma. It is hardly surprising that people facing multiple potential sources of stress, present pain, functional incapacity, typical demands from hospitable environment or that come from their interaction with sanitary personnel and treatments they are receiving; additionally, adverse effects produced from medicaments, diet restrictions and schedules, among others.

So as to face this multiplicity of stressors, PCVS activate those known as "coping skills" (CS). These ones are referred to capacity each person has to evaluate both the situation and personal resources available to response adjustably to adverse (Lazarus and Folkman, 1986). In the specific case of HIV infection, such strategies are essential in order to predict how probable is PCVS: a) shall be adapted to those new life conditions recently mentioned; b) if shall practice or not consistently and efficiently adherence behaviors to ART, and c) if finally it shall become or not in a substantial recovery of survival quality and time. (Bottonari, Safren, McQuaid, Hsiao, and Roberts, 2010; Vosvick, Gore-Felton, Koopman, Thoresen, Krumboltz, and Spiegel, 2002).

Coping

Lazarus and Folkman (1986) define coping as those constantly changing cognitive and behavioral efforts, developed to handle specific demands (external and/or internal), evaluated as exceeding or boundless, from resources. For his part, Gard (1999) perceives them as a dynamic group of answers whose expression is based on stressing and environmental situations, as well as on individual factors.

Role of different coping styles in view of potentially stressing situations has been an important topic of psychology studies during the last 50 years. Bibliographical revision shows a diversity of areas where it has been studied, until to be the central problem in health field (Aldwin, 1994; Burish and Bradley, 1983; Heckman, Sikkema, Hansen, Kochman, Heh, Neufeld et al., 2011; Levine and Ursin, 1980; Moos, 1989; Pelechano, 1992, 1999; Snyder and Ford, 1987).

After a long evolution in coping study, nowadays new stances favoring individual differences analysis are arising from personality theories integration, under clinical and social approaches (Rueda-Ruiz and Aguado-Diaz, 2003). It is in this context where Pelechano proposal acquires a special importance (1992), which, from our point of view, has been constituted as the first theoretical development regarding coping, framed in an explanatory model of personality and total human functioning.

According to this author, convergence between personality theories and stress studies in health field would allow to advance in searching solutions to all theoretical gaps of explanatory models about coping and lack of consensus, or about existing contradictions. Many of current controversies about entity, stability and functionality of coping skills acquire a new meaning in parameters model distinguishing personality dimensions and interpersonal aptitudes-skills.

Both subjects (personality and aptitudes-skills) are hierarchically organized according to consolidation grade and generalization power. In this general model, coping skills would be an important part of personality abilities-aptitudes, together with interpersonal problems solving dimensions (Pelechano, 1992).

From this consideration concerning coping as personality ability, it is rejected situational nature of coping skills, meanwhile these ones would provoke general tendencies to face potentially stressing events; that is why their interaction with and in a concrete situation would make possible the use of some skills instead of others.

From Pelechano (1991) coping model of chronic physical illnesses, certain stability in coping and person's interaction with environment is defended, understanding there exist previous manners to cope with stressing situation that are influenced both by illness course and own environmental events.

Based on the foregoing, it could be concluded coping constitutes the results from personal decisions and environmental demands combination, in such a way that only from its interaction we could explain individual differences lying in different modes to cope illness. From there, a global understanding of this phenomenon demands a coping skills study related to personality variables, as well as to carry out specific coping studies in some situations that are emerging and which persons need to face.

In this way, and based on Pelechano proposal, this study was proposed, its goal was to find possible associations between different coping skills with ART adherence, as well as other variables of interest, among which some socio-demographic and biological variables are highlighted (i.e., age, knowledge of viral charge levels and CD4 cell count), level of physical discomfort produced by antiretroviral medicaments and social support perceived.

METHOD

Participants

Sample was formed by 158 PCVS, who were receiving specialized attention at Immunodefficient Help Foundation (FUNDAI, in Spanish) of Municipal Hospital of Infectious Diseases "Dr. Francisco J. Muñiz", in Ciudad Autonoma de Buenos Aires, Argentina.

Participants' age varied from 24 and 65 years old (X = 40.3; DE = 8.8), 109 out of them were males (69%) and 49 women (31%). 51.9% was living as a couple; meanwhile, 49.4% had children. On the other hand, 75.3% (n = 119 patients) were under any ART scheme, meanwhile most of participants (n = 33; 27.7%) took 3 pills, followed by those taking 5 (n =

20; 16.8%) and 4 (n = 19; 16%); the amount of pills they must consume varied from 2 and 18 (X= 5.69) per day.

Table 1. Socio-demographic, clinical and behavioral characteristics of the entire sample (n = 158)

	X	SD	Range	N	%
Age	40.3	8.8	24-65	158	
Sex					
Men				109	69
Women				49	31
Marital status					
Single Married/with couple				76 82	48.1 51.9
Children					
Yes				78	49.4
No				80	50.6
PWHA under ART					
Yes				119	75.3
No				39	24.7
Amount of pills (daily consumption) PWHA that sometime stopped using ART	5.7	3.6	2-18	36	22.8
CD4 and CV values knowledge					
Yes				100	63.3
No				58	36.7

Instruments

A questionnaire constructed a*d hoc,* in which it was inquired about socio-demographic data and aspects referred accurately antiretroviral treatment, adherence and abandon such treatment in any moment of process. It was composed of a first part with information about: age, sex, if the person lives alone or in couple, number of months he/she was living in couple, if he/she had children and how many, levels of viral charge and CD4 cell count. The second part collected information of antiretroviral treatment, by questions concerning if they were under treatment, since when, amount of pills taken daily, adverse effects produced by medicaments, grade of discomfort perceived regarding adverse effects, treatment voluntary abandon and his/her motives, time they have been exposed to treatment, and if abandon, since when.

In second place, Moss Coping Scale (B form) was used, validated and adapted by Aduna (1998) to chronic illness patients. It is a questionnaire composed of 34 questions: from 1 to 29 found out about coping skills in daily life that were defined in a Likert type scale with optional answers going from 1 (never) to 6 (always). Questions from this part were grouped in strategies oriented to solution and prevention of problems (behavioral, cognitive and emotional). It is understood here as *oriented behaviors to problems solving*: all those concrete acts a person accomplishes to solve problems he/she is facing (question no. 12):"I think about an action plan and I carry it out"). As *behaviors oriented to problems prevention*: all those concrete acts the person accomplish to prevent problems resolution (question no. 23: "I prefer to be distant from people"). As *cognitions oriented to problems solving:* all those thoughts-cognitions addressed to problems solving (question no. 17: "I analyze the problem and to see things objectively").

As *cognitive avoidance-resignation:* all those thoughts tending to resignation or avoidance in problems solving (question no. 11: "I do other things in order to avoid thinking about the problem"). As *emotions oriented to problems solving:* all those emotions the person perceives as tendency to problems solving (question no. 20: "I tell myself things in order to feel me better"). As *emotional avoidance-release:* all the avoiding acts and emotional releases toward objects that are not real problems (question no. 27: "I try to remain insensitive, avoiding it affects me"). On the other hand, question 30 deals with stress handling strategies ("I try to relax and to take things easy"), meanwhile questions from 31 to 34 questions related to social support, evaluated by a Likert type scale with level- answers going from 1 (none) to 6 (more than four); the following is an example: How many close friends with whom you can talk to about your problems, do you have?

Procedure

Previously to instrumentation, research protocol was submitted to consideration of FUNDAI Management Commission of Municipal Hospital of Infectious Diseases "Dr. Francisco J. Muñiz". Once corresponding authorization is granted, all PCVS were individually contacted, who were exposed all the objectives pursued by this study. Those who accepted to cooperate voluntarily, read and signed the informed consent, and then to give them both instruments and provide them instructions about how to answer. It was explained their answers were anonymous and confidential, besides results would be used for research purposes. Finally, no economic remuneration was paid.

Statistical Analysis

First of all, frequencies and percentages of study variables were obtained. Next, Student t test was used in order to identify possible differences in independent variables behavior from PCVS comparison, which reported to have abandoned or not the treatment voluntarily at any moment. So as to explore possible associations between dependent variable (adherence behaviors) and independent ones, Pearson r statistics was used, by which it is possible to determine both direction (sign of relation) and magnitude (grade) which correlates two or more variables each other.

Finally, and in order to identify possible differences among PCVS that had knowledge about biological markers (viral load levels and CD4 cells count) and their even eventual relation with coping skills, Student t test (Siliva, 1998) was used. So as to process data, version 12.0 Windows SPSS statistical program (Statistical Packages for Social Sciences) was employed.

RESULTS

At the time study was applied, 119 (75.3 %) participants were under any antiretroviral treatment scope; from such percentage, 36 (22.8%) reported they have failed in one or more occasion, through treatment process. In general, pills average consumed per day were between 2 and 18, with more than half consuming between 3 and 5 pills: 33 (27.7%) consumed 3 pills per day; 20 (16.8%), 5 pills and 19 (16%), 4 pills.

For purposes of the following analysis, univariate statistics (frequencies, medians and standard deviations from different independent variables are described in Table 2. Student *t* test values are summarized, by which differences among PCVS were reported to have or not abandoned the treatment voluntarily. As such, it can be observed only two significant statistically differences: in CD4 cell counts ($t = -1.94$; $p = .05$) and in the problems avoidance skills ($t = 2.61$; $p = .01$), in the sense PCVS who reported to have abandoned the treatment obtained as a result in its laboratory studies, a less CD4 cell count, and in coping scale, a higher score in skills practice.

On the other side, correlations obtained by Pearson *r* correlation coefficient were presented in Table 3. Numerical value located in the upper part of each box belongs to correlation (*r*) coefficient and the lower one indicates statistical significance level (p). It was found that age variable correlated positively ($r = .23$; $p = .01$) with the number of years of treatment carried out by PCVS; on the other hand, viral load levels correlated toward a negative direction ($r = -.23$; $p = .02$) with CD4 cell count, suggesting that as circulating virus amount is increased in the body, CD4 cell count amount is reduced. These ones, in turn, were positively correlated ($r = .22$; $p = .05$) with ART years; consequently, when treatment exposition time is higher, CD4 cell count is higher.

On the other hand, these ones are correlated in a positive direction ($r = .23$; $p = .04$) with the number of pills PCVS must consume. An interesting correlation was observed among CD4 cell count and time of treatment abandon ($r = -.57$; $p = .00$), indicating that as more time treatment was abandoned, CD4 cell count was reduced. Finally, it was also carried out, but in a negative direction ($r = -.25$; $p = .01$) with behaviors oriented to prevent problems and the avoidance ($r = -.21$; $p = .04$), where it constitutes a variable by averaging behaviors, cognitions and emotions oriented to problems avoidance, so it can be inferred that as avoidance behaviors, cognitions and emotions are more evident, CD4 cell counts are reduced.

It should emphasized as well stress handling strategies that were significantly correlated, in a positive way, with behaviors oriented to problems solving ($r = .64$; $p = .00$), with cognitions oriented to problems solving ($r = .49$; $p = .00$), with cognitive avoidance-resignation ($r = .16$; $p = .04$), with emotions oriented to problems solving ($r = .25$; $p = .00$), as well as social support ($r = .26$; $p = .00$). From these results, it can be said stress handling strategies used by PCVS of this sample, are addressed to problems solving, and measured by behavioral, cognitive or emotional processes. Nonetheless, such skills are used sometime to "forget" and/or "get away" from problems by cognitive avoidance; finally, social support is very frequently used to reduce stress potential effects.

Table 2. Univariate statistics and medians comparison of "ART voluntary giving up "with the rest of independent variables

Variables	ART voluntary giving up	N	Median	*t*	P
Viral load	Yes	22	4020.73	-.76	.45
	No	78	13027.26		
CD4	Yes	22	375.82	-1.94	.05
	No	78	497.47		
Stress management strategies	Yes	36	4.57	.85	.39
	No	122	4.28		
Years since treatment started	Yes	28	5.46	.80	.42
	No	91	4.71		
Pills amount	Yes	28	5.79	.16	.87
	No	91	5.66		
Adverse effects	Yes	28	1.75	.03	.98
	No	91	1.75		
Level of malaise perceived by medication	Yes	7	1.86	1.46	.15
	No	23	1.43		
Problem-solving behaviors	Yes	36	3.98	-1.50	.13
	No	122	4.26		
Problem-avoidance behaviors	Yes	36	3.84	2.61	.01
	No	122	3.42		
Cognition oriented to problem-solving	Yes	36	4.54	.28	.78
	No	122	4.49		
Cognitive avoidance-resignation	Yes	36	4.05	-.05	.96
	No	122	4.06		
Emotions oriented to problem-solving	Yes	36	4.06	-1.46	.14
	No	122	4.42		
Variables	ART voluntary giving up	N	Median	*t*	P
Emotional avoidance/release	Yes	36	2.79	.49	.62
	No	122	2.67		
Social support	Yes	36	3.74	-.46	.65
	No	122	3.84		
Avoidance (index)	Yes	36	3.56	1.45	.15
	No	122	3.38		

Table 3. Matrix of correlations between different variables of study

		Age	Viral load	CD4	Stress management strategies	Level of malaise	Problem-solving behaviors	Problem-avoidance behaviors	Cognition of solving-problems	Emotional avoidance-release	Social support
CD4	*r*	.03	-.23	---	-.16	-.34	.09	-.25	-.16	-.05	.11
	p	.72	.02		.12	.14	.37	.01	.12	.58	.26
Years of treatment	*r*	.23	-.18	.22	-.08	-.25	.05	-.00	.02	-.17	-.07
	p	.01	.11	.05	.36	.19	.58	.95	.87	.07	.47
Amount of pills	r	-.11	-.13	.23	-.14	-.03	-.05	.05	-.17	-.17	.06
	p	.22	.25	.04	.12	.89	.60	.60	.07	.06	.52
Level of malaise	*r*	.22	.19	-.34	.23	---	-.30	.11	.11	.54	-.07
	p	.23	.41	.14	.21		.11	.56	.57	.00	.71
Time of giving up	*r*	-.19	.10	-.57	.17	-.61	.18	.22	.05	-.14	-.22
	p	.24	.60	.00	.27	.04	.25	.16	.77	.38	.16
COSP	*r*	.13	.01	.09	.64	-.30	---	.00	.61	-.12	.38
	p	.11	.89	.37	.00	.11		.92	.00	.12	.00
CEP	*r*	.04	.04	-.25	.14	.11	.01	---	.10	-.01	-.26
	p	.58	.72	.01	.08	.56	.92		.22	.90	.00
CogOSP	*r*	.11	.05	-.16	.49	.11	.61	.10	---	-.02	.16
	p	.16	.57	.12	.00	.57	.00	.22		.77	.05
EC-R	*r*	-.02	-.13	-.05	.16	.01	.17	.14	.27	.15	-.05
	p	.78	.21	.59	.04	.95	.03	.08	.00	.07	.56
EOSP	*r*	.02	-.10	.04	.25	.03	.43	-.03	.40	.08	.15
	p	.81	.33	.70	.00	.89	.00	.69	.00	.34	.06
E-DE	*r*	-.10	.01	-.06	.16	.54	-.12	-.01	-.02	---	-.21
	p	.20	.88	.58	.04	.00	.12	.90	.77		.01
Social support	*r*	.10	.07	.11	.26	-.07	.38	-.26	.16	-.21	---
	p	.21	.46	.26	.00	.71	.00	.00	.05	.01	
Avoidance index	*r*	-.05	-.03	-.21	.06	.41	-.01	.61	.15	.69	-.30
	p	.54	.80	.04	.46	.02	.93	.00	.07	.00	.00

Note: COSP (Solving-problem Behaviors). CEP (Problems-avoidance behaviors). CogOSP (Cognitions oriented to problem-solving). EC-R (Cognitive avoidance-resignation). EOSP (Emotions oriented to problem-solving). E-DE (Emotional avoidance-release).

Meanwhile, discomfort grade perceived with treatment only correlated with two variables: avoidance-emotional release (r = .54; p = .00) and with avoidance (r = .41; p = .02). In both cases, it means higher discomfort perceived, higher probability to put in practice avoidance skills in both modalities. On the other hand, behaviors oriented to problems solving significantly correlated and positively with (r = .61; p = .00) and with emotions oriented to problems solving (r = .43; p = .00), as well as a good social support perceived (r = .38; p = .00). It is understood, then, as instrumental practice of behaviors oriented to problems solving is increased, at the same extent it is preceded by cognitive and emotional skills use addressed to problems solving and an increase in social support search.

Behaviors oriented to avoidance correlated negatively (r = -.26; p = .00) with social support perceived and in an opposite sense with avoidance (r = .61; p = .00). Therefore, it can be said persons counting on higher social support present a minor tendency to respond by preventing difficulties, nonetheless when they do it persistently is more probable to adopt a general practice of avoidance mediated by behavioral, cognitive and emotional processes.

Additionally, there were found correlations between cognitions oriented to problems solving (r = .61; p = .00), with cognitive avoidance-resignation (r = .27; p = .00), with emotions oriented to problems solving (r = .40; p = .00) and with social support (r = .16; p = .00). That is, persons orienting their cognitions toward problems solving are logic, by practicing behaviors and by expressing their emotions in that same direction, even though they eventually tend to avoid problems by using determined cognitions; lastly, those who employ such skills used to look for support more frequently from other significant persons. On the other hand, those who use skills of avoidance-emotional release do not look for social support sources with higher frequency (r = -.21; p = .01) and, consequently, used to avoid situations implying behavioral, cognitive and emotional skills use (r = .69; p = .00).

Table 4. Comparison of Median of "Viral load and CD4 cell values knowledge" variable with "coping modes"

	Does it know CV y CD4 values?	N	X	*T*	P
Problem-avoidance behaviors	Yes	100	3.46	-2.10	.04
	No	58	3.61		
Emotions oriented to problem-solving	Yes	100	4.37	2.01	.04
	No	58	4.28		

Finally, social support correlated positively with behaviors oriented to problems solving (r = .38; p = .00), with cognitions oriented to problems solving (r = .16; p = .05), and in a negative sense with behaviors of problems avoidance (r = -.26; p = .00), with Avoidance-emotional release (r = -.21; p = .00) and with avoidance (r = -.30; p = .00).

Then, if it is perceived a good social support, there exist a higher probability PCVS practice problems solving behaviors, meanwhile if such support is not perceived as favorable, the implementation of coping skills of avoidance in behavioral, cognitive and emotional levels is facilitated.

Concerning Student t test analysis to evaluate possible differences between PCVS, who had or not knowledge of the two main biological markers and the use of determined coping skills, results are described in Table 4. Here, it is important to notice result of statistically significant differences are submitted only for discussion: on the other hand, PCVS who had a better and a more complete knowledge about the two clinic markers made a minor use of skills in their problems avoidance modality (t = -2.10; p = .04), nonetheless that at the same time they were supported more in emotional skills oriented to problems solving (t = 4.37; p = .04).

Discussion

This study had as objective, to explore the association between ART adherence and coping skills in a group of 158 PCVS who were receiving attention at the Hospital Muñiz, in Ciudad Autonoma de Buenos Aires, Argentina. 75.3% (n = 119) was found under any ART scope, and 22.8% (n = 36) reported not being one hundred percent adherent.

According to results exposed, it stands out, in first place, the association between ART abandon variables, both CD4 cell count and with coping skills oriented to problems avoidance. Meaning, those persons who were not 100% adherent to ART showed a minor CD4 cell count, besides presenting a statistically significant difference when using avoidance under its problems coping modality. These results are consisted with those ones reported by Weaver, Llabre, Duran, Antoni, Ironson, and Penedo et al. (2005), who found a relation between lack of adherence and coping strategies use oriented to avoidance, so everything seems to indicate these one function as mediators influencing a negative state of mind, and a minor probability of counting on social support in PCVS; even though a direct relation between coping and adherence strategies were not researched, in general and in a direction similar to the one supported by Fleishman, Sherbourne, Cleary, Wu, Crystal, and Hays (2003), who were also included in its PCVS studies.

Likewise, problems avoidance variable (which averages variables referred behavioral, cognitive and emotional coping oriented problems avoidance) correlated with CD4 cell count inversely. Meaning, as first ones increase, the second ones are reduced, which could mean to be tightly bonded with expositions about association between no ART adherence and an increase in coping oriented to avoidance. Although, it could not be possible to corroborate a correlation between coping styles addressed to problems solving (behavioral, cognitive or emotional) and ART adherence. Again, our results match with those exposed by Weaver et al. (2005), where it was not possible as well to observe such association. This last situation lead us to propose that those persons distinguished by their coping style addressed to avoidance, use very specific resources and well centered on starting behaviors, cognitions and emotions, that in this case have as a consequence the non-adherence to treatments; understanding adherence not only fulfill medical prescription, but from all those factors going beyond it, meaning, personal, social/interpersonal ones, those concerning sickness and health services, etc. (Hotz, Kaptein, Pruitt, Sanchez-Sosa, and Willey, 2003; Varela, Salazar, and Correa, 2008).

In contrast, those behaviors, cognitions and emotions that would be linked to a direct approach to problem and that must have as a consequence an adherence to ART; apparently they are not so specific. This would make suppose appropriate instruments detecting coping stales oriented to avoidance in persons who need to start an ART, we would dispose of better elements to predict adherence or non-adherence, and based on this knowledge, to take the necessary measures for to hinder in a short, medium and long terms the therapeutic failure; it would happen the same to those persons with coping styles oriented to problems resolution, since in these cases a prediction attempt would be uncertain.

It was observed as well a correlation between strategies called stress handling (i.e., to drink more, eat more, smoke more, sleep more, to exercise more, etc.) with coping strategies (behavioral, cognitive and emotional) oriented to problems solving. Here, the discussion is addressed to the concern of researching deeper up to the extent everything implies an "active coping", prone to solve a problem (for example, to collect information about what is HIV, what is AIDS, why it is important to know the serologic markers and how to construe such markers, among other issues), used to be accompanied with stress handling strategies that have all the configuration characteristics as avoidance strategies, up to the point of having as well a positive correlation with cognitive avoidance-resignation, like a kind of "mental escape" of problems.

A very important aspect in most of the studies referred to psychosocial factors linked to HIV is social support. The perception about it is considered as a facilitator factor of therapeutic adherence, meanwhile a low level of support perceived is related to an obstacle or a variable that at least limits it in a considerable percentage (Gonzalez and Piña, 2011; Martos and Pozo, 2011; Varela et al., 2008). In this sample of social support correlated positively with three modalities of coping oriented to problems solving, even though it is not associated directly to ART adherence, and in turn, it did it inversely with coping avoidance index. Therefore, we can conclude that for this sample, there is a direct relation between coping skills oriented to problems resolution and social support perceived, which it does not imply that it necessarily deals with a support eventually facilitating psychosocial adjustment of PCVS, or that even improves adherence to ART (Sun, Zhang, and Fu, 2007). It is stated, then, heterogeneity of samples of HIV patients sometime shows results are not extrapolative to other populations (Ruiz-Perez, Labry-Lima, Prada-Pardal, Rodriguez-Baño, Causse-Prados, Lopez-Ruz et al., 2006).

Other important aspect is the one referred to knowledge of biological markers (viral load levels and CD4 cell counts), which has been widely studied because of its relation to antiretroviral adherence treatment (Kalichman, Rompa, DiFonzo, Simpson, Austin, Luke et al., 2001; Kumarasamy, Safren, Raminani, Pickard, James, Krishnan et al., 2005; Piña, Garcia, Ybarra, and Fierros, 2012; Reynolds, 2003; Sanchez-Sosa, Fierros, Cázares, and Piña, 2011). This knowledge is expected to be expressly linked to an appropriate knowledge of illness, of ART and instructions to take it, as well as non pharmacological recommendation, etc., (Hotz, et al., 2003; Piña et al., 2012). Otherwise, PCVS will be characterized by adherence problems, in percentages referred at the beginning of this work (Catz, Kelly, Bogart, Benotsch, and McAuliffe, 2000; Knobel, Codina, Miro, Carmona, Garcia, Antela et al., 2000; Sternhell and Corr, 2002; Tucker, Orlando, Burnman, Sherbourne, Kung, and Guifford, 2004; Veinot, Flicker, Skinner, McClelland, Saulnierd, Read et al., 2006).

An interesting issue having to de with the foregoing, is that in population studied here, it was found that those who knew their viral load indicators and CD4 cell count, use less the avoidance as coping skills; nonetheless, and it is important to emphasize it, it could be possible to establish the association between these variables and adherence. Concerning CD4 cell count, it correlated positively with the number of pills had to be taken, according to prescription to each one of the patients; meaning, higher number of pills that must be taken, higher CD4 cell count. Although it is a statistically significant result, there exist currently evidence showing a direct association between non termination of antiretroviral treatment and pills overload (Rodriguez-Torne, Iranzu, Berrocal, and Gomez-Serranillo, 2009). Consequently, these are aspects that must be reviewed by treating physician who prescribe medical cares, having decided if it is more important an increase of serologic progress indicators or therapeutic adherence maintenance through time.

Although it was possible to corroborate some of hypothesis proposed and important correlations between variables were found, this work had to face different limitations. Among them, there is the impossibility to collect more accurate and specific information due to the heterogeneity of socio-cultural resources of population attending health centers—which in general belong to more economic vulnerable groups, and in indicators such as educational level—, failing optimum conditions in the health institutions themselves and services they offer. On the other hand, a limitation clearly reflected in results was the lack of an instrument that would allow us to measure in a more direct and wide manner the factors influencing adherence to antiretroviral treatments, especially those having to do with accurate aspects of personality, or with emotional states like anxiety and depression, to mention just two cases.

For such reasons, it will be necessary to design a research program proposing variables considered by Pelechano in his theoretical model about coping, by incorporating these last variables mentioned in the previous paragraph. Once more reliable and valid information is available, we will be in an excellent position so, in turn, to design, instrument and evaluate intervention programs tending to promote consistent and efficient practice of adherence behaviors in PCVS and to promote a substantial improvement in quality and time of survival.

REFERENCES

Aduna, A. (1998). Afrontamiento, apoyo social y solución de problemas en estudiantes universitarios. Estudio experimental. Tesis de Maestría en Psicología no publicada. México: Universidad Nacional Autónoma de México.

Aldwin, C.M. (1994). *Stress, coping and development.* Londres: The Guilford Press.

Bangbserg, D.R. (2006). Less than 95% adherence to nonnucleoside reverse-transcriptase inhibitor therapy can lead to viral suppression. *Clinical Infectious Diseases, 43,* 939-941.

Bottonari, K.A., Safren, S.A., McQuaid, J.R., Hsiao, C-B., and Roberts, J.E. (2010). A longitudinal investigation of the impact of life stress on HIV treatment adherence. *Journal of Behavioral Medicine, 33,* 486-495.

Burish, T.G. and Bradley, L.A. (1983). *Coping with chronic disease.* New York, NY: Academic Press.

Catz, S.L., Kelly, J.A., Bogart, L.M., Benotsch, E.G., and McAuliffe, T.L. (2000). Patterns, correlates, and barriers to medication adherence among persons prescribed new treatments for HIV disease. *Health Psychology, 19*, 124-133.

Fleishman, J.A., Sherbourne, C.D., Cleary, P.D., Wu, A.W., Crystal, S., and Hays, R.D. (2003). Patterns of coping among persons with HIV infection: Configurations, correlates, and change. *American Journal of Community Psychology, 32,* 187-204.

Gard, T. (1999). The importance of intimacy and use of avoidance coping in predicting depression among HIV+ individuals. Unpublished Doctoral Thesis. Albany, New York: State University of New York.

González, M.T. and Piña, J.A. (2011). Motivos, apoyo social y comportamientos de adhesión en personas con VIH: modelamiento con ecuaciones estructurales. *Universitas Psychologica, 10,* 597-607.

Heckman, T.G., Sikkema, K.J., Hansen, N., Kochman, A., Heh, V., and Neufeld, S. (201q). A randomized clinical trial of a coping improvement group intervention for HIV-infected older adults. *Journal of Behavioral Medicine, 34,* 102-111.

Hotz, S., Kaptein, A., Pruitt, S., Sánchez-Sosa, J.J., and Willey, C. (2003). Behavioural mechanism explaining adherence. In E. Sabaté (Ed.), *Adherence to long-term therapies* (pp. 157-171). Geneva: World Health Organization.

Kalichman, S.C., Rompa, D., DiFonzo, K., Simpson, D., Austin, J., Luke, W., et al. (2001). HIV treatment adherence in women living with HIV/AIDS: research based on the information-motivation-behavioral skills model of health behaviour. *Journal of the Association of Nurses in AIDS Care, 12*, 58-67.

Knobel, H., Codina, C., Miró, J.M., Carmona, A., Garcia, B., Antela, A., et al. (2000). Recomendaciones GESIDA/SEFH/PNS para mejorar la adherencia al tratamiento antiretroviral. *Enfermedades Infecciosas y Microbiología Clínica, 18,* 27-39.

Krueger, K.P., Berger, B.A., and Felkey, B. (2005). Medication adherence and persistence: A comprehensive review. *Advances in Therapy, 22,* 313-356.

Kumarasamy, N., Safren, S.A., Raminani, S.R., Pickard, R., James, R., Krishnan, S., et al. (2005). Barriers and facilitators to antiretroviral medication adherence among patients with HIV in Chennai, India: a qualitative study. *AIDS Patient Care and STDs, 19,* 526-537.

Lazarus, R.S. and Folkman, S. (1986). *Estrés y procesos cognitivos.* Barcelona: Martínez Roca.

Levine, S. and Ursin, H. (1980). *Coping and health.* New York, NY: Plenum Press.

Martos, M.J. and Pozo, C. (2011). Apoyo social funcional *vs.* disfuncional en una muestra de pacientes crónicos. Su incidencia sobre la salud y el cumplimiento terapéutico. *Anales de Psicología, 27,* 47-57.

Moos, R.H. (1989). *Coping with physical illness 2: New perspectives.* New York, NY: Plenum Medical Book Company.

Pelechano, V. (1991). La personalidad desde la perspectiva de los parámetros. *Psicologemas, 10*, 53-176.

Pelechano, V. (1992). Personalidad y estrategias de afrontamiento en pacientes crónicos (1) (2). *Análisis y Modificación de Conducta, 18*, 167-201.

Pelechano, V. (1999): Calidad de vida, familia y afrontamiento en la enfermedad física crónica: Datos y sugerencias para un modelo. En J. Buendía (Dir.), *Familia y psicología de la salud* (pp. 133-180). Madrid: Pirámide.

Piña, J.A., Garcia, C.H., Ybarra, J.L., and Fierros, L.E. (2012). Psychological and biological variables among 100% adherent patients: A path analysis. In C.H. Garcia, R. Ballester, and J.A. Piña (Eds.), *Chronic diseases and medication adherence behaviors: Psychological research in Ibero-American countries* (pp. 203-220). Hauppauge, NY: Nova Science Publishers.

Reynolds, N.R. (2003). The problem of antiretroviral adherence: a self-regulatory model for intervention. *AIDS Care, 15*, 117-124.

Rodríguez-Torné, G., Iranzu, M.C., Berrocal, M.A., and Gómez-Serranillo, M. (2009). Adherencia al tratamiento antirretroviral: repercusión del número de tomas diarias. *Revista Cubana de Farmacia, 43*, 1 (Published online April 2009).

Rueda-Ruiz, M.B. and Aguado-Díaz, A.L. (2003). *Estrategias de Afrontamiento y Proceso de Adaptación a la Lesión Medular*. Madrid: IMSERSO.

Ruiz-Pérez, I., Labry-Lima, A., Prada-Pardal, J., Rodríguez-Baño, J., Causse-Prados, M., López-Ruz, M., et al. (2006). Impacto de los factores demográficos y psicosociales en la no adherencia a los fármacos antirretrovirales. *Enfermedades Infecciosas y Microbiología Clínica, 24*, 373-378.

Sánchez-Sosa, J.J., Fierros, L.E., Cázares, O., and Piña, J.A. (2011). Estudio longitudinal de variables psicológicas y conductas de adhesión en personas VIH+: efectos sobre los niveles de carga viral. In J.L. Ybarra, J.J. Sánchez-Sosa, and J.A. Piña (Eds.), *Trastornos y enfermedades crónicas: una aproximación psicológica* (pp. 137-154). México: Universidad Autónoma de Tamaulipas/El Manual Moderno.

Silva, A. (1998). *La investigación asistida por computadora.* México: Universidad Nacional Autónoma de México.

Simpson, S.H., Eurich, D.T., Majumdar, S.R., Padwal, R.S., Tsuyuki, R.T., Varney, J., et al. (2006). A meta-analysis of the association between adherence to drug therapy and mortality. *British Medical Journal, 333(7557)*, 15.

Snyder, C.R. and Ford, C.E. (1987). *Coping with negative life events.* New York, NY: Plenum Press.

Sternhell, P.S., and Corr, M.J. (2002). Psychiatric morbidity and adherence to antiretroviral medication in patients with HIV/AIDS. *Australian and New Zealand Journal of Psychiatry, 36,* 528-533.

Tucker, J.S., Orlando, M., Burnam, A., Sherbourne, C.D., Kung, F.Y., and Gifford, A. L. (2004). Psychosocial mediators of antiretroviral nonadherence in HIV-positive adults with substance use and mental health problems. *Health Psychology, 23*, 363-370.

Varela, M.T., Salazar, I., and Correa, D. (2008). Adherencia al tratamiento en la infección por VIH/SIDA. Consideraciones teóricas y metodológicas para su abordaje. *Acta Colombiana de Psicología, 11*, 101-113

Veinot, T.C., Flicker, S.E., Skinner, H.A., McClelland, A., Saulnierd, P., Read, S.E., et al. (2006). "Supposed to make you better but it doesn't really": HIV-positive youths' perceptions of HIV treatment. *Journal of Adolescent Health, 38*, 261-267.

Vosvick, M., Gore-Felton, C., Koopman, C., Thoresen, C., Krumboltz, J., and Spiegel, D. (2002). Maladaptative coping strategies in relation to quality of life among HIV+ adults. *AIDS and Behavior, 6,* 97-106.

Weaver, K., Llabre, M., Durán, R., Antoni, M., Ironson, G., Penedo, F., et al. (2005). A stress and coping model of medication adherence and viral load in HIV-positive men and women on highly active antiretroviral therapy (HAART). *Health Psychology, 24,* 385–392.

(Manuscript received on October 13, 2011. Revised version accepted for publication on May 31, 2012)

In: Recent Hispanic Psychological Research ... ISBN: 978-1-62948-919-3
Editors: C. H. Garcia Cadena, A. Lopez-Espinoza et al.

Chapter 16

HOMOPHOBIA AND QUALITY OF LIFE AMONG PEOPLE LIVING WITH HIV IN CHILE*

Jaime Barrientos[1,#], Manuel Cárdenas[1] and Francisco Vidal[Z]
[1]Escuela de Psicología, Universidad Católica del Norte, Chile
[2]Universidad Metropolitana de Ciencias de la Educación, Chile

ABSTRACT

The convenience sample consisted of 325 gay men whose ages range from 18 to 64 years (X = 32.8; SD = 9.81). Of the total number of participants, 17.8% (n = 58) had been diagnosed with HIV and 78.8% (n = 265) had not. People living with HIV (PLWHIV) were compared with non-living HIV people. This study included different measures of homophobia (minority stress events, perceived discrimination and perceived victimization, stigma perceived by homosexual people), HIV stigma, and different measures concerning quality of life. Results show that the homophobia measures of the two groups may be regarded as similar. For general measures concerning quality of life, statistically meaningful differences were found in satisfaction with life and in some dimensions of psychological and social well-being. As to psychological and social well-being, significant differences were found in autonomy levels ($t_{[306]} = -3.82$; $p < .005$; $d = .50$) and social integration ($t_{[312]} = -2.34$; $p < .05$; $d = .35$) in the social well-being scale. Concerning clinical symptomatology, differences were found only in dimensions referring to somatization and depression, indicating that PLWHIV are more prone to show their discomfort in bodily dysfunctions and mood disorder. Finally, participants with high scores on the HIV stigma scale report significant higher levels of victimization and discrimination, lower levels of social well-being and high levels of clinical symptomatology.

Keywords: Gay Men, Homophobia, PLWHIV, Quality of Life, Chile

---

* This paper was supported by FONDECYT Project number 1110423, entitled "Homophobia and psychosocial effects in homosexuals' quality of life in Chile: Toward a comprehensive model."
# Address for correspondence: Avenida Angamos 0610, Escuela de Psicología, Universidad Católica del Norte, Antofagasta, Chile. Email: jbarrien@ucn.cl.

Introduction

Male-to-male sexual contact (MSM) has been an important route of HIV spread since HIV/AIDS was first identified some 25 years ago. MSM have a markedly greater risk of being infected with HIV, as compared with general population samples from low- and middle-income countries. Recent reports of high HIV prevalence among MSM in different low- and middle-income countries indicate high levels of HIV infection among MSM (Baral, Sifakis, Cleghorn, and Beyrer, 2007). For example, in Chile, the main way to get infected with HIV is sex, mainly affecting homo-bisexual population (MINSAL, 2011). A recent study in the country reported 21.1% prevalence in the MSM population, including gay men population (CHIPREV, 2009).

At present, HIV has become a more chronic and manageable illness. HIV is now considered a chronic disease requiring complex medication regimes, often including multiple co-morbidities that influence all aspects of an individual's well-being (Henderson, et al., 2010). Today, HIV people may live 20 to 30 years beyond the time of diagnosis (Henderson et al., 2008) Recent studies have shown that overall assessments of quality of life among PLWHIV have also become a major focus of interest as more efficacious and simpler regime treatments are available. Antiretroviral therapy is highly effective and can bring about significant benefits; however, these therapies have unpleasant side effects and interfere with daily social activities. Despite these negative effects, antiretroviral therapy has a positive general outcome for quality of life and general health (Nogueira, Cominic, and Crosland, 2009).

Psychosocial behavior among people living with HIV (PLWHIV) probably varies as a function of sexual identity (Mosack et al., 2009). For example, among MSM a gay sexual identity has been associated with less loneliness and isolation, less depression, and better social support. Similarly, higher levels of distress and depression have been associated with not identifying as gay, queer, or homosexual among MSM in the Urban Men's Health Study (Mosack, et al., 2009). Heterosexual men and women tend to have different social support experiences, coping mechanisms, and stressors than gay men or women. Social support from the family is more readily available and satisfactory for HIV-positive heterosexual women than for HIV-positive heterosexual men or gay men.

For HIV, health behavior plays a very important role in the process the disease follows. In addition, factors that might influence health motivation are important variables. The HIV pandemic is global, affecting people's quality of life and care costs. Quality of life is an existential concept with multiple definitions (Greeff et al., 2010).

Studies in different countries have shown that stigma and discrimination continue affecting PLWHIV, their quality of life and well-being, and their health care providers. Stigma has also become an important barrier to access primary and secondary HIV and AIDS care and prevention services (Greeff et al., 2010). These studies have also revealed that PLWHIV experience a great deal of stigma and discrimination. For example, research on HIV stigma has described the psychosocial experiences of PLWHIV who have been stigmatized (Maman et al., 2009). Stigma has been associated with stress, depression, and lower perceived quality of life among PLWHIV (Maman et al., 2009). According to the authors, some researchers have also focused on how stigma affects HIV prevention and treatment efforts, including the condom use, HIV testing and mother-to-child transmission prevention programs, describing how stigma can negatively affect people's acceptance of and adherence to antiretroviral therapy.

In addition, studies on PLWHIV have revealed its impact on quality of life, health, and other activities. Although some studies have shown that, despite sex, income, and mental and immunological differences, PLWHIV have a better quality of life —both physical and psychological— than patients who suffer other diseases, PLWHIV experience many difficulties regarding their social relations. This is associated with stigma and discrimination processes and difficulties in revealing HIV in various social environments. Some studies have shown that levels of satisfaction with life are lower in PLWHIV, resulting from levels of stigma and discrimination perceived (Greeff et al., 2010). Also, PLWHIV often experience chronic challenges that may affect coping resources and negatively impact their mental health (Mavandadi, Zanjani, Have, and Oslin, 2009). The quality of life and well-being among PLWHIV are determined not only by their health status and response to treatment, but also by other social and psychological dimensions (Rüütel, Pisarev, Loit, and Uusküla, 2009). Thus, the identification of psychological and social factors that determine quality of life is important in order to better tailor health and social care services, therefore improving the HIV people behavior and well-being. In this regard, studies have shown that, although variables such as age, gender, education, income, and employment status play an important role in PLWHIV's quality of life, they are also relevant physical and mental health-related factors (Rüütel et al., 2009). Several studies have reported the negative effect HIV plays on HIV people's mental health. For example, depression is one of the main psychiatric disorders affecting PLWHIV, that is, about 37%, two or three times higher than the general population (Wolff, Alvarado, and Wolff, 2010).

Thus, it is essential to improve HIV people's quality of life. It is also important to identify factors related to reducing psychical and psychosocial symptoms and sustained social well-being. Although this is important, few studies have empirically explored the relationship between quality of life and perceived homophobia and HIV stigma in PLWHIV in Chile. Following this assumption the purpose of this paper is to report and examine how homophobia affects the quality of life among PLWHIV versus non-HIV people in a gay men sample in Chile.

METHOD

Participants and Procedure

The convenience sample consisted of gay men, whose ages range between 18 and 64 years (X = 32.8; SD = 9.81). Of all participants, 17.8% (n = 58) had been diagnosed with HIV and 78.8% (n = 265) had not been diagnosed. The remaining percent (3.4%) corresponds to lost data of people who did not answer this question (n = 11). Participants were recruited through snowball sampling beginning with three seeds belonging to each city. The data collection process included the cities of Arica (25.1%), Valparaiso (24.5%), and Santiago (50.5%). It was done from May through July 2011. Participation was voluntary and non-paid. To be included, participants had to sign an "informed consent" letter explaining study objectives, guaranteeing response anonymity and confidentiality. The ethical criteria of the National Commission for Scientific and Technological Research (CONICYT, for its acronym in Spanish) were used. Once participants signed their agreement to take part in the study, they completed a paper-and-pencil questionnaire individually. The study was presented as a piece of research aiming at evaluating homophobia effects on gay men quality of life.

Sample Description

Table 1 shows some socio-demographic features of the sample, which are included in the study, separating groups formed by PLWHIV and without HIV diagnosis.

Table 1. Sample description: socio-demographic variables

Variables	Gay men (% over the total)	Gay men + HIV (% over the total)
Age		
18-24 years	90 (28.6)	5 (1.6)
25-35 years	108 (34.3)	18 (5.7)
36-44 years	29 (9.2)	22 (6.9)
45-54 years	15 (4.8)	9 (2.8)
55 or more	15 (4.8)	4 (1.3)
City		
Santiago	114 (37.0)	39 (12.7)
Arica	72 (23.4)	5 (1.6)
Valparaíso	65 (21.1)	13 (4.2)
Socio-economic level		
High	37 (12.7)	9 (3.1)
Middle	164 (56.2)	38 (13.0)
Low	38 (13.0)	6 (2.0)

Measures

The measures consisted of two parts. The first one referred to variables describing and segmenting the sample in sub-groups: a) age ("How old are you"); b) socioeconomic level (measured with ESOMAR system from the World Association of Market Research), and c) HIV diagnosis ("Are you diagnosed with HIV). The question on HIV diagnosis helps group segmentation. It is necessary to detect differences in the dependent variable scores of these groups. The second part includes scales used as dependent variables:

Measures of Homophobia and HIV Stigma

Minority Stress Events (Rosario, Schrimshaw, Hunter, and Gwadz, 2002). This scale was translated and adapted for this study. It consists of 12 items referring to different stressful events associated with homosexuality. Responses for each item have a dichotomy format ("Yes" and "No"). This scale has been adapted for use on a national basis.

Perceived Discrimination (Barrientos, Silva, Catalán, Gómez, and Longueira, 2010). This 10-item scale enquires about discrimination events against homosexual people, which are directly attributed to their sexual orientation ("Think about a moment in your life when you were involved in one of the following events due to your homosexuality"). It includes discrimination in the family, at school, or other public places, among others (e.g., "Not being hired or being fired from a job" or "access or permanence prohibited in a shop or recreation place"). Response options are dichotomy (yes/no) and a graded scale is used to highlight the importance of each event. Response options range from 1 ("nothing at all") to 6 ("very much"). High scores in this scale show high discrimination levels.

Perceived Victimization (Barrientos, Silva, Catalán, Gómez, and Longueira, 2010). A 10-item scale was used to enquire about victimization events against homosexual people, which are attributed to their sexual orientation ("Think about a moment in your life when you were involved in one of the following events due to your homosexuality"). It includes mockery, insult, threat, attempt of physical and sexual aggression, blackmail or extortion, assault or non-violent robbery, and assault and violent robbery. Response options are dichotomy (yes/no).

Stigma Perceived by Homosexual People (Barrientos, Cárdenas, Vidal, Berendsen, and Meneses, 2011). This scale was created in Chile to evaluate stigma and discrimination perceived by homosexual people. It consists of 23 Likert-type items with response options ranging from 1 ("completely in disagreement") to 6 ("Completely in agreement"). The scale includes 6 dimensions: Stigma and discrimination experiences (5 items), Lack of protection in front of authorities (3 items), Discrimination at work (6 items), Expression of sexual identity (3 items), Institutional exclusion and negation of rights (3 items), and Discrimination at the religious community (3 items). The reliability coefficient of the total scale in this application was high (α = .94). Reliability coefficients for the scale dimensions were as follows: Stigma and discrimination experiences (α = .92); Lack of protection in front of authorities (α = .90); Discrimination at work (α = .88); Expression of sexual identity (α = .77); Institutional exclusion and negation of rights (α = .83), and Discrimination at the religious community (α = .67).

HIV Stigma (Berger, Ferrans, and Lashley, 2001). This scale was translated into Spanish and adapted for use in a national sample (Barrientos and Cardenas, 2011). The scale includes 40 items ranging from 1 ("completely in disagreement") to 6 ("Completely in agreement"), measuring stigma perception due to HIV/AIDS. Higher scores show higher stigma perception. The reliability coefficient for this application was high (α = .97).

Quality of Life Measures

Satisfaction with Life (Diener, Emmons, Larsen, and Griffin, 1985). This scale has 5 items to evaluate general satisfaction with life by means of statements comparing expectations with achievements. Response options range from 1 ("Completely in disagreement") to 6 ("Completely in agreement"). The greater scores mean greater satisfaction with life. The reliability coefficient for the scale was good (α = .89) in this application. An adapted version used in a previous study in a national sample (Cárdenas et al., in press) was used in this research.

Subjective Happiness Scale (Lyubomirsky and Lepper, 1999). This is a general subjective happiness measure consisting of 4 Likert-type items with response options ranging from 1 ("Completely in disagreement") to 6 ("Completely in agreement"). Higher scores indicate higher levels of subjective happiness. A moderate internal consistency index was obtained in this application (α = .65). We used Chilean adapted version (Vera-Villarroel, Celis-Atenas, and Córdoba-Rubio, 2011).

Psychological Well-Being (Ryff, 1989). A translated version adapted for a Spanish sample (Díaz et al., 2006) was used on a national basis (Cárdenas and Barrientos, 2011). The instrument included 6 scales and 39 items, whose scores range from 1 ("Completely in disagreement") to 6 ("Completely in agreement"). Higher scores indicate good psychological adjustment. The reliability coefficient of the total scale was .91 (Cronbach alpha) in this application. The reliability coefficients for the scale dimensions were as follows: Self-acceptance (α = .59); Positive relations (α = .58); Autonomy (α = .65); Environmental mastery (α = .56); Growth (α = .70), and Purpose in life (α = .72).

Social Well-Being (Keyes, 1998). A translated version validated for Spanish speakers (Blanco and Díaz, 2005) was used in a national sample (Cárdenas and Barrientos, 2011). The scale consists of 33 items distributed in 5 dimensions: Social integration (7 items), Social acceptance (8 items), Social contribution (6 items), Social actualization (6 items), and Social coherence (6 items). Response options range from 1 ("Completely in disagreement") to 5 ("Completely in agreement"). High scores indicate good social adjustment. The reliability coefficient for the total scale was .89 (Cronbach alpha) in this application. The reliability coefficients for the scale dimensions were: Social integration (α = .63); Social acceptance (α = .83); Social contribution (α = .38); Social actualization (α = .64), and Social coherence (α= .86). Symptom inventory SCL-90 (Derogatis, 1975). This inventory consists of 90 items whose objective is to make up a representative sample of the most characteristic psychiatric symptoms of the syndromes evaluated by the inventory. Scores range from 0 to 4 points ("Nothing" = 0; "Very little" = 1; "Little" = 2; "Quite a lot" = 3; "Much" = 4). All items are direct, so it is not necessary to reverse scores in none of them. A high score in an item shows that the corresponding syndrome occurs with high frequency. Only somatization, anxiety, depression, hostility, and phobic anxiety dimensions were included in this application. Only these dimensions are used since they are the most representative of the symptomatology reported by people belonging to minorities (Cárdenas and Yáñez, 2012; Díaz et al., 2005). A translated version validated for Gempp and Avendaño (2008) was used in this study.

Data Analysis

Data obtained were analyzed with SPSS 15.0. An analysis of descriptive statistics (mean and typical deviation) was made for sociodemographic variables and all the measured used, for both the gay men and HIV gay men groups. Later, several t-tests were made for independent samples, comparing the means obtained for each group to variables concerning quality of life and stigma, discrimination, and victimization perception. The effect size of these comparisons (Cohen d) was calculated in order to check if the magnitude of the differences detected are really significant, confirming our conclusions. Finally, correlations between HIV-associated stigma and stigma, discrimination, and victimization perception measures were calculated.

RESULTS

Homophobia Measures

Descriptive statistics (mean and typical deviation) are shown below for each group (gay men population with and without HIV) concerning minority stress, perceived discrimination, perceived victimization, and stigma perceived. Table 2 shows that there are no significant differences for the four variables compared, thus indicating that the perception and experiences of these two groups may be regarded as similar. This was expected since the knowledge of living with HIV is private, unless the individual affected reveals this situation to others. Therefore, discrimination and stigma perception, along with the stress resulting from the participants' sexual practices, does not result from HIV diagnosis, but from their homosexual orientation.

Table 2. Descriptive statistics and measure comparison for minority stress, discrimination perceived, victimization, and stigma perceived

	Gay men X (SD)	Gay men + HIV X (SD)	*t*-test	Effect size (d)
Minority stress	2.02 (3.22)	2.20 (3.42)	0.37	.05
Victimization	3.35 (1.45)	3.77 (1.96)	1.70	.24
Discrimination	3.41 (1.41)	3.73 (1.64)	1.20	.21
Stigma perceived	4.06 (1.08)	4.20 (0.93)	0.86	.14

A dimensional analysis reveals that there are significant differences ($t_{[312]} = 2.31$; $p < .05$; $d = .35$), only in the exclusion dimension of the scale concerning stigma perceived by gay men, showing that PLWHIV scores the highest in this dimension. So, a greater capacity to perceive exclusion events and attribute them to their diagnosis may be assume. Questions in this dimension aim at detecting experiences related to exclusion in different ambits such as family, school, and public places. However, general stigma perception by the PLWHIV cannot be statistically differentiated. Finally, effect size values may confirm the slight differences between both groups.

Quality of Life Measures

Next, a comparison is made between both groups as to quality of life, that is, happiness, satisfaction with life, and psychological and social well-being. Table 3 shows the descriptive statistics for these variables. As shown in the Table below, statistically significant differences for general measures of quality of life are found only in satisfaction with life. This means that PLWHIV evaluate their lives as less satisfactory. When comparing their achievements in life with their expectations, the gap is smaller for PLWHIV.

If attention is put only on general results, differences in psychological and social well-being could be minimized. If attention is put on psychological and social well-being dimensions, significant differences can be observed concerning autonomy dimensions of psychological well-being ($t_{(306)} = -3.82$; $p < .005$; $d = .50$) and social integration dimensions of social well-being ($t_{(312)} = -2.34$; $p < .05$; $d = .35$). Autonomy refers to people's capacity to resist social pressure and stick to their own convictions. Social integration refers to the individual's evaluation of the quality of his/her relation with the community. In this sense, the fact that PLWHIV may perceive less integration with their community is coherent due to the rejection that HIV ignorance and prejudice still produce in many people. In addition, the internalization of such prejudice may reduce autonomy and make people more susceptible to social pressures.

Table 3. Descriptive statistics and measure comparison of variables concerning with quality of life

Variables	Gay men X (SD)	Gay men + HIV X (SD)	*t*-test	Effect size (d)
Subjective Happiness	4.19 (0.98)	4.02 (1.09)	-1.19	.16
Satisfaction with life	4.40 (1.08)	3.93 (1.32)	-2.77**	.39
Social well-being	3.58 (0.76)	3.40 (0.71)	-1.93	.24
Psychological well-being	3.93 (0.66)	3.77 (0.55)	-1.67	.26

**$p < .01$.

Concerning clinical symptomatology of the groups, Table 4 shows the descriptive statistics of the five SCL-90 dimensions included in this study. Differences are shown in dimensions referring to somatization and depression, indicating that PLWHIV are more susceptible to show their discomfort through symptoms related to bodily dysfunctions and mood disorders. For example, the people can perceive more corporal cardiovascular and, gastrointestinal dysfunctions.

Table 4. Descriptive statistics and measure comparison for SCL-90 dimensions

	MSM X (SD)	MSM+HIV X (SD)	*t*-test	Effect size (d)
Somatization	2.16 (1.02)	2.47 (1.05)	2.04*	.30
Anxiety	2.06 (1.01)	2.28 (1.14)	1.45	.20
Depression	2.22 (0.98)	2.56 (1.02)	2.30*	.34
Hostility	2.04 (1.15)	2.06 (1.14)	0.11	.02
Phobic anxiety	1.80 (1.02)	1.58 (0.79)	-1.52	.26

*$p < .05$

HIV Stigma Scale

Finally, The HIV sample was divided into high and low, considering HIV stigma and using the mean score of the scale (X = 3.57; SD = 1.24). In this case, the objective is to corroborate if HIV is an additional discomfort source for participants and a relevant factor when determining an increase in stigma and discrimination perception. The group of individuals with the lowest score amounts to 54.4% (n = 31), and those with the highest punctuation total 45.6% (n = 26).One of the PLWHIV have not agreed to answer HIV stigma scale. The mean for the scale of stigma in people living with HIV was 3.36 (SD = 1.03). Significant differences were detected between two groups (t (55) = -10.27; $p < .001$; d =

2.31), indicating that these two groups are distinct in reported levels of stigma. In comparing these two groups, there are significant differences in victimization ($t_{(48)} = -2.61$; $p < .05$; $d = .59$), discrimination ($t_{(35)} = -4.02$; $p < .001$; $d = .89$), stigma perceived ($t_{(55)} = -2.88$; $p < .005$; $d = 1.17$), and social well-being ($t_{(55)} = -2.55$; $p < .05$; $d = .59$), along with the five SCL-90 dimension included: somatization ($t_{(55)} = -2.36$; $p < .05$; $d = .56$) , anxiety ($t_{(55)} = -1.97$; $p < .05$; $d = .46$), depression ($t_{(55)} = -2.36$; $p < .05$; $d = .55$), hostility ($t_{(55)} = -3.19$; $p < .005$; $d = .74$), and phobic anxiety ($t_{(55)} = -2.63$; $p < .05$; $d = .58$). In addition, correlations were detected between the scores of the HIV stigma scale, victimization measures ($r = .25$), and stigma perceived ($r = .63$). Thus, HIV diagnosis plays a key role in determining well-being and quality-of-life levels, negatively influencing the individual's perception of his/her environment and encouraging an anticipated rejection which will finally be harmful for the individual himself/herself.

Discussion

This study confirms the high levels of discrimination and victimization perceived by the HIV and non-HIV gay population in Chile. So, it is necessary to make progress in the concretion of an anti-discrimination law, which is still being discussed in Congress. This law should include sexual minority particularities so as to ensure the country's LGTB population rights.

This study also confirms that the epidemic is concentrated on the gay men population, a fact that makes prevention focused on this group mandatory. An 18.5% reports HIV infection, thus supporting previous studies on seroprevalence in the country, a 21.1% following CHIPREV report (2009).

In addition, this study strengthens the idea that the gay men and other MSM population are inadequately studied in many countries, including Chile and that despite well-characterized risks for HIV acquisition and transmission, probably gay men and other MSM population continues being under-represented in national HIV surveillance systems, targeted prevention programs, and care.

This study also provides hints about some psychological and social factors influencing HIV people's quality of life. Thus, health actions should be improved by including these factors in order to make HIV people's quality of life better.

However, this study has some disadvantages that must be considered. Sampling populations difficult to access is currently a huge challenge for social research. This study tried to approach this population by using snowball sampling, which starts with "seeds" (people having a big contact network), thus allowing less intrusive access to the target population.

However, this type of sampling has some limitations. For example, it does not allow a random selection of participants, which makes findings difficult to be generalized for the whole Chilean gay men population. This introduces bias resulting from the sample selection, a fact attempting against result validity. Therefore, further sampling methods should be included for difficult access populations, such as respondent-driven sampling (Cárdenas and Yañez, 2012; Mantecón, Calafat, Becoña, and Román, 2008) or those taking place in meeting places and schedules of group members (Muhib et al., 2001; Salganik and Heckathorn, 2004).

In the same way, progress must be made by doing studies on population estimation (in order to work with, at least, pseudo representative gay men populations), thus ensuring the possibility of generalizing findings.

REFERENCES

Baral, S., Sifakis, F., Cleghorn, F., and Beyrer, C. (2007). Elevated risk for HIV infection among men who have sex with men in low- and middle-income countries 2000–2006: A Systematic Review. *PLoS Med*, 4, 12: e339. doi:10.1371/journal.pmed.0040339

Barrientos, J., Cárdenas, M., Vidal, F., Berendsen, P., and Meneses, A. (2011). *Development and validation of a standardized measure of the perceived stigma of a gay population.* Santiago: Universidad Católica del Norte (Unpublished document).

Barrientos, J. and Cárdenas, M. (2011). *Adaptación y validación chilena de la Escala de estigma al HIV.* Antofagasta: Universidad Católica del Norte (Unpublished document).

Barrientos, J., Silva, J., Catalán, S., Gómez, F., and Longueira, J. (2010). Discrimination and victimization: parade for lesbian, gay, bisexual, and transgender (LGTB) pride, in Chile. *Journal of Homosexuality*, *57*, 760-775.

Berger, B., Ferrans, C., and Lashley, F. (2001) Measuring stigma in people with HIV: Psychometric assessment of the HIV Stigma Scale. *Research in Nursing and Health, 24,* 518-529.

Blanco, A. and Díaz, D. (2005) El bienestar social: su concepto y medición. *Psicothema, 17,* 582-589.

Cárdenas, M. and Yáñez, S. (2012). Nuevas formas de muestreo para minorías y poblaciones ocultas: muestras por encuestado conducido en una población de inmigrantes sudamericanos. *Universitas Psychologica, 11,* 2, in press.

Cárdenas, M., Barrientos, J., Bilbao, M., Páez, D., Gómez, F., and Asún, D. Estructura Factorial de la Escala de Satisfacción con la Vida en una Muestra de Estudiantes Universitarios Chilenos. *Revista Mexicana de Psicología, in press.*

Cárdenas, M. and Barrientos, J. (2011). *Adaptación y validación chilena de la Escala de Bienestar Social).* Santiago: Universidad Católica del Norte (Unpublished document).

CHIPREV (2009). *Estudio de prevalencia de VIH y factores asociados en hombres que tienen sexo con hombres. Informe final del estudio* Chile: MUMS (Unpublished document). Retrieved November 25, 2011, available in: http://es.scribd.com/doc/34664715/Estudio-de-Prevalencia-de-VIH-y-Factores-Asosidados-en-Hombres-que-tienen-Sexo-con-Hombre-Chile-Enero-2009.

Derogatis, L. (1975). *The SCL-90-R.* Baltimore, MD: Clinical Psychometric Research.

Díaz, C., Cogollo, Z., Bánquez, J. Luna-Salcedo, LL., Fontalvo, K., Arrieta-Puello, M., and Campo, A. (2005) Síntomas depresivos y la orientación sexual en adolescentes estudiantes: un estudio transversal. *MedUNAB (Revista Medicina Universidad Autónoma de Bucaramangna)*, 8, 3, 183-190.

Díaz, D., Rodríguez, R., Blanco, A., Moreno-Jiménez, B., Gallardo, I., Valle, C., and van Dierendonck, D. (2006) Adaptación española de las escalas de bienestar psicológico de Ryff. *Psicothema*, *18*, 572-577.

Diener, E., Emmons, R., Larsen, R., and Griffin, S. (1985). The Satisfaction with Life Scale. *Journal of Personality Assessment*, *49*, 71-75.

Gempp, R. and Avendaño, C. (2008) Datos Normativos y Propiedades Psicométricas del SCL-90-R en Estudiantes Universitarios Chilenos. *Terapia Psicológica, 26,* 39-58.

Greeff, M., Uys, L., Wantland, D., Makoae, L., Chirwa, M., Dlamini, P., Kohi, T., Mullan, J., Naidoo, J., Cuca, Y., and Holzemer, W. (2010). Perceived HIV stigma and life satisfaction among persons living with HIV infection in five African countries: A longitudinal study. *International Journal of Nursing Studies, 47*, 475-486.

Henderson, W., Fall-Dickson, J., Schlenk, E., and Kim, K., Matthews, J., and Erlen, J. (2000). Effects of liver disease on the well-being of persons living with HIV. *Journal of the Association of Nurses in AIDS Care, 19*, 368-374.

Henderson, W., Schlenk, E., Kim, K., Hadigan, C., Martino, A., Sereika, S., and Erlen, J. (2010). Validation of the MOS-HIV as a Measure of Health-Related Quality of Life in persons living with HIV and liver disease. *AIDS Care, 22*, 483-490.

Keyes, C. (1998). Social well-being. *Social Psychology Quarterly, 61*, 121-140.

Lyubomirsky, S. and Lepper, H. (1999). A measure of subjective happiness: Preliminary reliability and construct validation. *Social Indicators Research, 46,* 137-155.

Maman, S., Abler, L., Parker, L., Lane, T., Chirowodza, A., Ntogwisangu, J., Srirak, N., Modiba, P., Murima, O., and Fritz, K. (2009). A comparison of HIV stigma and discrimination in five international sites: The influence of care and treatment resources in high prevalence settings. *Social Science and Medicine, 68*, 2271-2278.

Mantecón, A., Juan, M., Calafat, A., Becoña, E., and Román, E. (2008). Respondent-driven sampling: un nuevo método de muestreo para el estudio de poblaciones visibles y ocultas. *Adicciones, 20*,161-170.

Mavandadi, S., Zanjani, F., Have, T., and Oslin, D. (2009). Psychological wellbeing among individuals living with HIV: The value of social relationships. *Journal of Acquired Immune Deficiency Syndromes, 51*, 91-98.

MINSAL (2011). *Circular B/51, Núm. 35 del 14 octubre de 2010. Vigilancia epidemiológica de VIH/SIDA*. Chile: Autor.

Morandi dos Santos, E., França, I., and Lopes, F. (2007). Qualidade de vida de pessoas vivendo com HIV/Aids em São Paulo. *Revista de Saúde Pública,* 41 (Supl. 2), S64-S71.

Mosack, K., Weinhardt, L., Kelly, J., Gore-Felton, Ch., McAuliffe, T., Johnson, M., Remien, R., Rotheram-Borus, M., Ehrhardt, A., Chesney, M., and Morin, S. (2009). Influence of coping, social support, and depression on subjective health status among HIV-positive adults with different sexual identities. *Journal of Behavioral Medicine, 34*, 133-144.

Muhib, F., Lin, L., Stueve, A., Miller, R., Ford, W., Johnson, W., Smith, P., and Community Intervention Trial for Youth Study Team (2001). A venue-based method for sampling hard-to-reach populations. *Public Health Reports, 116*, 216-222.

Nogueira, L., Cominic, C., and Crosland, M. (2009). Quality of life among HIV-infected patients in Brazil after initiation of treatment. *Clinics, 64*, 867-75.

Rosario, M., Schrimshaw, E., Hunter, J., and Gwadz, M. (2002). Gay-related stress and emotional distress among gay, lesbian, and bisexual youths: A longitudinal examination. *Journal of Consulting and Clinical Psychology, 70*, 967-975.

Ryff, C. (1989). Beyond Ponce de Leon and life satisfaction: New directions in quest of successful aging. *International Journal of Behavioral Development, 12,* 35-55.

Rüütel, K., Pisarev, H., Loit, H., and Uusküla, A. (2009). Factors influencing quality of life of people living with HIV in Estonia: a cross-sectional survey. *Journal of the International AIDS Society,* 12: 13.

Salganik, M., and Heckathorn, D. (2004). Sampling and estimation in hidden population using respondent-driven sampling. *Sociological Methodology, 4*,193-239.

Vera-Villarroel, P., Celis-Atenas, K., and Córdova-Rubio, N. (2011). Evaluación de la felicidad: análisis psicométrico de la Escala de Felicidad Subjetiva en población chilena. *Terapia Psicológica*, *29*,127–133.

Wolff, C., Alvarado, R., and Wolff, M. (2010). Prevalencia, factores de riesgo y manejo de la depresión en pacientes con infección por VIH: Revisión de la literatura. *Revista Chilena de Infectología*, *27,* 65-74.

(Manuscript received on 23 October 2011. Revised version accepted for publication on 15 February 2012)

INDEX

A

D

E

F

G

H

I

J

K

L

M

N

Q

R

S

T

U

V

W

Y

Z